Geriatric Medicine and Gerontology

Geriatric Medicine and Gerontology

Editor: Mason Button

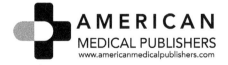

AMERICAN
MEDICAL PUBLISHERS
www.americanmedicalpublishers.com

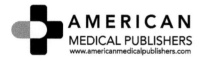

AMERICAN
MEDICAL PUBLISHERS
www.americanmedicalpublishers.com

Cataloging-in-Publication Data

Geriatric medicine and gerontology / edited by Mason Button.
     p. cm.
Includes bibliographical references and index.
ISBN 978-1-63927-675-2
1. Geriatrics. 2. Gerontology. 3. Older people--Diseases.
4. Older people--Health and hygiene. 5. Aging. I. Button, Mason.
RC952 .G47 2023
618.97--dc23

American Medical Publishers,
41 Flatbush Avenue,
1st Floor, New York,
NY 11217, USA

ISBN 978-1-63927-675-2 (Hardback)

Contents

Permissions

List of Contributors

Index

Preface

This book aims to highlight the current researches and provides a platform to further the scope of innovations in this area. This book is a product of the combined efforts of many researchers and scientists, after going through thorough studies and analysis from different parts of the world. The objective of this book is to provide the readers with the latest information of the field.

Geriatrics, or geriatric medicine, is a specialized branch of medical science that focuses on serving the health care needs of the elderly. The objective of this speciality is to prevent and treat diseases and disabilities in older adults for promoting their overall well-being. Geriatrics deals with the prevention, cure, and rehabilitation of the elderly. The study of the social, cultural, psychological, cognitive and biological aspects of aging is called gerontology. Aging is a biological process that causes a steady physiologic deterioration accompanied with disability and disease. It is characterized by the development of wrinkles, decline in fertility, reduced body mass, decreased mobility and strength, and gray hair. Adult stem cell transplantation, cloning, tissue transplantation, and gene therapy are currently being investigated as potential treatments for aging related diseases. Common diseases caused due to aging include diabetes, cancer, stroke, Alzheimer's disease, and cardiovascular disease. This book presents the upcoming researches on geriatric medicine and gerontology. It is appropriate for students seeking detailed information in this area as well as for experts.

I would like to express my sincere thanks to the authors for their dedicated efforts in the completion of this book. I acknowledge the efforts of the publisher for providing constant support. Lastly, I would like to thank my family for their support in all academic endeavors.

Editor

Behavioral Factors Related to the Incidence of Frailty in Older Adults

Hiroyuki Shimada [1],*[iD], Takehiko Doi [1], Kota Tsutsumimoto [1], Sangyoon Lee [1], Seongryu Bae [1] and Hidenori Arai [2]

[1] Center for Gerontology and Social Science, National Center for Geriatrics and Gerontology, 7-430 Morioka-cho, Obu City, Aichi Prefecture 474-8511, Japan; take-d@ncgg.go.jp (T.D.); k-tsutsu@ncgg.go.jp (K.T.); sylee@ncgg.go.jp (S.L.); bae-sr@ncgg.go.jp (S.B.)

[2] National Center for Geriatrics and Gerontology, 7-430 Morioka-cho, Obu City, Aichi Prefecture 474-8511, Japan; harai@ncgg.go.jp

* Correspondence: shimada@ncgg.go.jp

Abstract: Frailty is a widely prevalent geriatric condition whereby individuals experience age-related functional declines. This study aimed to identify behavioral factors related to the incidence of frailty in older adults. Participants were 2631 older adults (average age: 71) without physical frailty at a baseline assessment in 2011–2012 who took part in a second-wave assessment in 2015–2016. Physical frailty was defined as having limitations in at least three of the following domains: weight loss, low physical activity, exhaustion, slow walking speed, and muscle weakness. Participants completed a 16-item questionnaire examining cognitive, social, and productive activity as well as instrumental activities of daily living (IADL) as varying dimensions of lifestyle activity. During the follow-up period, 172 participants (6.5%) converted from nonfrail to frail. Logistic regression showed that the odds ratios (ORs) for conversion were significantly lower in the participants who had high IADL scores (OR: 0.78; 95% confidence interval (CI): 0.64–0.96), cognitive activity (OR: 0.74; 95% CI: 0.62–0.89), social activity (OR: 0.52; 95% CI: 0.43–0.63), and total activity (OR: 0.81; 95% CI: 0.75–0.87). There was no significant association between frailty and productive activity. Health care providers should recommend an active lifestyle to prevent frailty in older adults.

Keywords: frailty; older adults; cohort study; lifestyle; prevention; instrumental activities of daily living; cognitive activities; nonfrail; prefrail

1. Introduction

The clinical condition of frailty is among the most prevalent and problematic expressions of population aging. Frailty is a multifaceted geriatric syndrome and an effect of age-related physiological decline reflecting multisystem functional decline and a reduced capacity to cope with stressors. Individuals experiencing frailty become more vulnerable to sudden shifts in health status triggered by even minor stressor events such as an infection [1]. As such, frailty is a complex concept involving a state of greater vulnerability to adverse health factors, including long-term care, disability, and an overall negative state of health. Frailty may also involve psychological, emotional, and social dimensions in addition to physical symptoms such as deterioration of motor performance [2].

Between a quarter and a half of people older than 85 years are estimated to be frail, and thus, have a considerably increased risk of long-term care, disability, and death [3,4]. Reducing or eliminating risk factors and increasing protective factors are potential actions for minimizing the chances of frailty. Regular physical, cognitive, social, and productive activities promote improvements in both physical and psychological health and contribute to the reversal of detrimental effects of chronic diseases as well as the maintenance of functional autonomy in older adults [5–7].

In 2019, individuals who were 65 years of age or older comprised 28.6% of Japan's population [8]. Faced with an increasingly aging population, the Japanese government has been reforming its policies to provide for the needs of the elderly population and to prevent the need for long-term care. Among such efforts, the National Center for Geriatrics and Gerontology-Study of Geriatric Syndromes (NCGG-SGS) has been striving to identify behavioral factors that contribute to healthy aging. Using the NCGG-SGS database, it was confirmed that reversible factors such as lifestyle activities are associated with mild cognitive impairment (MCI) reversion in elderly individuals. A logistic regression model showed significantly higher odds ratios (ORs) for MCI reversion in participants who had an active lifestyle compared to the inactive participants [7].

This study examined the relationship between behavioral factors and the incidence of frailty in community-living older adults. The reduction in risk factors and the promotion of protective factors are essential to developing and implementing effective interventions to sustain successful aging and prevent disability. Observational studies have indicated several common factors related to disability prevention. Specifically, older persons who regularly participate in activities of daily life have shown a lower risk of disability and dementia [9–17]. Such findings indicate that lifestyle activities could be intermediaries in the incidence of frailty. Accordingly, the study also examined the relationship between frailty and lifestyle activities, including cognitive activity, social activity, productive activity, and instrumental activities of daily living (IADL). In this study, the hypothesis was that individuals with a loss of lifestyle activities would have a higher risk of frailty incidence than those with an active lifestyle.

2. Methods

2.1. Participants

The current study is part of a national study that assessed 5104 individuals, aged 65 years and older (average age: 71 years), enrolled in the NCGG-SGS [18]. Participants were recruited from Obu, a residential suburb of Nagoya. The inclusion criteria were residing in Obu and being 65 years or older during the baseline assessment (2011 or 2012). Some participants were excluded based on previous reports that certain conditions could produce characteristics of disability [19]. Accordingly, participants with a functional decline in basic activities of daily living (ADL) ($n = 39$), certified long-term care insurance ($n = 126$), and a history of Parkinson's disease ($n = 21$) or Alzheimer's disease ($n = 8$) were excluded. The study also excluded participants with missing data values of confounding factors ($n = 323$) or activity measurements ($n = 81$) and participants with frailty at baseline ($n = 326$). The study also excluded participants without follow-up measurements ($n = 1549$, reason unknown). This study analyzed data from a total of 2631 eligible older adults (mean age: 71.0 ± 4.7 years; 49.5% male) from the initial 5104 participants who took part in a follow-up assessment between August 2015 and August 2016. Table 1 shows the baseline characteristics of the participants, both included and excluded in the study. The study protocol was approved by the ethics committee of the National Center for Gerontology and Geriatrics (numbers 523 and 791), and participants gave written informed consent prior to their inclusion.

Table 1. Baseline characteristics of the included and excluded participants.

	Included Participants (n = 2631)	Excluded Participants (n = 2473)	p
Age (years) [†]	71.0 (4.7)	73.6 (6.4)	<0.01
Sex (% male)	49.5	48.2	0.34
Education (years) [†]	11.7 (2.5)	10.9 (2.6) [*14]	<0.01
BMI > 27.5 (% yes)	7.6	10.7	<0.01
BMI < 18.5 (% yes)	3.3	5.8	<0.01
Stroke (% yes)	4.0	7.1	<0.01
Heart disease (% yes)	15.6	18.4	<0.01
Pulmonary disease (% yes)	10.9	12.1	0.20
Osteoarthritis (% yes)	13.8	15.4	0.11
Diabetes mellitus (% yes)	11.4	15.6	<0.01
History of falls (% yes)	13.1	17.9	<0.01
Medication (number) [†]	1.9 (1.9)	2.4 (2.4)	<0.01
Minimental state examination (points) [†]	26.6 (2.5)	25.6 (3.0) [*13]	<0.01
Geriatric depression scale (points) [†]	2.4 (2.4)	3.5 (2.9) [*18]	<0.01
Serum albumin (g/dL) [†]	4.3 (0.2)	4.3 (0.3) [*39]	<0.01
Instrumental activities of daily living (% yes)			
Going outdoors using bus and train	93.1	84.5	<0.01
Cash handling and banking	90.7	86.6	<0.01
Driving a car	76.7	60.2	<0.01
Using map to go unfamiliar places	67.6	53.9	<0.01
Cognitive activity (% yes)			
Reading of book or newspaper	97.1	93.3	<0.01
Cognitive stimulation such as board game and learning	53.7	42.2	<0.01
Culture lesson	46.8	32.6	<0.01
Using personal computer	39.6	25.2	<0.01
Social activity (% yes)			
Daily conversation	97.1	93.9	<0.01
Giving someone a helping hand	93.7	87.3	<0.01
Attending a meeting in the community	55.5	44.3	<0.01
Hobby or sports activity	79.9	61.5	<0.01
Productive activity (% yes)			
Housecleaning	87.7	84.2	<0.01
Field work or gardening	75.5	66	<0.01
Taking care of grandchild or pet	57.8	50.1	<0.01
Working	32.2	25.5	<0.01
Activity score (points) [†]			
Instrumental activities of daily living	3.3 (0.8)	2.9 (1.1) [*40]	<0.01
Cognitive activity	2.4 (1.1)	1.9 (1.0) [*31]	<0.01
Social activity	3.3 (0.8)	2.9 (1.0) [*71]	<0.01
Productive activity	2.5 (0.9)	2.3 (1.0) [*38]	<0.01
Total	11.4 (2.4)	9.9 (2.9) [*151]	<0.01

* number of missing values; [†] average (standard deviation); BMI: body mass index.

2.2. Operational Definition of Physical Frailty

The assessments were performed by well-trained assessors with nursing, allied health, or similar statements. Prior to commencement, all assessors acquired training from the authors in the correct protocols for administering the measurements.

The physical frailty phenotype was defined as existing limitations in three or more of the following domains: strength, mobility, physical activity, exhaustion, and weight loss. Grip strength was assessed using a handheld dynamometer (GRIP-D; Takei Ltd., Niigata, Japan). Low grip strength was determined according to a sex-specific cutoff (male: <26 kg; female: <17 kg) [20]. Walking speed as an indicator of mobility was measured using a stopwatch. The participants were asked to walk at a comfortable pace on a flat, straight surface of a 2.4 m path with a 2 m section to be traversed prior to the start marker. Low mobility was established as <1.0 m/s [21,22]. Physical activity was assessed with the following questions: (1) "Do you engage in moderate levels of physical exercise or sports aimed at health?" and (2) "Do you engage in low levels of physical exercise aimed at health?"

If participants answered "no" to both, they were considered to engage in low levels of activity [21]. Exhaustion was evaluated as being present if the participant responded "yes" to the following question included on the Kihon Checklist [23], a self-reported health checklist developed by the Japanese Ministry of Health, Labour and Welfare: "In the last two weeks, have you felt tired without a reason?" Weight loss was determined as a response of "yes" to the question "Have you lost 2 kg or more in the past six months?" [23]. The participants with impairments in one or two of the five domains were considered prefrail.

2.3. Measurements of Lifestyle Activity

The participants completed a 16-item questionnaire examining cognitive, social, and productive activities as well as IADL as varying dimensions of lifestyle activity [7]. The following questions measured IADL: (1) "Do you go outdoors using the bus and train?", (2) "Do you engage in cash handling and banking?", (3) "Do you drive a car?", and (4) "Do you use maps to go to unfamiliar places?" The following items measured cognitive activity: (5) "Do you read books or newspapers?", (6) "Do you engage in cognitive stimulation such as board games and learning?", (7) "Do you engage in cultural classes?", and (8) "Do you use a personal computer?" The following questions measured social activity: (9) "Do you talk with other people every day?", (10) "Are you sometimes called on for advice?", (11) "Do you attend meetings in the community?", and 12) "Do you engage in hobbies or sports activities?" Finally, the following items measured productive activity: (13) "Do you engage in housecleaning?", (14) "Do you engage in fieldwork or gardening?", (15) "Do you take care of grandchildren or pets?", and (16) "Do you engage in paid work?" Answers of "yes" were considered positive responses. The total score for the 16 items (range 0–16) was calculated along with subscore totals (range 0–4) for IADL, cognitive activity, social activity, and productive activity.

2.4. Potential Confounding Factors

Possible confounding factors of ADL limitations were demographic variables (age, sex, and education), overweight or underweight, primary diseases or health conditions, Mini-mental State Examination (MMSE) scores [24], scores on the 15-item version of the Geriatric Depression Scale (GDS-15) [25,26], and serum albumin levels (Table 2) [27–29]. The overweight and underweight were determined by measuring body mass index (BMI), and the Asian cut points of overweight and underweight were set at 27.5 and <18.5 kg/m^2, respectively [29]. Primary diseases and other health conditions—namely, stroke, heart disease, pulmonary disease, osteoarthritis hypertension, diabetes mellitus, history of falls, and medication—were acquired via self-reporting and interview surveys.

2.5. Statistical Analysis

The study calculated incidence rates of frailty per 1000 person-years, and compared incidence of frailty between the participants categorized as robust and prefrail at baseline using chi-square tests. Baseline characteristics were compared according to frailty status using Student's t-tests and Pearson's chi-square tests. Baseline characteristics were also compared between included and excluded participants using Student's t-tests and Pearson's chi-square tests to evaluate possible selection bias. Chi-square tests were used to compare frailty incidence between age group and sex, and adjusted standardized residuals were used to identify the impact of age on the incidence of frailty. The adjusted standardized residuals followed the t distribution: >1.96, $p < 0.05$ and >2.56, $p < 0.01$.

Associations between each lifestyle activity status and incidence of frailty were analyzed with multiple logistic regression models adjusted for confounding factors (model 1). The logistic models included estimated adjusted ORs and their 95% confidence intervals (95% CIs). To determine which lifestyle activities are independently associated with frailty development, another logistic model was created including all types of activities and confounding factors (model 2). All data management and statistical computations were performed using the IBM SPSS Statistics 24.0 software package (IBM Japan, Tokyo). The significance threshold was set at 0.05.

Table 2. Comparisons of baseline characteristics according to frailty status.

	Participants without Frailty ($n = 2459$)	Participants with Frailty ($n = 172$)	p Value
Age (years) *	70.8 (4.5)	73.9 (5.9)	<0.01
Sex (% male)	49.8	44.8	0.20
Education (years) *	11.8 (2.5)	10.7 (2.4)	<0.01
BMI > 27.5 (% yes)	7.1	15.7	<0.01
BMI < 18.5 (% yes)	3.3	3.5	0.89
Stroke (% yes)	3.6	9.9	<0.01
Heart disease (% yes)	15.5	16.9	0.63
Pulmonary disease (% yes)	10.7	15.1	0.07
Osteoarthritis (% yes)	13.8	13.4	0.87
Diabetes mellitus (% yes)	11.0	16.9	0.02
History of falls (% yes)	12.3	25.0	<0.01
Medication (number) *	1.8 (1.9)	2.5 (2.1)	<0.01
Mini-mental state examination (points) *	26.7 (2.4)	25.3 (3.2)	<0.01
Geriatric depression scale (points) *	2.3 (2.3)	3.6 (2.7)	<0.01
Serum albumin *	4.3 (0.2)	4.3 (0.2)	<0.01
Activity score (points) *			
Instrumental activities of daily living	3.3 (0.8)	2.9 (1.0)	<0.01
Cognitive activity	2.4 (1.0)	1.9 (1.0)	<0.01
Social activity	3.3 (0.8)	2.7 (1.0)	<0.01
Productive activity	2.5 (0.9)	2.3 (0.9)	<0.01
Total	11.6 (2.3)	9.7 (2.7)	<0.01

* average (standard deviation); BMI: body mass index.

3. Results

At baseline, the frailty status of the participants was 1340 (50.9%) nonfrail participants and 1291 (49.1%) prefrail participants. Among people without frailty at baseline who survived during the 4-year follow-up, 172 participants (6.5%) became frail. The incidence rate of frailty was 16.3 (95% CI: 14.1–19.0) cases per 1000 person-years. During the follow-up, 33 participants (2.5%) who were robust at baseline and 139 participants (10.8%) who were prefrail at baseline developed frailty. The frailty incidence rates among the robust and prefrail participants were 6.2 (95% CI: 4.4–8.6) and 26.9 (95% CI: 22.8–31.8) cases per 1000 person-years, respectively. There was a significant difference in the incidence rates based on the baseline status ($p < 0.01$). The comparison of the baseline characteristics of the excluded participants showed that they had higher age, lower education, higher rates of abnormal body composition, chronic diseases, history of falls, higher number of medications, lower MMSE score, higher depressive mood, lower albumin level, and lower activity status than the included participants (Table 1).

Table 2 presents potential confounding factors for frailty incidence among the participants. Significant differences based on frailty status were found for age, educational level, overweight, stroke, diabetes, fall history, medications, MMSE scores, GDS scores, serum albumin levels, and all lifestyle activities (Table 2).

Results showed that 172 participants (6.5%) had incident frailty during the 4-year follow-up period. It was found that the incidence of physical frailty increased with age ($p < 0.01$) (Figure 1A). In the residual analyses, the participants aged 65 to 69 years showed low incidence ($p < 0.01$), and the participants aged 75 to 79 years, 80 to 84 years, and 85 years and over showed a high incidence of frailty. However, there were no significant sex-specific differences in the incidence of frailty (Figure 1B). Chi-square tests identified a significantly lower incidence of prefrailty in the participants who performed all IADL activities (all activities vs. 0 to 3 activities: 42.6% vs. 55.2%, $p < 0.001$), cognitive activities (all activities vs. 0 to 3 activities: 32.6% vs. 52.3%, $p < 0.001$), and social activities (all activities vs. 0 to 3 activities: 39.4% vs. 57.2%, $p < 0.001$). However, there was no significant difference based on productive activities (all activities vs. 0 to 3 activities: 46.0% vs. 49.6%, $p = 0.205$).

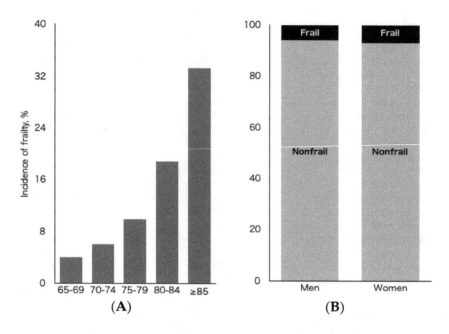

Figure 1. Incidence of frailty by age and sex during the 4-year follow-up period. (**A**) showed the incidence of frailty by age group. (**B**) showed sex-specific differences in the incidence of frailty.

The regression identified several significant relations between frailty incidence and lifestyle activities (Table 3). The individuals engaging in the following activities had lower ORs for frailty incidence in model 1: going out using the bus or train (OR: 0.47; 95% CI: 0.28–0.81), using maps to go to unfamiliar places (OR: 0.66; 95% CI: 0.46–0.95), cognitive stimulation (OR: 0.69; 95% CI: 0.48–0.98), culture lessons (OR: 0.64; 95% CI: 0.45–0.93), personal computer use (OR: 0.57; 95% CI: 0.36–0.90), daily conversation (OR: 0.48; 95% CI: 0.25–0.95), giving advice (OR: 0.52; 95% CI: 0.31–0.86), community meetings (OR: 0.49; 95% CI: 0.35–0.69), and hobbies and sports (OR: 0.32; 95% CI: 0.22–0.46). Furthermore, the multiple logistic model included all types of activities; the regression model identified several significant relationships between frailty incidence and lifestyle activities. The individuals engaging in the following activities had lower ORs for frailty incidence: community meetings (OR: 0.61; 95% CI: 0.42–0.88) and hobbies and sports (OR: 0.35; 95% CI: 0.23–0.52) (Table 3).

Frailty incidence was also significantly associated with each total score in the following activity domains: IADL (OR: 0.78; 95% CI: 0.64–0.96), cognitive activity (OR: 0.74; 95% CI: 0.62–0.89), social activity (OR: 0.52; 95% CI: 0.43–0.63), and all activities (OR: 0.81; 95% CI: 0.75–0.87). However, there was no significant association between productive activity and frailty incidence (Table 4). The multiple logistic model included all types of activities; the regression model identified that total scores of social activities remained significant relationships with frailty incidence (OR: 0.55; 95% CI: 0.44–0.67) (Table 4).

Table 3. Relationships between frailty status and lifestyle activities.

	Model 1		Model 2	
	Odds Ratio (95% CI)	p Value	Odds Ratio (95% CI)	p Value
Instrumental activities of daily living (% yes)				
Going outdoors using bus and train	0.47 (0.28–0.81)	<0.01	0.66 (0.37–1.18)	0.16
Cash handling and banking	0.72 (0.42–1.21)	0.21	0.86 (0.49–1.51)	0.60
Driving a car	1.09 (0.72–1.65)	0.68	1.33 (0.86–2.05)	0.20
Using map to go unfamiliar place	0.66 (0.46–0.95)	0.02	0.81 (0.55–1.18)	0.27
Cognitive activity (% yes)				
Reading of book or newspaper	0.99 (0.42–2.32)	0.98	1.40 (0.57–3.44)	0.47
Cognitive stimulation such as board game and learning	0.69 (0.48–0.98)	0.04	1.04 (0.7–1.55)	0.86
Culture lessons	0.64 (0.45–0.93)	0.02	1.12 (0.73–1.72)	0.61
Using personal computer	0.57 (0.36–0.90)	0.02	0.68 (0.42–1.09)	0.11
Social activity (% yes)				
Daily conversation	0.48 (0.25–0.95)	0.03	0.66 (0.32–1.37)	0.27
Giving someone advice	0.52 (0.31–0.86)	0.01	0.71 (0.41–1.22)	0.22
Attending a meeting in the community	0.49 (0.35–0.69)	<0.01	0.61 (0.42–0.88)	0.01
Hobby or sports activity	0.32 (0.22–0.46)	<0.01	0.35 (0.23–0.52)	<0.01
Productive activity (% yes)				
Housecleaning	0.82 (0.49–1.38)	0.45	1.04 (0.60–1.80)	0.90
Field work or gardening	0.82 (0.57–1.18)	0.53	0.99 (0.67–1.46)	0.97
Taking care of grandchild or pet	0.83 (0.60–1.16)	0.28	0.94 (0.66–1.33)	0.73
Working	0.93 (0.63–1.39)	0.74	0.88 (0.58–1.33)	0.54

Model 1 included each lifestyle activity and confounding factors which were age, sex, education, and overweight or underweight, stroke, heart disease, pulmonary disease, osteoarthritis hypertension, diabetes mellitus, history of falls, medication, Mini-mental State Examination, Geriatric Depression Scale, and serum albumin levels. Model 2 included all types of activities and confounding factors.

Table 4. Relationships between frailty status and lifestyle activities.

	Model 1		Model 2	
	Odds Ratio (95% CI)	p Value	Odds Ratio (95% CI)	p Value
Total score of IADL (point)	0.78 (0.64–0.96)	0.02	0.92 (0.74–1.14)	0.44
Total score of cognitive activity (point)	0.74 (0.62–0.89)	<0.01	0.92 (0.75–1.11)	0.38
Total score of social activity (point)	0.52 (0.43–0.63)	<0.01	0.55 (0.44–0.67)	<0.01
Total score of productive activity (point)	0.86 (0.72–1.04)	0.12	0.98 (0.81–1.19)	0.87
Total score of all activity (point)	0.81 (0.75–0.87)	<0.01		

Model 1 included each total score of lifestyle activity and confounding factors which were age, sex, education, and overweight or underweight, stroke, heart disease, pulmonary disease, osteoarthritis hypertension, diabetes mellitus, history of falls, medication, Mini-mental State Examination, Geriatric Depression Scale, and serum albumin levels. Model 2 included all types of activities and confounding factors. IADL: instrumental activities of daily living.

4. Discussion

This study presents original findings regarding physical vulnerability with age and lifestyle activities among 2631 older adults in Obu, Japan. It was revealed that the incidence of physical frailty was associated with IADL, cognitive activity, and social activity and that individuals with high social activity scores had the lowest risk of frailty.

In this Japanese national cohort, 172 (6.5%) older adults developed frailty during the 4-year follow-up, and the incidence rate of frailty was 16.3 (95% CI: 14.1–19.0) cases per 1000 person-years. A previous meta-analysis that compared the incidence of frailty estimates based on different frailty definitions reported 43.4 (95% CI: 37.3–50.4) cases per 1000 person-years [30]. The participants of the present study showed a lower incidence rate of frailty than participants included in the meta-analysis [30]. A subanalysis in the meta-analysis identified that the incidence of frailty was higher in prefrail persons than in robust individuals (pooled incidence rates: 62.7 (95% CI: 49.2–79.8) vs. 12.0

(95% CI: 8.2–17.5) cases per 1000 person-years), respectively [30]. In this study, the frailty incidence rates among the prefrail and robust participants were 26.9 (95% CI: 22.8–31.8) and 6.2 (95% CI: 4.4–8.6) cases per 1000 person-years, respectively. Considering frailty status at baseline, the participants in this study had a lower incidence of frailty than previous studies. It was considered that participants in this study included a large number of healthy elderly people who lived independently in the community and that the survival effect impacted the difference in incidence. The principal difference between Fried's frailty criteria and the frailty criteria of NCGG-SGS is the cutoff point for walking speed: in Fried's criteria, it is set at 0.65 m/s (height ≤ 173 cm), whereas in NCGG-SGS, it is 1.0 m/s. Walking speed has been found to be a strong predictor of adverse events such as recurrent falls [31,32], disability [33–39], mortality [40,41], and hospitalization [34,35,37,42]. Previous studies have identified that the crucial point for predicting functional decline was 1.0 m/s in comfortable walking speed in community-dwelling older adults [34,35,37–39]. These findings also suggest that walking speed could be the most useful indicator for specifying frailty and the most reliable predictor of functional decline among older adults [43,44]. The low prevalence of physical frailty in participants of this study despite the higher cut-off point for walking speed may have been due to the participants' better functional status than that of participants in the previous studies.

A growing body of evidence has indicated a close relationship between physical frailty and activity. A systematic review has stated that physical activity has a beneficial effect on muscle mass and strength or physical performance in healthy adults aged ≥ 60 years; however, an additional effect of dietary supplementation has been reported in only a limited number of studies [45]. A randomized controlled trial compared the effects of physical and cognitive training, nutritional supplementation, and combination treatments vs. control in reducing frailty among prefrail and frail older adults. The results showed that frailty status over a year-long period was reduced in all groups, including the control group (15%), but was significantly higher in the physical (OR: 4.05), cognitive (OR: 2.89), nutritional (OR: 2.98), and combination (OR: 5.00) intervention groups [46]. Luger and colleagues reported that frailty prevalence decreased to the same extent for participants who received volunteer-administered cognitive training and social support (−16%) and home-based physical training and nutrition programs (−17%) [47]. The study suggested that employing robust older people as volunteers could potentially foster community empowerment and contribute to a sustainable, beneficial health intervention for frail older people. Engagement in productive activities has been positively associated with older adults' physical and psychological health and survival [48], and such activities that require complex physical and cognitive functioning may help postpone declines in physical performance, as well as induce psychosocial changes that could impact functioning in domains related to measures of frailty [49].

The multiple logistic regression analyses identified some significant relations between frailty and lifestyle activities in our cohort. Measurements of IADL, cognitive activity, and social activity were significantly associated with frailty incidence, although there was no significant relationship between productive activity and frailty. Regarding the baseline prefrailty status, chi-square tests identified a significantly lower incidence of prefrailty in the participants who performed all activities in the IADL, cognitive activity, and social activity domains, although there was no significant difference in productive activity domain. It was considered that the prevalence of prefrailty at baseline was similar for the older adults with and without all the productive activities, which have an impact on the future incidence of frailty.

A meta-analysis of longitudinal studies identified the biological, sociodemographic, physical, psychological, and lifestyle-related risk and protective factors that have been associated with frailty among older adults [50]. Significant sociodemographic factors included age, ethnicity, neighborhood, and access to private insurance; significant lifestyle factors included a better diet quality, particularly higher habitual dietary resveratrol exposure, and higher fruit/vegetable consumption; significant psychological factors included depressive symptoms; important physical factors included obesity and ADL functional status; and significant biological factors included serum uric acid [50]. The present findings revealed that, in addition to these factors identified in previous studies, the implementation of activities such as IADL and cognitive or social activities has a preventive effect on frailty incidence in older adults. Furthermore, the multiple logistic model included all types of activities; the model identified that the individuals engaging in the community meetings or hobbies and sports had a lower risk of frailty incidence than those who were not engaged in such activities. These results suggest that specific social activities may be effective to prevent frailty. Future intervention studies will need to verify whether the implementation of these activities is effective in preventing the incidence of frailty in older adults.

An important limitation of the study is that NCGG-SGS participants were not randomly recruited, which could have led to an underestimation of frailty prevalence, as the participants were relatively healthy older persons who could access health checkups from their homes. Second, the study could not perform a follow-up survey in 1549 individuals (30.3%) who enrolled in the NCGG-SGS, which could have led to an underestimation of frailty incidence due to survival effects and poor health conditions at baseline. Moreover, the comparison of the baseline characteristics of the excluded participants showed that they were older, had a lower education, had higher rates of abnormal body composition, chronic diseases, and a history of falls, used a higher number of medications, and had a lower MMSE score, higher depressive mood, lower albumin level, and lower activity status than the included participants. The nonrandom missing data could have biased the study's findings and decreased its statistical power. A simulation study suggested that the missing not-at-random mechanism provided seriously biased estimates of the OR that moved toward zero as loss to follow-up increased. With merely 20% of the data lost to follow-up, the true odds ratio was underestimated by approximately half its value [51]. This underestimation may be the reason for no significant association between productive activity and frailty incidence in the present study. Third, participants were restricted to the Nagoya area and may not reflect national trends. Living environments were also not addressed, such as urban vs. rural or suburban and assisted living vs. living on one's own. Finally, this study failed to address covariates related to biological factors (e.g., cytokines) and social support that could contribute to the incidence of frailty. Future studies should include these potential covariates for frailty. However, an important strength of the study is the large size of the cohort and that the findings are supported by comprehensive geriatric assessments used as indicators of frailty. In addition, to our knowledge, this is the first study to use a large population-based sample to identify the relationships between frailty incidence and lifestyle activity in an Asian population. This study suggests that modifiable lifestyle activities may be useful for preventing the incidence of frailty in older adults.

5. Conclusions

During a follow-up period from 2011–2012 to 2015–2016, 172 participants (6.5%) converted from nonfrail to frail. The incidence of frailty was related to lifestyle activities. The incidence of frailty was associated with IADL, cognitive activities, and social activities; therefore, it was considered that activity assessments could be used in research fields of gerontology and in primary health care settings as an indicator of disability prevention in older adults. Further intervention studies using these activities are required to determine the validity of these measures as correlates of physical frailty. Health care providers should recommend an active lifestyle, such as conducting IADL and cognitive or social activities, to prevent frailty in older adults without frailty.

Author Contributions: Conceptualization, H.S.; methodology, H.S.; formal analysis, H.S.; investigation, T.D., K.T., S.L., and S.B.; writing—original draft preparation, H.S.; writing—review and editing, T.D., K.T., S.L., S.B. and H.A.; visualization, H.S.; supervision, H.A.; project administration, H.S.; funding acquisition, H.S. All authors have read and agreed to the published version of the manuscript.

Acknowledgments: We wish to thank the following healthcare staff for their assistance with the study assessments: Sho Nakakubo, Keitaro Makino, Kenji Harada, SungChul Lee, Kazuhiro Harada, Ryo Hotta, Daisuke Yoshida, and Yuya Anan. We thank Editage for editing a draft of this manuscript.

References

1. Clegg, A.; Young, J.; Iliffe, S.; Rikkert, M.O.; Rockwood, K. Frailty in elderly people. *Lancet* **2013**, *381*, 752–762. [CrossRef]
2. Rodriguez-Manas, L.; Feart, C.; Mann, G.; Vina, J.; Chatterji, S.; Chodzko-Zajko, W.; Gonzalez-Colaco Harmand, M.; Bergman, H.; Carcaillon, L.; Nicholson, C.; et al. Searching for an operational definition of frailty: A Delphi method based consensus statement. The frailty operative definition-consensus conference project. *J. Gerontol. A Biol. Sci. Med. Sci.* **2013**, *68*, 62–67. [CrossRef] [PubMed]
3. Song, X.; Mitnitski, A.; Rockwood, K. Prevalence and 10-year outcomes of frailty in older adults in relation to deficit accumulation. *J. Am. Geriatr. Soc.* **2010**, *58*, 681–687. [CrossRef] [PubMed]
4. Fried, L.P.; Tangen, C.M.; Walston, J.; Newman, A.B.; Hirsch, C.; Gottdiener, J.; Seeman, T.; Tracy, R.; Kop, W.J.; Burke, G.; et al. Frailty in older adults: Evidence for a phenotype. *J. Gerontol. A Biol. Sci. Med. Sci.* **2001**, *56*, M146–M156. [CrossRef] [PubMed]
5. Paulo, T.R.; Tribess, S.; Sasaki, J.E.; Meneguci, J.; Martins, C.A.; Freitas, I.F., Jr.; Romo-Perez, V.; Virtuoso, J.S., Jr. A Cross-Sectional Study of the Relationship of Physical Activity with Depression and Cognitive Deficit in Older Adults. *J. Aging Phys. Act.* **2016**, *24*, 311–321. [CrossRef]
6. Shimada, H.; Makizako, H.; Lee, S.; Doi, T.; Lee, S. Lifestyle activities and the risk of dementia in older Japanese adults. *Geriatr. Gerontol. Int.* **2018**, *18*, 1491–1496. [CrossRef]
7. Shimada, H.; Doi, T.; Lee, S.; Makizako, H. Reversible predictors of reversion from mild cognitive impairment to normal cognition: A 4-year longitudinal study. *Alzheimers Res. Ther.* **2019**, *11*, 24. [CrossRef]
8. Statistics Bureau of Japan. Population Estimates Monthly Report. Available online: http://www.stat.go.jp/english/data/jinsui/tsuki/index.html (accessed on 31 March 2020).
9. Fabrigoule, C.; Letenneur, L.; Dartigues, J.F.; Zarrouk, M.; Commenges, D.; Barberger-Gateau, P. Social and leisure activities and risk of dementia: A prospective longitudinal study. *J. Am. Geriatr. Soc.* **1995**, *43*, 485–490. [CrossRef]
10. Wang, H.X.; Karp, A.; Winblad, B.; Fratiglioni, L. Late-life engagement in social and leisure activities is associated with a decreased risk of dementia: A longitudinal study from the Kungsholmen project. *Am. J. Epidemiol.* **2002**, *155*, 1081–1087. [CrossRef]
11. Karp, A.; Paillard-Borg, S.; Wang, H.X.; Silverstein, M.; Winblad, B.; Fratiglioni, L. Mental, physical and social components in leisure activities equally contribute to decrease dementia risk. *Dement. Geriatr. Cogn. Disord.* **2006**, *21*, 65–73. [CrossRef]
12. Laurin, D.; Verreault, R.; Lindsay, J.; MacPherson, K.; Rockwood, K. Physical activity and risk of cognitive impairment and dementia in elderly persons. *Arch. Neurol.* **2001**, *58*, 498–504. [CrossRef]
13. Scarmeas, N.; Levy, G.; Tang, M.X.; Manly, J.; Stern, Y. Influence of leisure activity on the incidence of Alzheimer's disease. *Neurology* **2001**, *57*, 2236–2242. [CrossRef] [PubMed]
14. Wilson, R.S.; Mendes De Leon, C.F.; Barnes, L.L.; Schneider, J.A.; Bienias, J.L.; Evans, D.A.; Bennett, D.A. Participation in cognitively stimulating activities and risk of incident Alzheimer disease. *JAMA* **2002**, *287*, 742–748. [CrossRef] [PubMed]
15. Wilson, R.S.; Bennett, D.A.; Bienias, J.L.; Aggarwal, N.T.; Mendes De Leon, C.F.; Morris, M.C.; Schneider, J.A.; Evans, D.A. Cognitive activity and incident AD in a population-based sample of older persons. *Neurology* **2002**, *59*, 1910–1914. [CrossRef] [PubMed]
16. Sorman, D.E.; Sundstrom, A.; Ronnlund, M.; Adolfsson, R.; Nilsson, L.G. Leisure activity in old age and risk of dementia: A 15-year prospective study. *J. Gerontol. B Psychol. Sci. Soc. Sci.* **2014**, *69*, 493–501. [CrossRef]
17. Akbaraly, T.N.; Portet, F.; Fustinoni, S.; Dartigues, J.F.; Artero, S.; Rouaud, O.; Touchon, J.; Ritchie, K.; Berr, C. Leisure activities and the risk of dementia in the elderly: Results from the Three-City Study. *Neurology* **2009**, *73*, 854–861. [CrossRef]
18. Shimada, H.; Tsutsumimoto, K.; Lee, S.; Doi, T.; Makizako, H.; Lee, S.; Harada, K.; Hotta, R.; Bae, S.; Nakakubo, S.; et al. Driving continuity in cognitively impaired older drivers. *Geriatr. Gerontol. Int.* **2015**, *16*, 508–514. [CrossRef]

19. Miller, E.A.; Weissert, W.G. Predicting elderly people's risk for nursing home placement, hospitalization, functional impairment, and mortality: A synthesis. *Med. Care Res. Rev.* **2000**, *57*, 259–297. [CrossRef]

20. Chen, L.K.; Liu, L.K.; Woo, J.; Assantachai, P.; Auyeung, T.W.; Bahyah, K.S.; Chou, M.Y.; Chen, L.Y.; Hsu, P.S.; Krairit, O.; et al. Sarcopenia in Asia: Consensus report of the Asian Working Group for Sarcopenia. *J. Am. Med. Dir. Assoc.* **2014**, *15*, 95–101. [CrossRef]

21. Shimada, H.; Makizako, H.; Doi, T.; Yoshida, D.; Tsutsumimoto, K.; Anan, Y.; Uemura, K.; Ito, T.; Lee, S.; Park, H.; et al. Combined Prevalence of Frailty and Mild Cognitive Impairment in a Population of Elderly Japanese People. *J. Am. Med. Dir. Assoc.* **2013**, *14*, 518–524. [CrossRef]

22. Shimada, H.; Suzuki, T.; Suzukawa, M.; Makizako, H.; Doi, T.; Yoshida, D.; Tsutsumimoto, K.; Anan, Y.; Uemura, K.; Ito, T.; et al. Performance-based assessments and demand for personal care in older Japanese people: A cross-sectional study. *BMJ Open* **2013**, *3*, e002424. [CrossRef] [PubMed]

23. Fukutomi, E.; Okumiya, K.; Wada, T.; Sakamoto, R.; Ishimoto, Y.; Kimura, Y.; Chen, W.L.; Imai, H.; Kasahara, Y.; Fujisawa, M.; et al. Relationships between each category of 25-item frailty risk assessment (Kihon Checklist) and newly certified older adults under Long-Term Care Insurance: A 24-month follow-up study in a rural community in Japan. *Geriatr. Gerontol. Int.* **2014**, *15*, 864–871. [CrossRef]

24. Folstein, M.F.; Folstein, S.E.; McHugh, P.R. "Mini-mental state." A practical method for grading the cognitive state of patients for the clinician. *J. Psychiatr. Res.* **1975**, *12*, 189–198. [CrossRef]

25. Sheikh, J.I.; Yesavage, J.A. Geriatric Depression Scale (GDS): Recent evidence and development of a shorter version. *Clin. Gerontol.* **1986**, *5*, 165–173. [CrossRef]

26. Lesher, E.L.; Berryhill, J.S. Validation of the Geriatric Depression Scale–Short Form among inpatients. *J. Clin. Psychol.* **1994**, *50*, 256–260. [CrossRef]

27. Stuck, A.E.; Walthert, J.M.; Nikolaus, T.; Bula, C.J.; Hohmann, C.; Beck, J.C. Risk factors for functional status decline in community-living elderly people: A systematic literature review. *Soc. Sci. Med.* **1999**, *48*, 445–469. [CrossRef]

28. Ishizaki, T.; Watanabe, S.; Suzuki, T.; Shibata, H.; Haga, H. Predictors for functional decline among nondisabled older Japanese living in a community during a 3-year follow-up. *J. Am. Geriatr. Soc.* **2000**, *48*, 1424–1429. [CrossRef]

29. WHO Expert Consultation. Appropriate body-mass index for Asian populations and its implications for policy and intervention strategies. *Lancet* **2004**, *363*, 157–163. [CrossRef]

30. Ofori-Asenso, R.; Chin, K.L.; Mazidi, M.; Zomer, E.; Ilomaki, J.; Zullo, A.R.; Gasevic, D.; Ademi, Z.; Korhonen, M.J.; LoGiudice, D.; et al. Global Incidence of Frailty and Prefrailty Among Community-Dwelling Older Adults: A Systematic Review and Meta-analysis. *JAMA Netw. Open* **2019**, *2*, e198398. [CrossRef]

31. Beauchet, O.; Annweiler, C.; Allali, G.; Berrut, G.; Herrmann, F.R.; Dubost, V. Recurrent falls and dual task-related decrease in walking speed: Is there a relationship? *J. Am. Geriatr. Soc.* **2008**, *56*, 1265–1269. [CrossRef]

32. Kang, H.G.; Dingwell, J.B. Effects of walking speed, strength and range of motion on gait stability in healthy older adults. *J. Biomech.* **2008**, *41*, 2899–2905. [CrossRef]

33. Guralnik, J.M.; Ferrucci, L.; Pieper, C.F.; Leveille, S.G.; Markides, K.S.; Ostir, G.V.; Studenski, S.; Berkman, L.F.; Wallace, R.B. Lower extremity function and subsequent disability: Consistency across studies, predictive models, and value of gait speed alone compared with the short physical performance battery. *J. Gerontol. A Biol. Sci. Med. Sci.* **2000**, *55*, M221–M231. [CrossRef] [PubMed]

34. Cesari, M.; Kritchevsky, S.B.; Penninx, B.W.; Nicklas, B.J.; Simonsick, E.M.; Newman, A.B.; Tylavsky, F.A.; Brach, J.S.; Satterfield, S.; Bauer, D.C.; et al. Prognostic value of usual gait speed in well-functioning older people—Results from the Health, Aging and Body Composition Study. *J. Am. Geriatr. Soc.* **2005**, *53*, 1675–1680. [CrossRef]

35. Cesari, M.; Kritchevsky, S.B.; Newman, A.B.; Simonsick, E.M.; Harris, T.B.; Penninx, B.W.; Brach, J.S.; Tylavsky, F.A.; Satterfield, S.; Bauer, D.C.; et al. Added value of physical performance measures in predicting adverse health-related events: Results from the Health, Aging And Body Composition Study. *J. Am. Geriatr. Soc.* **2009**, *57*, 251–259. [CrossRef]

36. Onder, G.; Penninx, B.W.; Ferrucci, L.; Fried, L.P.; Guralnik, J.M.; Pahor, M. Measures of physical performance and risk for progressive and catastrophic disability: Results from the Women's Health and Aging Study. *J. Gerontol. A Biol. Sci. Med. Sci.* **2005**, *60*, 74–79. [CrossRef] [PubMed]

37. Studenski, S.; Perera, S.; Wallace, D.; Chandler, J.M.; Duncan, P.W.; Rooney, E.; Fox, M.; Guralnik, J.M. Physical performance measures in the clinical setting. *J. Am. Geriatr. Soc.* **2003**, *51*, 314–322. [CrossRef] [PubMed]

38. Simonsick, E.M.; Newman, A.B.; Visser, M.; Goodpaster, B.; Kritchevsky, S.B.; Rubin, S.; Nevitt, M.C.; Harris, T.B. Mobility limitation in self-described well-functioning older adults: Importance of endurance walk testing. *J. Gerontol. A Biol. Sci. Med. Sci.* **2008**, *63*, 841–847. [CrossRef]

39. Shinkai, S.; Watanabe, S.; Kumagai, S.; Fujiwara, Y.; Amano, H.; Yoshida, H.; Ishizaki, T.; Yukawa, H.; Suzuki, T.; Shibata, H. Walking speed as a good predictor for the onset of functional dependence in a Japanese rural community population. *Age Ageing* **2000**, *29*, 441–446. [CrossRef]

40. Nofuji, Y.; Shinkai, S.; Taniguchi, Y.; Amano, H.; Nishi, M.; Murayama, H.; Fujiwara, Y.; Suzuki, T. Associations of Walking Speed, Grip Strength, and Standing Balance With Total and Cause-Specific Mortality in a General Population of Japanese Elders. *J. Am. Med. Dir. Assoc.* **2016**, *17*, 184 e181–187. [CrossRef]

41. Liu, B.; Hu, X.; Zhang, Q.; Fan, Y.; Li, J.; Zou, R.; Zhang, M.; Wang, X.; Wang, J. Usual walking speed and all-cause mortality risk in older people: A systematic review and meta-analysis. *Gait Posture* **2016**, *44*, 172–177. [CrossRef]

42. Montero-Odasso, M.; Schapira, M.; Soriano, E.R.; Varela, M.; Kaplan, R.; Camera, L.A.; Mayorga, L.M. Gait velocity as a single predictor of adverse events in healthy seniors aged 75 years and older. *J. Gerontol. A Biol. Sci. Med. Sci.* **2005**, *60*, 1304–1309. [CrossRef]

43. Volpato, S.; Guralnik, J.M.; Ferrucci, L.; Balfour, J.; Chaves, P.; Fried, L.P.; Harris, T.B. Cardiovascular disease, interleukin-6, and risk of mortality in older women: The women's health and aging study. *Circulation* **2001**, *103*, 947–953. [CrossRef] [PubMed]

44. Shimada, H.; Makizako, H.; Doi, T.; Tsutsumimoto, K.; Suzuki, T. Incidence of Disability in Frail Older Persons with or Without Slow Walking Speed. *J. Am. Med. Dir. Assoc.* **2015**, *16*, 690–696. [CrossRef] [PubMed]

45. Beaudart, C.; Dawson, A.; Shaw, S.C.; Harvey, N.C.; Kanis, J.A.; Binkley, N.; Reginster, J.Y.; Chapurlat, R.; Chan, D.C.; Bruyere, O.; et al. Nutrition and physical activity in the prevention and treatment of sarcopenia: Systematic review. *Osteoporos. Int.* **2017**, *28*, 1817–1833. [CrossRef] [PubMed]

46. Ng, T.P.; Feng, L.; Nyunt, M.S.; Feng, L.; Niti, M.; Tan, B.Y.; Chan, G.; Khoo, S.A.; Chan, S.M.; Yap, P.; et al. Nutritional, Physical, Cognitive, and Combination Interventions and Frailty Reversal Among Older Adults: A Randomized Controlled Trial. *Am. J. Med.* **2015**, *128*, 1225.e1–1236.e1. [CrossRef] [PubMed]

47. Luger, E.; Dorner, T.E.; Haider, S.; Kapan, A.; Lackinger, C.; Schindler, K. Effects of a Home-Based and Volunteer-Administered Physical Training, Nutritional, and Social Support Program on Malnutrition and Frailty in Older Persons: A Randomized Controlled Trial. *J. Am. Med. Dir. Assoc.* **2016**, *17*, 671.e9–671.e16. [CrossRef]

48. Glass, T.A.; de Leon, C.M.; Marottoli, R.A.; Berkman, L.F. Population based study of social and productive activities as predictors of survival among elderly Americans. *BMJ* **1999**, *319*, 478–483. [CrossRef]

49. Jung, Y.; Gruenewald, T.L.; Seeman, T.E.; Sarkisian, C.A. Productive activities and development of frailty in older adults. *J. Gerontol. B Psychol. Sci. Soc. Sci.* **2010**, *65*, 256–261. [CrossRef]

50. Feng, Z.; Lugtenberg, M.; Franse, C.; Fang, X.; Hu, S.; Jin, C.; Raat, H. Risk factors and protective factors associated with incident or increase of frailty among community-dwelling older adults: A systematic review of longitudinal studies. *PLoS ONE* **2017**, *12*, e0178383. [CrossRef]

51. Kristman, V.; Manno, M.; Cote, P. Loss to follow-up in cohort studies: How much is too much? *Eur. J. Epidemiol.* **2004**, *19*, 751–760. [CrossRef]

Mortality- and Health-Related Factors in a Community-Dwelling of Oldest-Older Adults at the Age of 90: A 10-Year Follow-Up Study

Yoshiaki Nomura [1],*[ID], Mieko Shimada [2], Erika Kakuta [3], Ayako Okada [1], Ryoko Otsuka [1], Yasuko Tomizawa [4], Chieko Taguchi [5], Kazumune Arikawa [5], Hideki Daikoku [6], Tamotsu Sato [6] and Nobuhiro Hanada [1][ID]

[1] Department of Translational Research, School of Dental Medicine, Tsurumi University, Yokohama 230-8501, Japan; okada-a@tsurumi-u.ac.jp (A.O.); otsuka-ryoko@tsurumi-u.ac.jp (R.O.); hanada-n@tsurumi-u.ac.jp (N.H.)
[2] Department of Dental Hygiene, Chiba Prefectural University of Health Sciences, Chiba 261-0014, Japan; mieko.shimada@cpuhs.ac.jp
[3] Department of Oral Bacteriology, School of Dental Medicine, Tsurumi University, Yokohama 230-8501, Japan; kakuta-erika@tsurumi-u.ac.jp
[4] Department of Cardiovascular Surgery, Tokyo Women's Medical University, Tokyo 162-8666, Japan; tomizawa.yasuko@twmu.ac.jp
[5] Department of Preventive and Public Oral Health, School of Dentistry at Matsudo, Nihon University, Matsudo 470-2101, Japan; taguchi.chieko@nihon-u.ac.jp (C.T.); arikawa.kazumune@nihon-u.ac.jp (K.A.)
[6] Iwate Dental Association, Morioka 020-0045, Japan; dai-koku@nifty.com (H.D.); tamosato-dent@k-2inc.jp (T.S.)
* Correspondence: nomura-y@tsurumi-u.ac.jp

Abstract: Mortality is obviously intended for epidemiological studies of community-dwelling older adults. There are several health-related factors associated with nutritional status and mortality. The aim of this study was to elucidate the risk factor for mortality in community-dwelling oldest-older adults at the age of 90 and clarify the structure of health-related factors associated with mortality. A 10-year follow-up study was performed for 93 subjects at the age of 90. The mean and median of their survival days were 2373 and 2581 days for women, and 1694 and 1793 days for men. By Cox's proportional hazards model, health-related factors associated with mortality were self-assessed for chewing ability, activities of daily living (ADLs), serum albumin, total cholesterol, serum creatinine, and gripping power for women but not for men. These factors interacted with each other, and the association of these factors was different in women and men. Self-assessed chewing ability was a powerful risk factor for mortality in women at the age of 90. It acted independently from nutritional status. For older adults, addressing healthy food choices together with improved oral functions is useful. However, risk factors for mortality may depend on the life stage of subjects. To investigate the risk factor for the mortality, the life course approach is necessary.

Keywords: mortality; self-assessed chewing ability; serum albumin; ADL; physical performance

1. Introduction

Mortality is obviously intended for epidemiological studies of community-dwelling older adults. Many health-related factors associated with mortality interact with each other [1–6]. Therefore, health-related factors associated with mortality comprise a complex structure.

Sufficient nutritional status is essential for maintaining health in older adults. A positive ageing process depends on adequate nutritional status [7]. Poor nutritional status leads to adverse health outcomes [8,9]. It results in functional decline and frailty [10,11] and has been suggested to be a risk for mortality [8,9].

Oral health status has a recondite impact on nutritional status. Food consistency and food choice have been adapted to oral status [12]. The association between impaired masticatory function and deficient dietary intake has been suggested [13,14]. Suboptimal nutritional status after impaired oral function can result in chronic diseases [15]. In addition, impaired oral function and dysphagia increases the risk of aspiration pneumonia and choking [16,17]. Several studies have suggested that self-assessed chewing ability or mastication deficiency is a risk for mortality [18–21]. However, for addressing oral health and nutrition, well-designed studies are still not enough [22].

Nutritional status and diet quality effect the physical performance and activities of daily living (ADLs) [9,23,24], as well as oral health-related to physical performance and ADLs [25–27]. Therefore, health-related factors can interact with each other and impact mortality.

Regarding community-dwelling older adults, evidence has been accumulated for the numerous risk factors associated with mortality. Studies have found that specific health-related factors are regarded as risks after adjustment for common risk factors. An investigation was performed within specific health-related factors, including nutrition [28,29], oral health [30–38], and physical performance [39–45]. In addition to this risk evaluation, a comprehensive assessment for the risk factors for mortality is necessary for planning health promotion for older adults [46,47], decision of priority of intervention [48–50], and health-related political decision-making.

In 1997, the Japanese Ministry of Labor and Health directed and supported a survey of 80-year-old people residing in four areas of Japan. The aims of the survey were to investigate the relationship between oral health and systemic health in 80-year-old adults. Iwate Prefecture, located in the northern region of Japan, was one of the areas participating in this survey. The survey items were common to the baseline study. Then, four areas were independently carried out in the follow-up study. Iwate Prefecture conducted the 5-year follow-up (85 years of age), 10-year follow-up (90 years of age), and 20-year follow-up (100 years old). Previous reports had shown the importance of chewing ability for mortality [51,52]. In this study, all the data in the 10-year follow-up study (90 years of age) were analyzed, including chewing ability.

We assessed the association between mortality and health status via blood tests, including reflection of nutritional status, oral health status via self-assessed chewing ability, physical performance, and activities of daily living (ADLs). The magnitude of health-related factors pertinent to mortality were investigated. In addition, the correlation between mortality and these health-related factors were summarized.

The aim of this study was to elucidate the risk factor for mortality in community-dwelling oldest-older adults at the age of 90 and clarify the structure of health-related factors associated with mortality.

2. Materials and Methods

2.1. Setting

A 20-year follow-up survey was conducted on 80-year-old subjects living in 10 districts managed by one health center in Iwate Prefecture in northern Japan. For 20 years, heath examinations were conducted three times in 1997 for the 80-year-old subjects, in 2002 at the age of 85, and 2007 at the age of 90. Oral examination, physical performance measures, blood tests and questionnaire surveys were conducted as health examinations. Other than these three-times survey, no health examinations were conducted. In this study, data of subjects at the age of 90 were analyzed in a 10-year follow-up survey (2007–2017).

of reproductive age, and this is affecting the health of future generations [1]. Early-life nutrition plays a key role in infant growth and development and has a programming effect related to the appearance of future non-communicable diseases, such as obesity, diabetes and others [2,3]. Breast milk composition and breastfeeding practice are some of the most influential factors of child outcomes [4–6]. Even though lactation comprises a relatively short period in the average person's lifespan, the exposure to breast milk in the first months of life occurs during a very critical period of rapid growth and development [2,7–9]. Maternal obesity influences the nutritional status of the child through different mechanisms, breastfeeding being one of them. If the mother of the child has obesity, the fatty acid (FA) profile in breast milk can be different, with a prevalence of pro-inflammatory FAs beyond those critical for neurodevelopment [10]. Thus, the early nutritional status and future health of the child can be affected.

Breast milk contains long-chain (LC) polyunsaturated fatty acids (PUFAs), which are crucial nutrients—especially docosahexaenoic (DHA) and arachidonic acid (AA)—involved in growth, the immune system, vision, and cognitive and motor development [11]. These nutrients are associated with the prevention of obesity [12,13] and other infectious and chronic diseases in the future life [14]. However, maternal characteristics, such as diet [15] or obesity [10], may alter the FA content in human milk. Studies have shown that the breast milk of mothers with overweight and obesity have higher levels of n6 FAs and lower levels of n3 FAs than the breast milk of normal-weight mothers [16–18], and a high ratio of n6:n3 LC-PUFAs in red blood cells membrane phospholipids has been reported as a risk factor for obesity [19]. In fact, in high-fat rodent models of maternal obesity, lowering the maternal n6:n3 ratio using a novel genetic model or supplemental fish oil has been shown to prevent offspring obesity [20]. Nevertheless, the results appear to be inconsistent [18,21].

The direct impact of maternal weight on the infant cognition has also been studied [21–24]. Mostly, observational, prospective and longitudinal studies correlate a high pre-pregnancy maternal body mass index (BMI) with poorer cognitive performance [24]. High gestational weight gain (GWG) seems to augment this correlation, as well [25]. However, three studies have failed to find an association between maternal obesity and cognitive infant deficits [26–28].

Although there are studies that have analyzed the influence of maternal weight on breast milk FA composition [10,18,29–35], none of these studies have further assessed its effect on infant cognition and growth. Furthermore, there is a lot of variability regarding the timing of breastmilk collection in the existing studies, and most of them focus on the analysis of mature breastmilk, without considering the evolution of the different FAs from colostrum to mature milk. Therefore, the current study aims to analyze the implications of maternal obesity on FA levels in colostrum and mature milk and their association with infant growth and cognition, to raise awareness about the programming effect of maternal nutrition and promote a healthy weight in women.

2. Materials and Methods

2.1. Statement of Ethics

This study was carried out in accordance with the ethical standards recognized by the Declaration of Helsinki (2004), the EEC Good Clinical Practice guidelines (document 111/3976/88 of July 1990) and current Spanish legislation governing clinical research in humans (Royal Decree 561/1993 on clinical trials). Additionally, the study was approved by San Cecilio University Hospital Ethics Committee and the Faculty of Medicine at the University of Granada. Written informed consent was obtained from all participants at the beginning of the study.

2.2. Study Population and Design

For the present study, a subsample of mother–child pairs ($n = 78$) from the PREOBE cohort was selected and classified according to maternal pre-pregnancy BMI: normal-weight (BMI = 18.5–24.99 Kg/m^2, $n = 34$), overweight (BMI = 25–29.99 Kg/m^2, $n = 27$) and obese (BMI > 30 Kg/m^2, $n = 17$).

The PREOBE study (Role of Nutrition and Maternal Genetics on the Programming of Development of Fetal Adipose Tissue) is an observational cohort study of a total of 331 pregnant women that analyzes the impact of maternal obesity and gestational diabetes. The information regarding the PREOBE study has been published elsewhere [34] and was registered at www.ClinicalTrials.gov (NCT01634464). Figure 1 presents the study design and information of the PREOBE study.

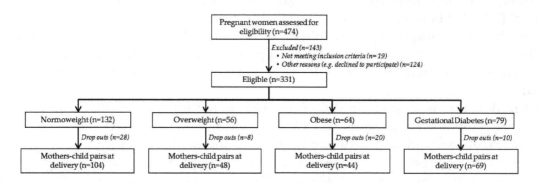

Figure 1. Participants in the PREOBE cohort and classification following BMI and gestational diabetes criteria.

Briefly, the study and recruitment of participants were carried out at San Cecilio University Hospital and the Mother-Infant Hospital in the city of Granada, Spain. The inclusion criteria were: singleton pregnancy, gestation between 12 and 20 weeks at enrollment, and an intention to deliver in one of the two obstetrics centers mentioned above. Women were excluded if they were participating in other research studies, receiving drug treatment or supplements of DHA or folate for more than the first three months of pregnancy, suffering from disorders such as hypertension, pre-eclampsia, fetal intrauterine growth retardation, infections, hypo- or hyperthyroidism and hepatic renal diseases, or following an unusual or vegan diet. Maternal age, pre-pregnancy BMI, parity, smoking status, diet, alcohol habits, socio-demographic information, education, gestational weight gain, infant anthropometry, gender and feeding practices were recorded. After birth, the women were encouraged to breastfeed their infants.

2.3. Breast Milk Sample Collection

Colostrum and mature milk were collected at 2–4 and 28–32 days postpartum, respectively, by an experienced nurse at the hospitals or by the mother at home (after receiving training by the nurse). Samples were collected over the course of an entire day (24 h) from both breasts before and after each feed. Milk samples were gathered in sterile polypropylene tubes by mechanically expressing each breast with a breast pump. Mothers were given 14 tubes with a capacity of 5 mL and the total volume obtained from each mother ranged from 45 to 70 mL. The samples collected at each time were frozen at −20 °C at home, and mothers brought them to the 3-month offspring follow-up visit. Each time, the samples were transported in ice boxes to the laboratory, where they were stored at −80 °C until analysis. All samples from each woman were mixed and aliquoted prior to analysis.

2.4. Fatty Acid Analysis of Breast Milk

The FA composition of breast milk was determined according to the method described by Chisaguano et al. [35]. 50 μL human milk samples were used for the analysis. FA methyl esters (FAMEs) were prepared with sodium methylate in methanol (0.5 M) and boron trifluoride methanol solution (14% v/v). They were then separated and quantified by fast gas chromatography (GC)using a HP-6890 Series GC System (Hewlett-Packard, Waldbronn, Germany) equipped with a flame ionization detector (FID), a split/splitless injector, a HP-7683B Series autoinjector, and a fused-silica SP-2560 capillary column (75 m 0.18 mm internal diameter, 0.14 μm thickness) coated with a 100% bis-cyanopropyl polysiloxane stationary phase (Supelco, Saunderton, UK). The chromatographic conditions used were: hydrogen as the carrier gas at a constant linear velocity of 22 cm/s (which gave an initial pressure of 39 psi). The detector and injector temperatures were set at 300 °C and 250 °C, respectively; the split ratio was at 1:50 and the injection volume was 1 μL. Oven temperatures were programmed as follows: the initial temperature was set at 120 °C, which was increased at a rate of 25 °C min^{-1} to 180 °C. This temperature was held for 6 min and finally increased to 240 °C at a rate of 25 °C min^{-1}, and held for 9 min.

FAs were identified by a comparison of the peak retention times of those of the standard solution Supelco 37-component FAME mix (Sigma-Aldrich, St. Louis, MO, USA). FAs were then quantified by standard normalization (% total fatty acids), and they are therefore expressed as a percentage of the total amount of FAs. FA summatories were derived by adding the corresponding single FAs to saturated FAs (SFAs), monounsaturated FAs (MUFAs), PUFAs, n6 PUFAs, n3 PUFAs, n6 LC-PUFAs and n3 LC-PUFAs. Moreover, n6 to n3 ratios were created for analysis.

2.5. Assessment of Anthropometric Infant Outcomes

After birth, the infants received a medical examination during which anthropometric measurements were recorded. Data, such as weight, length and BMI at 6, 18 and 36 months of age were included in the present study. Length and weight (with light clothing and no shoes) were recorded using a Harpenden Infantometer (Model 702) calibrated stadiometer (Holtain, Wales, United Kingdom) and a Multina Comfort calibrated balance scale (SOEHNLE, Backnang, Germany), respectively. Weight, length and BMI measurements were ultimately converted to weight-for-age z-scores (WAZ), length-for-age z-scores (LAZ) and BMI-for-age z-scores (BMIZ) (SD scores), according to World Health Organization (WHO) child growth standards [36,37].

2.6. Assessment of Infant Cognitive Development

Infant cognitive development was assessed at 18 months of age using the Bayley Scales of Infant Development III (BSID III) [38], by trained psychologists in the presence of the mother of the child. These scales measure the level of motor, language and cognitive or mental development. The present study uses the Cognitive Composite score, which is the global score of the scales and represents the overall cognitive development of the children.

2.7. Statistical Analysis

Statistical analyses were performed using the SPSS statistical software package for Windows (version 23.0; SPSS Inc., Chicago, IL, USA). The Kolmogorov-Smirnov test was used to study the normal distribution of the data and non-normally distributed data were natural log-transformed. Means and standard deviations (SD) were used to describe continuous variables. The characteristics of the population were analyzed using the ANOVA and Bonferroni post-hoc test. To analyze the FA evolution from colostrum to mature milk, a paired Student's *t*-test was used. The independent Student's *t*-test was used to compare the breast milk FA composition between maternal weight groups. The associations between breast milk FAs and child anthropometric measurements and cognitive scores were determined using linear regression analyses and corrected for potential confounders such as maternal BMI, smoking, education, GWG and parity, and infant characteristics, such as gender and feeding practices. The Bonferroni correction (0.05/(48 FAs × 3 study groups = 144 analyses)) was applied to take multiple testing into account and *p*-value thresholds were set at 0.002. In the tables, *p*-values ≤ 0.05 are highlighted in bold, while those ≤0.002 are additionally marked by stars.

3. Results

3.1. Characteristics of the Population

The characteristics of the population are shown in Table 1. Normal-weight women presented the highest GWG, followed by overweight and finally mothers with obesity. The latter group had the highest n6:n3 ratio in dietary intake, while normal-weight mothers had the lowest intake of AA. No significant differences were found in infant characteristics according to maternal BMI.

Table 1. Characteristics of the population.

Characteristic		Normal-Weight		Overweight		Obesity	p
		Mean (SD)		Mean (SD)		Mean (SD)	
Maternal characteristics	n		n		n		
Age (years)	34	31 (4)	27	32 (4)	17	32 (4)	0.492
Pre-pregnancy BMI (kg/m^2)	34	22.14 (1.54) [a]	27	27.59 (1.35) [b]	17	33.40 (2.65) [c]	**<0.001 ***
Weight Gain (kg)	25	13.17 (3.55)	23	10.32 (5.20)	15	9.14 (7.06)	**0.042**
Education (%)							0.660
<High school	26	14.71	19	11.11	11	23.53	
High school	3	8.82	5	18.52	2	11.76	
>High school	5	76.47	3	70.37	4	64.71	
Smoking during pregnancy (%)							0.415
No, never	17	77.27	15	71.43	10	73.68	
Yes	3	13.64	5	23.81	1	7.14	
Quit	2	9.09	1	4.76	3	21.43	
Maternal dietary intake							
Energy (Kcal/day)	27	2066.37 (261.93)	23	2089.59 (542.07)	12	2058.08 (469.97)	0.961
Lipids (g)	27	86.89 (17.29)	23	85.25 (25.86)	12	93.23 (20.95)	0.468
Lipids (%)	27	37.76 (5.26)	23	39.04 (7.73)	12	41.17 (5.38)	0.307
SFA (g/d)	27	30.81 (6.36)	23	30.05 (8.67)	12	34.19 (5.87)	0.203
MUFA (g/d)	27	36.53 (10.92)	23	39.33 (17.63)	12	36.32 (12.08)	0.926
PUFA (g/d)	27	12.10 (3.17)	23	13.34 (6.59)	12	14.63 (3.95)	0.285
n6 PUFA (g/d)	27	2.48 (1.95)	23	2.89 (2.53)	12	3.44 (1.50)	0.122
n3 PUFA (g/d)	27	0.18 (0.11)	23	0.21 (0.13)	12	0.20 (0.09)	0.427
n-3 from fish (g/d)	27	0.36 (0.31)	23	0.28 (0.34)	12	0.45 (0.34)	0.690
AA (g/d)	27	0.11 (0.06) [a]	23	0.17 (0.08) [b]	12	0.16 (0.08) [ab]	**0.005**
EPA (g/d)	27	0.12 (0.11)	23	0.09 (0.11)	12	0.16 (0.12)	0.213
DHA (g/d)	27	0.24 (0.18)	23	0.22 (0.21)	12	0.31 (0.21)	0.269
n6:n3	27	12.99 (2.98) [a]	23	13.53 (3.40) [a]	12	19.12 (8.94) [b]	**0.004**
Infant characteristics							
Sex, male (%)	14	41.18	11	40.74	7	41.18	0.999
Birth weight (g)	32	3359.06 (352.35)	27	3340.37 (511.85)	16	3532.35 (389.61)	0.277
Birth length (cm)	31	50.52 (1.57)	27	50.30 (1.88)	16	51.22 (1.80)	0.245
Birth head Circumference (cm)	26	34.31 (1.36)	22	34.36 (1.39)	16	34.69 (1.40)	0.674
Placenta (g)	30	496.67 (144.11)	25	509.20 (130.25)	16	568.13 (143.17)	0.332
Newborn according Lubchenco curves [#] (%)							0.627
SGA	0	0.00	1	4.55	0	0.00	
AGA	26	81.25	16	72.73	11	73.33	
LGA	6	18.75	5	22.73	4	26.67	
Breastfeeding [†] (%)							0.290
Exclusive	16	53.33	16	66.67	8	50.00	
Mixt	10	33.33	3	12.50	3	18.75	
Artificial	4	13.33	5	20.83	5	31.25	

Different superscript letters indicate differences among BMI groups, according to ANOVA and the Bonferroni post-hoc test. Chi-square test was applied to qualitative variables. p-values ≤ 0.05 are highlighted in bold and those ≤0.002 are additionally marked by stars. [#] The newborns were divided into three groups according to the Lubchenco curves: SGA: Small for Gestational Age; AGA: Appropriate for Gestational Age; LGA: Large for Gestational Age (LGA). [†] Breastfeeding practice information was collected at 3 months of age of the child. SFA: Saturated Fatty Acids; MUFA: Monounsaturated Fatty Acids; PUFA: Polyunsaturated Fatty Acids; AA: Arachidonic Acid; EPA: Eicosapentaenoic Acid; DHA: Docosahexaenoic Acid.

3.2. Breast Milk Fatty Acid Evolution

The FA evolution from colostrum to mature milk is shown in Table 2. In spite of maternal pre-pregnancy BMI, mature breast milk presented lower levels of C16:1n9, C20:1n9, AA, C22:1n9, C22:4n6, C22:5n6, C22:5n3, DHA, C24:0, C24:1n6 and n3 LC-PUFAs, and higher levels of C8:0, C10:0, medium-chain FAs (MCFAs), eicosapentaenoic acid (EPA):AA and DHA:AA ratios than those found in colostrum.

Table 2. Human milk fatty acids profile according to maternal pre-pregnancy BMI.

	Normal-Weight			Overweight			Obesity		
	Colostrum (n = 26)	Mature Milk (n = 20)	p	Colostrum (n = 21)	Mature Milk (n = 23)	p	Colostrum (n = 16)	Mature Milk (n = 14)	p
	Mean (SD)	Mean (SD)		Mean (SD)	Mean (SD)		Mean (SD)	Mean (SD)	
C6:0	0.06 (0.04)	0.08 (0.03)	0.19	0.05 (0.03)	0.10 (0.04)	<0.001 *	0.05 (0.03)	0.08 (0.07)	0.002 *
C8:0	0.13 (0.09)	0.23 (0.07)	0.002 *	0.13 (0.08)	0.24 (0.09)	<0.001 *	0.08 (0.03) #	0.24 (0.10)	<0.001 *
C10:0	0.86 (0.57)	1.29 (0.37)	0.010	0.86 (0.47)	1.36 (0.33)	0.002 *	0.70 (0.57)	1.47 (0.32)	<0.001 *
C12:0	4.10 (2.07)	4.86 (1.80)	0.039	4.18 (1.97)	4.86 (1.92)	0.14	3.67 (2.49)	5.32 (1.65)	0.029
C14:0	5.15 (1.41)	4.79 (1.71)	0.88	5.38 (1.92)	4.67 (1.66)	0.38	5.04 (2.31)	5.23 (1.22)	0.32
C14:1	0.08 (0.02)	0.10 (0.03)	0.20	0.11 (0.03) †	0.11 (0.04)	0.51	0.10 (0.05)	0.12 (0.06)	0.10
C15:0	0.21 (0.03)	0.21 (0.06)	0.80	0.24 (0.04) †	0.20 (0.05)	0.016	0.19 (0.04) #	0.22 (0.08)	0.32
C16:0	21.13 (2.32)	19.56 (2.29)	0.006	21.24 (1.46)	19.53 (2.02)	0.001 *	21.96 (2.11)	21.20 (2.55) #	0.42
C16:1t	0.12 (0.03)	0.13 (0.04)	0.59	0.14 (0.04)	0.11 (0.05)	0.06	0.13 (0.04)	0.13 (0.06)	0.98
C16:1n9	0.50 (0.05)	0.43 (0.06)	<0.001 *	0.54 (0.13)	0.45 (0.07)	0.010	0.54 (0.10)	0.46 (0.10)	0.024
C16:1n7	1.48 (0.45)	1.83 (0.62)	0.11	1.63 (0.36)	1.80 (0.49)	0.014	1.78 (0.60)	1.88 (0.58)	0.61
C17:0	0.30 (0.04)	0.29 (0.08)	0.74	0.34 (0.03) †	0.29 (0.06)	0.026	0.29 (0.05) #	0.32 (0.07)	0.28
C17:1	0.15 (0.03)	0.17 (0.03)	0.28	0.18 (0.04) †	0.18 (0.04)	0.88	0.17 (0.07)	0.17 (0.05)	0.83
C18:0	5.74 (0.67)	5.74 (0.41)	0.20	5.58 (0.85)	5.88 (0.67)	0.12	5.44 (0.81) †	6.03 (0.49)	<0.001 *
C18:1n9	38.47 (3.51)	39.69 (4.23)	0.41	38.16 (4.57)	38.73 (5.53)	0.87	37.36 (3.11)	36.63 (0.96) †	0.30
C18:1n7t	0.33 (0.14)	0.28 (0.09)	0.12	0.31 (0.09)	0.26 (0.08)	0.24	0.24 (0.05) †#	0.22 (0.04) †	0.15
C18:1n7	1.69 (0.22)	1.58 (0.24)	0.02	1.69 (0.28)	1.63 (0.23)	0.81	1.89 (0.42)	1.59 (0.32)	0.022
C18:1n-7t11	0.28 (0.12)	0.30 (0.12)	0.95	0.28 (0.09)	0.26 (0.11)	0.15	0.27 (0.14)	0.24 (0.08)	0.72
C18:2n6 (LA)	13.03 (2.42)	13.60 (3.21)	0.31	13.31 (3.20)	15.20 (3.86)	0.050	12.98 (2.74)	13.90 (3.14)	0.49
C18:2n7c9t11	0.12 (0.03)	0.13 (0.05)	0.69	0.14 (0.04)	0.12 (0.04)	0.32	0.13 (0.05)	0.14 (0.06)	0.67
C18:3n6	0.09 (0.04)	0.17 (0.06)	0.010	0.11 (0.07)	0.18 (0.05)	<0.001 *	0.13 (0.09)	0.17 (0.05)	0.15
C18:3n3 (ALA)	0.54 (0.18)	0.59 (0.21)	0.61	0.53 (0.13)	0.58 (0.16)	0.14	0.41 (0.04) #	0.46 (0.08) †#	0.16
C20:0	0.20 (0.03)	0.18 (0.01)	0.012	0.18 (0.02)	0.17 (0.03)	0.005	0.19 (0.04)	0.18 (0.04)	0.75
C20:1n9	0.77 (0.20)	0.50 (0.07)	<0.001 *	0.74 (0.26)	0.46 (0.05)	<0.001 *	0.77 (0.24)	0.48 (0.06)	<0.001 *
C20:3n6	0.60 (0.15)	0.47 (0.11)	<0.001 *	0.65 (0.21)	0.48 (0.06)	0.004	0.68 (0.24)	0.52 (0.14)	0.05
C20:4n6 (AA)	0.67 (0.19)	0.49 (0.05)	0.005	0.66 (0.13)	0.49 (0.12)	<0.001 *	0.67 (0.23)	0.47 (0.10)	0.004
C20:5n3 (EPA)	0.05 (0.02)	0.07 (0.03)	0.07	0.04 (0.02)	0.06 (0.02)	<0.001 *	0.05 (0.03)	0.07 (0.02)	0.10

Table 2. *Cont.*

	Normal-Weight			Overweight			Obesity		
	Colostrum (n = 26)	Mature Milk (n = 20)	p	Colostrum (n = 21)	Mature Milk (n = 23)	p	Colostrum (n = 16)	Mature Milk (n = 14)	p
	Mean (SD)	Mean (SD)		Mean (SD)	Mean (SD)		Mean (SD)	Mean (SD)	
C22:0	0.08 (0.03)	0.06 (0.02)	**0.007**	0.09 (0.03)	0.08 (0.03)	0.20	0.08 (0.02)	0.07 (0.02)	**0.039**
C22:1n9	0.18 (0.06)	0.09 (0.02)	**<0.001 ***	0.19 (0.08)	0.09 (0.02)	**<0.001 ***	0.18 (0.06)	0.09 (0.01)	**<0.001 ***
C22:2n6	0.07 (0.03)	0.04 (0.01)	**0.003**	0.08 (0.03)	0.06 (0.03)	0.22	0.06 (0.02)	**0.06 (0.02)** †	0.22
C22:4n6	0.25 (0.13)	0.10 (0.02)	**<0.001 ***	0.28 (0.15)	0.12 (0.04)	**<0.001 ***	0.37 (0.27)	0.12 (0.03)	**<0.001 ***
C22:5n6	0.12 (0.04)	0.05 (0.01)	**<0.001 ***	0.12 (0.05)	0.07 (0.03) †	**0.048**	0.12 (0.05)	**0.09 (0.05)** †	**0.040**
C22:5n3	0.16 (0.08)	0.11 (0.03)	**0.012**	0.14 (0.05)	0.11 (0.03)	**0.002 ***	0.19 (0.09)	0.12 (0.04)	**0.007**
C22:6n3 (DHA)	0.41 (0.14)	0.28 (0.11)	**<0.001 ***	0.35 (0.08)	**0.22 (0.06)** †	**<0.001 ***	0.39 (0.13)	0.25 (0.07)	**0.002 ***
C23:0	0.12 (0.05)	0.05 (0.02)	**<0.001 ***	0.12 (0.05)	0.06 (0.03)	**<0.001 ***	0.13 (0.05)	0.09 (0.07) †	0.06
C24:0	0.10 (0.03)	0.05 (0.02)	**0.002 ***	0.10 (0.04)	0.06 (0.03)	**0.007**	0.09 (0.03)	0.06 (0.03)	**0.031**
C24:1	0.20 (0.11)	0.06 (0.02)	**<0.001 ***	0.19 (0.13)	0.06 (0.04)	**<0.001 ***	0.19 (0.09)	0.07 (0.03)	**<0.001 ***
EPA:AA	0.07 (0.03)	0.12 (0.03)	**0.005**	0.06 (0.03)	**0.09 (0.04)** †	**<0.001 ***	0.07 (0.03)	0.12 (0.07)	**0.004**
DHA:AA	0.63 (0.22)	0.77 (0.19)	**0.005**	0.55 (0.13)	0.76 (0.24)	**<0.001 ***	0.61 (0.21)	0.90 (0.34)	**0.004**
SFA	27.45 (2.66)	25.83 (2.48)	**0.008**	27.43 (1.93)	25.95 (2.49)	**0.004**	27.96 (2.34)	**27.80 (2.62)** †,#	0.96
MCFA	5.14 (2.69)	6.46 (2.19)	**0.021**	5.23 (2.46)	6.56 (2.27)	**0.037**	4.50 (3.06)	7.11 (1.99)	**0.010**
MUFA	42.80 (3.51)	43.73 (4.17)	0.87	42.61 (4.91)	42.76 (5.70)	0.74	42.17 (3.56)	**40.74 (1.37)** †	0.12
n6 PUFA	15.41 (2.53)	15.24 (3.31)	0.77	15.79 (3.23)	16.89 (3.93)	0.29	15.67 (3.01)	15.64 (3.19)	0.93
n3 PUFA	1.16 (0.30)	1.05 (0.24)	**0.018**	1.07 (0.15)	0.96 (0.21)	0.12	1.04 (0.23)	0.90 (0.13)	0.06
n6 LC-PUFA	2.30 (0.59)	1.48 (0.22)	**<0.001 ***	2.36 (0.63)	1.52 (0.24)	**<0.001 ***	2.56 (0.93)	1.58 (0.34)	**<0.001 ***
n3 LC-PUFA	0.62 (0.22)	0.45 (0.16)	**<0.001 ***	0.54 (0.12)	0.38 (0.11)	**<0.001 ***	0.63 (0.23)	0.44 (0.09)	**0.008**
n6:n3 PUFA	14.28 (4.76)	15.08 (3.91)	0.06	15.13 (4.37)	**18.28 (5.33)** †	**0.033**	15.67 (4.22)	17.80 (4.97)	0.15
n6:n3 LC-PUFA	4.00 (1.16)	3.62 (1.18)	0.08	4.49 (0.95)	4.28 (1.24)	0.41	4.23 (1.05)	3.73 (0.92)	0.14

Means are expressed as percentages of total FAs. The *p*-value shown refers to the breast milk evolution within each group of weight, according to Student's paired *t*-test. *p*-values ≤ 0.05 are highlighted in bold and those ≤0.002 are additionally marked by stars. † Indicates differences (*p* ≤ 0.05) compared with normal-weight group and its corresponding breast milk, according to Student's independent *t*-test. # Indicates differences (*p* ≤ 0.05) between overweight and obese groups and corresponding breast milk, according to Student's independent *t*-test; LA: Linoleic Acid; AA: Arachidonic Acid; ALA: α-linolenic Acid; EPA: Eicosapentaenoic Acid; DHA: Docosahexaenoic Acid; SFA: Saturated Fatty Acids; MCFA: Medium-chain Fatty Acids; MUFA: Monounsaturated Fatty Acids; PUFA: Polyunsaturated Fatty Acids; LC-PUFA: Long-Chain Polyunsaturated Fatty Acids.

Regarding other biologically important FAs, and always compared to colostrum levels, the mature milk of normal-weight mothers showed higher levels of C12:0 and C18:3n6, and lower levels of C16:0, C20:0, C20:3n6, C22:0, C22:2 n6, C23:0, saturated fatty acids (SFAs) and n3 PUFAs; the mature milk of overweight mothers showed increased levels of C6:0, C16:1n7, linoleic acid (LA), C18:3n6, EPA and n6:n3 ratio, and decreased concentrations of C15:0, C16:0, C17:0, C20:0, C23:0 and SFAs; and finally, the mature milk of mothers with obesity had higher levels of C6:0, C12:0 and C18:0 and lower levels of C18:1n7 and C22:0.

3.3. Breast Milk FAs According to Maternal Weight Group

Table 2 also shows the differences in breast milk FAs between weight groups. Compared to normal-weight women, the overweight group had higher levels of C14:1, C15:0, C17:0 and C17:1 in colostrum; and higher levels of C22:5n6 and n6:n3 ratio and lower levels of DHA and EPA:AA in mature milk.

On the other hand, compared to normal-weight mothers, mothers with obesity had lower levels of C18:0, C18:1n9t and ALA in colostrum; and lower levels of C18:1n9, C18:1n9t, ALA and MUFAs and higher levels of C22:2n6, C22:5n6, C23:0 and SFAs in mature milk.

We also compared overweight with mothers with obesity and found that the group with obesity had lower concentrations of C8:0, C15:0, C17:0, C18:1n9t, ALA in colostrum; and higher levels of C16:0 and SFAs and lower levels of ALA in mature milk.

3.4. Association of Breast Milk FAs with Infant Growth

Table 3 shows the associations between breast milk FAs and infant growth. All associations were observed after adjusting for potential confounders, which included maternal pre-pregnancy BMI, maternal smoking, weight gain during pregnancy, maternal education, gender of the child and type of infant feeding practice.

Table 3. Associations between breast milk PUFA levels and anthropometric measurements in infants.

	BMIZ				WAZ				LAZ			
	Colostrum		Mature Milk		Colostrum		Mature Milk		Colostrum		Mature Milk	
Fatty Acid	6mo $n = 37$ 18mo $n = 38$ 36mo $n = 16$		6mo $n = 39$ 18mo $n = 37$ 36mo $n = 13$		6mo $n = 37$ 18mo $n = 38$ 36mo $n = 16$		6mo $n = 39$ 18mo $n = 38$ 36mo $n = 13$		6mo $n = 38$ 18mo $n = 38$ 36mo $n = 18$		6mo $n = 39$ 18mo $n = 38$ 36mo $n = 14$	
	β	p	β	p	β	p	β	p	β	p	β	p
					C18:3n3 (ALA)							
6mo	−0.11	0.63	−0.15	0.40	−0.06	0.77	−0.22	0.24	0.05	0.80	−0.12	0.49
18mo	0.32	0.13	−0.11	0.57	0.11	0.63	−0.13	0.51	−0.20	0.26	−0.06	0.69
36mo	−0.44	0.21	0.01	0.99	−0.27	0.52	0.06	0.95	−0.17	0.63	−0.86	0.22
					C18:2n6 (LA)							
6mo	0.33	0.12	−0.13	0.43	**0.42**	**0.027**	0.16	0.36	0.15	0.40	0.09	0.60
18mo	−0.19	0.34	0.04	0.85	0.18	0.37	0.05	0.79	0.06	0.73	0.17	0.26
36mo	0.12	0.75	−0.22	0.50	0.02	0.96	−0.136	0.75	0.01	0.98	−0.33	0.41
					C20:4n6 (AA)							
6mo	**−0.44**	**0.016**	0.02	0.91	−0.20	0.26	0.04	0.84	0.25	0.13	0.03	0.86
18mo	−0.03	0.89	−0.12	0.57	0.06	0.77	−0.13	0.52	0.10	0.50	0.15	0.39
36mo	0.30	0.30	0.09	0.81	0.42	0.20	0.07	0.86	0.20	0.48	0.12	0.75
					C20:5n3 (EPA)							
6mo	**−0.51**	**0.012**	0.00	0.99	−0.36	0.07	−0.13	0.49	0.18	0.31	−0.18	0.29
18mo	−0.30	0.12	0.00	0.98	−0.13	0.51	0.08	0.66	0.15	0.35	0.09	0.62
36mo	−0.74	0.155	−1.08	0.30	−0.58	0.34	−1.13	0.28	0.14	0.69	−0.59	0.61

Table 3. *Cont.*

Fatty Acid	BMIZ Colostrum 6mo n=37 18mo n=38 36mo n=16 β	p	BMIZ Mature Milk 6mo n=39 18mo n=37 36mo n=13 β	p	WAZ Colostrum 6mo n=37 18mo n=38 36mo n=16 β	p	WAZ Mature Milk 6mo n=39 18mo n=38 36mo n=13 β	p	LAZ Colostrum 6mo n=38 18mo n=38 36mo n=18 β	p	LAZ Mature Milk 6mo n=39 18mo n=38 36mo n=14 β	p
C22:6n3 (DHA)												
6mo	**−0.37**	**0.043**	−0.16	0.38	−0.31	0.07	−0.29	0.10	0.00	0.99	−0.23	0.17
18mo	0.14	0.42	0.03	0.88	0.08	0.66	0.00	0.99	−0.05	0.74	−0.03	0.84
36mo	0.42	0.29	0.33	0.46	0.65	0.13	0.38	0.39	0.46	0.22	0.58	0.14
n6 PUFA												
6mo	0.21	0.32	0.13	0.45	0.34	0.07	0.16	0.35	0.20	0.27	0.10	0.55
18mo	0.16	0.41	−0.06	0.776	0.18	0.40	0.04	0.83	0.08	0.65	0.18	0.23
36mo	0.20	0.587	−0.19	0.64	0.15	0.72	−0.11	0.79	0.07	0.84	−0.31	0.44
n3 PUFA												
6mo	**−0.38**	**0.047**	−0.19	0.27	−0.33	0.07	−0.32	0.07	−0.00	0.991	−0.22	0.18
18mo	0.16	0.38	−0.11	0.56	0.04	0.84	−0.11	0.53	−0.12	0.427	−0.05	0.75
36mo	−0.20	0.60	0.17	0.78	0.05	0.90	0.21	0.74	0.05	0.897	−0.18	0.77
n6 LC−PUFA												
6mo	**−0.38**	**0.047**	−0.06	0.77	−0.17	0.36	0.00	0.98	0.19	0.253	0.09	0.65
18mo	−0.05	0.77	−0.27	0.19	0.03	0.88	−0.17	0.41	0.10	0.508	0.19	0.25
36mo	0.40	0.22	0.11	0.78	0.60	0.09	0.12	0.76	0.25	0.390	−0.03	0.95
n3 LC−PUFA												
6mo	**−0.43**	**0.020**	−0.19	0.28	−0.34	0.05	−0.33	0.06	0.03	0.866	−0.24	0.16
18mo	0.07	0.70	−0.04	0.82	0.05	0.78	−0.02	0.90	−0.01	0.955	0.02	0.89
36mo	0.28	0.44	0.19	0.63	0.53	0.18	0.21	0.59	0.42	0.211	0.40	0.31
n6:n3												
6mo	**0.42**	**0.031**	0.30	0.10	**0.45**	**0.011**	**0.45**	**0.013**	0.11	0.519	0.30	0.08
18mo	−0.04	0.82	0.05	0.78	0.06	0.74	0.14	0.47	0.14	0.369	0.21	0.19
36mo	0.30	0.34	−0.23	0.55	0.05	0.88	−0.18	0.65	0.01	0.978	−0.26	0.58
LC n6:n3												
6mo	0.12	0.56	0.14	0.41	0.22	0.24	0.29	0.09	0.15	0.373	0.24	0.13
18mo	−0.13	0.48	−0.08	0.66	−0.04	0.86	−0.05	0.77	0.11	0.490	0.07	0.65
36mo	0.35	0.54	−0.07	0.86	0.16	0.81	−0.08	0.85	−0.31	0.516	−0.30	0.46

Associations were evaluated using lineal regression analyses. β and p are corrected values after adjustment for potential confounders: maternal pre-pregnancy BMI, maternal smoking, weight gain during pregnancy, maternal education, sex of the child and type of infant feeding practice. p-values ≤ 0.05 are highlighted in bold and those ≤0.002 are additionally marked by stars. mo: month; LA: Linoleic Acid; AA: Arachidonic Acid; ALA: α-linolenic Acid; EPA: Eicosapentaenoic Acid; DHA: Docosahexaenoic Acid; PUFA: Polyunsaturated Fatty Acids; LC-PUFA: Long chain Polyunsaturated Fatty Acids.

At 6 months of age, we found that colostrum levels of AA, EPA, DHA, n3 PUFAs, n6 LC-PUFAs and n3 LC-PUFAs were inversely associated with infant BMIZ, while the n6:n3 ratio was positively associated with it. Also, at 6 months of age, LA and the n6:n3 ratio in both colostrum and mature milk were positively associated with WAZ. No associations were found between mature milk and any variable at 1.5 or 3 years of age.

3.5. Associations of Breast Milk FAs with Infant Cognition

Table 4 presents the associations between breast milk PUFAs and infant cognition at 18 months of age. When the whole population was analyzed, no associations were found. However, infants born to normal-weight mothers presented a positive association between cognition scores and LA and n6 PUFA levels in colostrum. On the other hand, the infants of overweight mothers presented a direct association of DHA and n3 LC-PUFA levels in colostrum with cognitive score, while the n6:n3 ratio in colostrum was inversely associated with it. With respect to infants born to mothers with obesity, a positive association was found between ALA levels in mature milk and cognition.

Table 4. Associations between breast milk PUFA levels and infant cognition score at 18 months of age, according to maternal pre-pregnancy BMI.

Fatty Acid	All				Normal-Weight				Overweight				Obesity			
	Colostrum (n = 75)		Mature Milk (n = 77)		Colostrum (n = 14)		Mature Milk (n = 12)		Colostrum (n = 11)		Mature Milk (n = 15)		Colostrum (n = 12)		Mature Milk (n = 11)	
	β	p	β	p	β	p	β	p	β	p	β	p	β	p	β	p
C18:3n3 (ALA)	0.08	0.718	0.01	0.942	0.29	0.581	0.82	0.212	0.44	0.393	-0.15	0.662	0.55	0.468	**2.34**	**0.008**
C18:2n6 (LA)	0.20	0.339	0.12	0.527	**0.84**	**<0.001** *	0.88	0.069	-0.95	0.061	-0.16	0.687	0.12	0.869	0.53	0.470
C20:4n6 (AA)	0.03	0.889	-0.20	0.333	-1.23	0.136	-0.56	0.270	0.32	0.594	-0.28	0.544	0.48	0.416	-0.87	0.405
C20:5n3 (EPA)	0.31	0.133	-0.11	0.580	0.00	0.996	0.59	0.428	-0.07	0.932	-0.18	0.635	0.80	0.233	-0.29	0.658
C22:6n3 (DHA)	-0.16	0.396	-0.27	0.161	-0.73	0.124	-0.19	0.720	**0.88**	**0.045**	0.33	0.362	-0.03	0.954	-1.16	0.104
n6 PUFA	0.24	0.251	0.13	0.495	**0.81**	**0.002** *	0.88	0.064	-0.97	0.111	-0.15	0.713	0.16	0.803	0.45	0.520
n3 PUFA	-0.01	0.966	-0.12	0.541	-0.23	0.687	0.37	0.512	0.70	0.057	-0.04	0.922	0.13	0.829	-0.78	0.489
n6 LC-PUFA	0.14	0.446	0.18	0.407	0.01	0.984	0.31	0.536	0.53	0.227	0.36	0.481	0.28	0.650	-0.09	0.924
n3 LC-PUFA	-0.11	0.563	-0.25	0.190	-0.71	0.113	-0.08	0.873	**1.01**	**0.004**	0.21	0.585	0.04	0.949	-0.89	0.189
n6:n3	0.13	0.489	0.22	0.255	0.74	0.067	0.29	0.639	**-0.97**	**0.002** *	-0.10	0.805	0.01	0.985	0.57	0.426
LC n6:n3	0.27	0.166	0.29	0.105	0.52	0.172	0.16	0.752	0.05	0.952	-0.08	0.830	0.22	0.696	0.83	0.286

Associations were evaluated using lineal regression analyses. β and p are corrected values after adjustment for potential confounders: maternal smoking, weight gain during pregnancy, maternal education, sex of the child and type of infant feeding practice. Cognition performance was analyzed at 1.5 years of age. p-values ≤ 0.05 are highlighted in bold and those ≤ 0.002 are additionally marked by stars. LA: Linoleic Acid; AA: Arachidonic Acid; ALA: α-linolenic Acid; EPA: Eicosapentaenoic Acid; DHA: Docosahexaenoic Acid; PUFA: Polyunsaturated Fatty Acids; LC-PUFA: Long chain Polyunsaturated Fatty Acids.

4. Discussion

The present study offers the evaluation of human breast milk FA composition during the first month postpartum according to maternal weight, and the impact on child outcomes from 6 months to 3 years of age. This is one of the very few studies analyzing the influence of maternal weight on breast milk FA composition and, to our knowledge, the second one to assess this parameter in both colostrum and mature breast milk. Moreover, we believe this is the first study to address its effect on both infant cognitive developmental parameters and growth all in one study.

Upon analysis of the population characteristics, we observed that women with obesity had the lowest GWG, even though no nutritional intervention was carried out. This finding is in line with the results of a systematic review about GWG in women with obesity where they concluded that GWG decreased with each higher BMI classification [39]. In fact, weight loss during pregnancy is more common in women with obesity than non-obese women [40] and GWG decreases as the severity of obesity increases [41]. Nonetheless, we observed that women with obesity had the highest n6:n3 ratio in their dietary intake, which suggests they had the lowest-quality dietary intake, as similarly demonstrated by other studies where a high weight status is related to a high dietary intake of n6 FAs and a low intake of n3 FAs [42].

We did not observe any differences in infant characteristics according to maternal BMI. Evidence suggests that infants born to mothers with obesity have an increased risk of having a higher weight and length at birth [1], but this was not the case in our population. Since GWG is directly associated with birth weight [43], a possible explanation for this finding is that women with obesity showed the lowest GWG, and therefore their offspring did not present increased weight at birth. This is in the line with the conclusions of the systematic review of Faucher and Barger, in which several studies reported a linear decrease in the prevalence of being large for gestational age (LGA) and less GWG [39], suggesting that women with obesity and low GWG would have some benefits on fetal growth. This could be the reason why in our study children from women with obesity did not present higher weight or length. Nevertheless, our data still showed a tendency in which formula-fed infants and those considered LGA represented a higher percentage in the groups of women with overweight and obesity, according to Lubchenco's curves [44].

Regardless of maternal weight, our data showed that when breast milk transitioned from colostrum (2–4 days postpartum) to mature milk (28–32 days postpartum), the levels of crucial FAs such as AA, DHA, and n3 LC-PUFA were decreased. Other authors have also demonstrated this finding [45,46]. The high content of crucial FAs in colostrum has biological relevance because it is highly associated with child outcomes, possibly because of the nutrient supply during the first few days of life, which are critical for infant health [47]. Nonetheless, we also found higher levels of EPA:AA and DHA:AA in mature milk, which are positively associated with health outcomes as well [48]. Analyzing the breast milk evolution within each weight group, we found that SFA concentrations decreased in the mature milk of women with normal-weight and overweight, but not in the mature milk of women with obesity. As described in other studies, the human milk of these women could present higher levels of SFA [17]. The factors attributed to this increased amount of SFA in breast milk of women with obesity could be the metabolic status and diet. It is well known that obesity is intrinsically a pro-inflammatory state influenced by dietary intake [49], where the ratio of n6:n3 PUFA is a clear factor affecting inflammation and obesity development [50]. In our study, the higher dietary intake of n6:n3 PUFA ratio in women with obesity, might be enhancing the pro-inflammatory state, and thereby affecting the levels of breast milk SFAs. Moreover, the fact that women with an increased BMI may have an increased intake of n6:n3 PUFA might also explain the higher n6:n3 PUFA ratio found in the mature milk of overweight women compared to their colostrum, although their increased intake of dietary n6:n3 was not significant.

To the best of our knowledge, eight studies have evaluated the FA composition of breast milk according to maternal BMI, but the results available in the literature are not entirely consistent and the studies differ in terms of the weight groups tested and the timing of sample collections. Out of these eight studies, only one shares the same collection timing for colostrum that we used [32]; another one used a similar timing for both colostrum and mature milk [16], but the other 6 studies collected the milk in different times ([10,17,18,29–31]). Regarding the weight groups used, 5 did not share the same groups that we used [10,16,17,29,31], and 2 out of the 3 studies that did [18,30,31] used a different criteria to classify weight according to BMI [30,32].

Although our results and the ones available in the literature suggest that a high maternal weight status alters human milk nutrient content, there is an inconsistency regarding which FAs are the most influenced according to BMI groups. This could be attributed to numerous factors, such as sample size, population, methods, FAs included in the analysis, weight group classification and the timing of breast milk collection. However, it is important to highlight that, even without a clear consistency among studies, an increased BMI is found to alter FA concentrations in breast milk, generally increasing SFA and n6 PUFAs and decreasing FAs from the n3 series. An important factor that could explain the differences found among weight groups could be related to dietary intake during late pregnancy, since several studies have demonstrated that this affects breast milk composition [51]. This suggests that women with overweight and obesity could have an increased dietary intake of n6 FAs and SFAs and a poor intake of n3 FAs. As previously mentioned, this happened in our population, where we found that the n6:n3 ratio of dietary intake was higher in women with an increased BMI, especially those with obesity. Since a maternal pro-inflammatory diet is positively associated with increased concentrations of SFA and MUFA in breast milk [10], specific maternal metabolic markers could be an interesting approach to predicting the predominance of certain FAs in breast milk.

This study also analyzed the possible association between breast milk FA composition and infant growth and cognition. It is well known that many nutrients are critical for proper infant growth and neurodevelopment. Animal models and epidemiological studies suggest that PUFAs such as AA and DHA are particularly important [52,53]. Thus, we evaluated the association between the PUFA levels in breast milk and infant anthropometric measurements at 6, 18 and 36 months of age. For this analysis, we used the z-score values WAZ, LAZ and BMIZ to evaluate with greater accuracy which children were within or outside the normal range [1,36,54]. Our findings showed that LC-PUFAs—especially AA, EPA, DHA, n3 and n6 LC-PUFAs—in colostrum had a negative association with infant BMIZ at 6 months. In accordance with these results, a recent review that analyzed the association between n3 PUFAs and growth suggested that DHA during pregnancy, lactation and early life may be associated with significant benefits in infant growth and development [55]. Similarly, Pedersen et al. observed a negative association between DHA levels in breast milk and BMI in children from 2 to 7 years of age. They also found an overall inverse association between breast milk DHA and body fat percentage [56]. Although it is important to mention that BMI is not the best method to quantify body composition, and especially to assess body fat in children [57,58], DHA content in breast milk could have some benefits in postponing the age of adiposity rebound [56], which is the second rise in adiposity that usually occurs between 3 and 7 years of age [59]. It is known that the age that rebound occurs predicts later fatness, meaning that an earlier rebound would be a risk factor for later obesity [59]. On the other hand, our data also indicated that n6 PUFA levels may contribute to a fat mass increase in children [59], since LA in colostrum and the n6:n3 ratio in both mature milk and colostrum could influence WAZ and BMIZ at 6 months of age. Since the n6 PUFAs in mature milk were generally increased in overweight and obese mothers, their children could be more susceptible to developing obesity [17,20,50]. Indeed, children from overweight and obese mothers presented a tendency to be LGA. In contrast, Much et al. found that AA and n6 PUFAs in mature breast milk were negatively associated with infant weight and BMI (up to 4 months of age) [33], suggesting that the role of these n6 FAs (including AA) might be age-dependent and serve as important regulating factors for growth in early postnatal life. Due to the low variability of AA contents in breast milk across populations (0.24–1% of FAs) [7], a possible explanation of this discrepancy could be the quantitative amount of milk intake by the breastfed infant, meaning that depending on the daily ingested volume of milk, AA would have its growth-regulatory effects or not [33]. Further studies are needed to look into such quantitative aspects. In our study, we only found significant associations between FAs and infant growth at 6 months of life, but not at 18 nor 36. This finding may be due to the child's own diet, lifestyle and metabolism. However, the associations found at 6 months are relevant, because it is a crucial age that represents a critical period in the child's development and programming [3]. A curious result that we found is that length was not correlated to any PUFA, which again is in disagreement with Much et al. They inversely correlated DHA, EPA and n3 PUFA with length at 1 year of age. Their milk collection was at 6 weeks and 4 months postpartum [33], whereas in our study it was at 2–4 days and 28–32 days postpartum. Therefore, the possible evolution of FA species over time would be a possible explanation for the different results. From our study and the evidence gathered, we can see that PUFAs in breastmilk influence infant growth; however, there is a high variability in existing results. Further studies are needed to obtain more conclusive outcomes [2].

PUFAs are also critical for an adequate brain growth and function in aspects such as neurogenesis, nerve impulse transmission, neuronal integrity, and vitality and gene expression in the brain [52,53,60]. Thus, we explored the association between breast milk PUFA levels and cognitive score at 18 months of life. On the one hand, when we analyzed the total population, we found no association between any FA in breast milk and child development. Similarly, there have been observational studies that found no strong evidence for a beneficial role of LC-PUFAs in order to explain the positive relationship between breastfeeding and cognition [61]. This raises the question as to whether LC-PUFA levels may only be beneficial in children's mental development when breastfeeding levels are high [62]. Although we corrected the analysis by the type of breastfeeding, this information was collected at 3 months of age, so we do not know which effect could have had a longer period of exclusive breastfeeding.

We also explored the association between breast milk FA levels and infant cognition according to maternal BMI. In general, we found a direct association between n3 and n6 PUFA levels in colostrum and infant cognition at 18 months of age. The colostrum from overweight mothers was the one that presented more relevant associations, specifically, a high n6:n3 ratio was negatively associated with cognition, whereas higher DHA concentrations were directly associated with better cognitive scores, which is in line with Bernard et al. [63]. This suggests that the cognition of infants born to overweight women could be enhanced by promoting n3 FAs, more specifically DHA, in the maternal diet. These results are in line with meta-analyses, animal and epidemiologic studies [60,64,65], and support WHO recommendations on breastfeeding for the two first years of life or beyond [66]. We must consider that, in our study, the cognitive score was assessed at 1.5 years of life, and at this age, there are many factors related to the child that could influence their cognition. The potential cofounders that we have used to adjust this analysis were mainly related to the mother, and only the gender and type of feeding practice were related to the child. Important factors such as infant diet or physical activity are lacking and could have a huge influence in the results because intake of micronutrients, such as n3 FAs, vitamin B12, folic acid, zinc, iron and iodine, together with malnutrition and general dietary patterns and other lifestyle habits, influence child cognitive development as well [67–69].

Overall, our study highlights the importance of the maternal health before, during and after pregnancy, since it could have a great impact in the breast milk FA composition and, in consequence, in the offspring's growth and cognition which affects their future health. Many women start developing healthy habits when they are pregnant or planning a pregnancy. However, as presented in our study, the pre-pregnancy health status has an important effect in the quality of the human milk, consequently affecting the health of the child. Therefore, bigger efforts must be put in place to promote and guarantee a healthier lifestyle and nutritional status in the general population to pursuit healthier future generations.

We acknowledge some limitations in our study, such as the small sample size. However, it is important to understand that, even though PREOBE is a larger cohort, we were not able to include all the participants in the present study due to lack of data or samples, possibly related to indisposition to participate given the complexity and sensitivity of the periods involved: childbirth and breastfeeding. Although risk factors, such as socio-demographic information and maternal diet, allowed us to adjust our statistical models for potential confounders, we cannot rule out residual confounding, especially coming from data related to the infants at 1.5 and 3 years of age because data on their dietary intake, lifestyle and other characteristics, could be greatly influencing the results. Another limitation is that women receiving supplements of DHA for over 3 months were excluded, but we do not know the possible effect of that initial supplementation in the breast milk FA profile. Moreover, recording the timing between sample collection or the last meal, collecting information on what was consumed before and after each sample was taken, and analyzing the different breast milk samples of one day without mixing them, would provide valuable data to assess the human milk nutrient content and impact. In general, further research is required to provide a better understanding of the role that FAs play in obesity development and management, paying special attention to the methods used for analysis and promoting the comparison of results between cohorts.

5. Conclusions

In conclusion, our results show that (1) the FA composition of colostrum and mature milk was different. Regardless of maternal weight, mature milk had lower levels of AA and DHA (among others) than colostrum; (2) Maternal obesity influenced the FA concentrations in breast milk. Overall, breast milk of mothers with a high BMI presented increased SFA levels and n6:n3 ratio, and decreased ALA, DHA and MUFA concentrations; and (3) The early supply of n6 and n3 PUFAs through colostrum influenced infant weight status and cognition, at 6 and 18 months of life, respectively. Infant BMIZ at 6 months of age was inversely associated with colostrum levels of n6 and n3 LC-PUFAs (e.g., AA and DHA) and positively associated with n6:n3 ratio. Depending on the maternal BMI, infant cognition may be positively affected by colostrum levels of LA, n6 PUFAs, DHA, n3 LC-PUFAs and ALA, and negatively affected by the n6:n3 ratio. Since the maternal pre-pregnancy weight can influence the breast milk FAs, which is related to the early nutritional status of the child and to health conditions throughout the life span, this study endorses the need for early preventive health care through diet and lifestyle. A healthy weight in women before, during and after pregnancy should be encouraged to promote beneficial FAs in breast milk and promote healthier future generations.

Author Contributions: The authors' responsibilities were as follows. C.C., M.C.L.-S. and A.I.C. designed the project. F.J.T.-E., L.G.-V., M.E.-M., M.T.S. were involved in participant recruitment, data and sample collection. A.I.C., A.M.A., A.d.l.G.P. and R.M.G. processed the samples. A.d.l.G.P. and A.M.A. conducted the data analysis and interpretation. A.d.l.G.P., A.M.A. and A.M.C. wrote the manuscript. All authors performed a critical review of the final manuscript.

Acknowledgments: The authors sincerely thank the women and children involved in the PREOBE study for their valuable participation. We are also grateful to personnel, scientists, staff and all people involved in the PREOBE team who have made this research possible. We acknowledge members of the Autonomous University of Barcelona for their assistance in statistical analysis. Members of the PREOBE team include: University of Granada. Spain: EURISTIKOS Excellence Centre for Paediatric Research. Department of Paediatrics: Cristina Campoy (PI), Luz Mª García-Valdés, Francisco J Torres-Espínola, Mª Teresa Segura, Cristina Martínez-Zaldívar, Tania Anjos, Antonio Jerez, Daniel Campos, Rosario Moreno-Torres, Mª José Aguilar, Iryna Rusanova, Jole Martino, Signe Altmäe; Department of Obstetrics and Gynecology: Jesús Florido, Carmen Padilla; Department of Biostatistics: Mª Teresa Miranda; Mind, Brain and Behavior International Research Centre: Andrés Catena, Miguel Pérez-García; Department of Legal Medicine: Jose A. Lorente, Juan C. Alvarez; Department of Pharmacology: Ahmad Agil; ICTAN-CSIC–Madrid. Spain: Ascensión Marcos, Esther Nova, Department of Nutrition and Bromatology. University of Barcelona. Spain: Mª Carmen López-Sabater; Lorgen, S.L.: Carmen Entrala; Rowett Institute, University of Aberdeen, UK: Harry McArdle, University of Nöttingham, UK: Michael Symonds; Ludwig-Maximiliam University of Munich, Germany: Berthold Koletzko, Hans Demmelmair, Olaf Uhl; University of Graz, Austria: Gernot Desoye; Abbott Laboratories: Ricardo Rueda; University of Umeå, Sweden: Staffan K Berglund.

References

1.   Poston, L.; Caleyachetty, R.; Cnattingius, S.; Corvalán, C.; Uauy, R.; Herring, S.; Gillman, M.W. Preconceptional and maternal obesity: Epidemiology and health consequences. *Lancet Diabetes Endocrinol.* **2016**, 4, 1025–1036. [CrossRef]

2.   Koletzko, B.; Godfrey, K.M.; Poston, L.; Szajewska, H.; van Goudoever, J.B.; de Waard, M.; Brands, B.; Grivell, R.M.; Deussen, A.R.; Dodd, J.M.; et al. Nutrition During Pregnancy, Lactation and Early Childhood and its Implications for Maternal and Long-Term Child Health: The Early Nutrition Project Recommendations. *Ann. Nutr. Metab.* **2019**, *74*, 93–106. [CrossRef]

3.   Langley-Evans, S.C. Nutrition in early life and the programming of adult disease: A review. *J. Hum. Nutr. Diet.* **2015**, *28*, 1–14. [CrossRef] [PubMed]

4.   Pérez-Escamilla, R.; Martinez, J.L.; Segura-Pérez, S. Impact of the Baby-friendly Hospital Initiative on breastfeeding and child health outcomes: A systematic review. *Matern. Child Nutr.* **2016**, *12*, 402–417. [CrossRef]

5.   Mosca, F.; Giannì, M.L. Human milk: Composition and health benefits. *La Pediatr. Med. Chir.* **2017**, *39*, 155. [CrossRef]

6.   Binns, C.; Lee, M.; Low, W.Y. The Long-Term Public Health Benefits of Breastfeeding. *Asia Pac. J. Public Health* **2016**, *28*, 7–14. [CrossRef] [PubMed]

7.   Brenna, J.T.; Varamini, B.; Jensen, R.G.; Diersen-Schade, D.A.; Boettcher, J.A.; Arterburn, L.M. Docosahexaenoic and arachidonic acid concentrations in human breast milk worldwide. *Am. J. Clin. Nutr.* **2007**, *85*, 1457–1464. [CrossRef] [PubMed]

8.   Savino, F.; Liguori, S.A.; Fissore, M.F.; Oggero, R. Breast milk hormones and their protective effect on obesity. *Int. J. Pediatr. Endocrinol.* **2009**, *2009*, 327505. [CrossRef]

9.   Lauritzen, L.; Carlson, S.E. Maternal fatty acid status during pregnancy and lactation and relation to newborn and infant status. *Matern. Child Nutr.* **2011**, *7*, 41–58. [CrossRef] [PubMed]

10. Panagos, P.G.; Vishwanathan, R.; Penfield-Cyr, A.; Matthan, N.R.; Shivappa, N.; Wirth, M.D.; Hebert, J.R.; Sen, S. Breastmilk from obese mothers has pro-inflammatory properties and decreased neuroprotective factors. *J. Perinatol.* **2016**, *36*, 284–290. [CrossRef] [PubMed]

11. Martin, C.; Ling, P.R.; Blackburn, G.; Martin, C.R.; Ling, P.R.; Blackburn, G.L. Review of Infant Feeding: Key Features of Breast Milk and Infant Formula. *Nutrients* **2016**, *8*, 279. [CrossRef] [PubMed]

12. Muhlhausler, B.S.; Ailhaud, G.P. Omega-6 polyunsaturated fatty acids and the early origins of obesity. *Curr. Opin. Endocrinol. Diabetes Obes.* **2013**, *20*, 56–61. [CrossRef] [PubMed]

13. Ailhaud, G.; Guesnet, P. Fatty acid composition of fats is an early determinant of childhood obesity: A short review and an opinion. *Obes. Rev.* **2004**, *5*, 21–26. [CrossRef] [PubMed]

14. Gertosio, C.; Meazza, C.; Pagani, S.; Bozzola, M. Breastfeeding and its gamut of benefits. *Minerva Pediatr.* **2016**, *68*, 201–212. [PubMed]

15. Barrera, C.; Valenzuela, R.; Chamorro, R.; Bascuñán, K.; Sandoval, J.; Sabag, N.; Valenzuela, F.; Valencia, M.P.; Puigrredon, C.; Valenzuela, A.; et al. The Impact of Maternal Diet during Pregnancy and Lactation on the Fatty Acid Composition of Erythrocytes and Breast Milk of Chilean Women. *Nutrients* **2018**, *10*, 839. [CrossRef] [PubMed]

16. Storck Lindholm, E.; Strandvik, B.; Altman, D.; Möller, A.; Palme Kilander, C. Different fatty acid pattern in breast milk of obese compared to normal-weight mothers. *Prostaglandins Leukot. Essent. Fat. Acids* **2013**, *88*, 211–217. [CrossRef] [PubMed]

17. Mäkelä, J.; Linderborg, K.; Niinikoski, H.; Yang, B.; Lagström, H. Breast milk fatty acid composition differs between overweight and normal weight women: The STEPS Study. *Eur. J. Nutr.* **2013**, *52*, 727–735. [CrossRef] [PubMed]

18. Marín, M.C.; Sanjurjo, A.; Rodrigo, M.A.; de Alaniz, M.J.T. Long-chain polyunsaturated fatty acids in breast milk in La Plata, Argentina: Relationship with maternal nutritional status. *Prostaglandins Leukot. Essent. Fat. Acids* **2005**, *73*, 355–360. [CrossRef] [PubMed]

19. Simopoulos, A.P. An Increase in the Omega-6/Omega-3 Fatty Acid Ratio Increases the Risk for Obesity. *Nutrients* **2016**, *8*, 128. [CrossRef]

20. Heerwagen, M.J.R.; Stewart, M.S.; de la Houssaye, B.A.; Janssen, R.C.; Friedman, J.E. Transgenic increase in N-3/n-6 Fatty Acid ratio reduces maternal obesity-associated inflammation and limits adverse developmental programming in mice. *PLoS ONE* **2013**, *8*, e67791. [CrossRef]

21. Edlow, A.G. Maternal obesity and neurodevelopmental and psychiatric disorders in offspring. *Prenat. Diagn.* **2017**, *37*, 95–110. [CrossRef] [PubMed]
22. Rivera, H.M.; Christiansen, K.J.; Sullivan, E.L. The role of maternal obesity in the risk of neuropsychiatric disorders. *Front. Neurosci.* **2015**, *9*, 194. [CrossRef]
23. Veena, S.R.; Gale, C.R.; Krishnaveni, G.V.; Kehoe, S.H.; Srinivasan, K.; Fall, C.H. Association between maternal nutritional status in pregnancy and offspring cognitive function during childhood and adolescence; a systematic review. *BMC Pregnancy Childbirth* **2016**, *16*, 220. [CrossRef] [PubMed]
24. Contu, L.; Hawkes, C.A. A Review of the Impact of Maternal Obesity on the Cognitive Function and Mental Health of the Offspring. *Int. J. Mol. Sci.* **2017**, *18*, 1093. [CrossRef] [PubMed]
25. Huang, L.; Yu, X.; Keim, S.; Li, L.; Zhang, L.; Zhang, J. Maternal prepregnancy obesity and child neurodevelopment in the Collaborative Perinatal Project. *Int. J. Epidemiol.* **2014**, *43*, 783–792. [CrossRef] [PubMed]
26. Heikura, U.; Taanila, A.; Hartikainen, A.L.; Olsen, P.; Linna, S.L.; Wendt, L.; Jarvelin, M.R. Variations in Prenatal Sociodemographic Factors associated with Intellectual Disability: A Study of the 20-Year Interval between Two Birth Cohorts in Northern Finland. *Am. J. Epidemiol.* **2007**, *167*, 169–177. [CrossRef] [PubMed]
27. Brion, M.J.; Zeegers, M.; Jaddoe, V.; Verhulst, F.; Tiemeier, H.; Lawlor, D.A.; Smith, G.D. Intrauterine effects of maternal prepregnancy overweight on child cognition and behavior in 2 cohorts. *Pediatrics* **2011**, *127*, e202–e211. [CrossRef]
28. Craig, W.Y.; Palomaki, G.E.; Neveux, L.M.; Haddow, J.E. Maternal Body Mass Index during Pregnancy and Offspring Neurocognitive Development. *Obstet. Med.* **2013**, *6*, 20–25. [CrossRef]
29. Kwon, M. Nutrient Content of Human Breast Milk from Overweight and Normal Weight Caucasian Women of Northeast Tennessee. Master's Thesis, East Tennessee State University, Johnson City, TN, USA, 2017.
30. Rudolph, M.C.; Young, B.E.; Lemas, D.J.; Palmer, C.E.; Hernandez, T.L.; Barbour, L.A.; Friedman, J.E.; Krebs, N.F.; MacLean, P.S. Early infant adipose deposition is positively associated with the n-6 to n-3 fatty acid ratio in human milk independent of maternal BMI. *Int. J. Obes. (Lond.)* **2017**, *41*, 510–517. [CrossRef]
31. Kim, H.; Kang, S.; Jung, B.M.; Yi, H.; Jung, J.A.; Chang, N. Breast milk fatty acid composition and fatty acid intake of lactating mothers in South Korea. *Br. J. Nutr.* **2017**, *117*, 556–561. [CrossRef]
32. Sinanoglou, V.J.; Cavouras, D.; Boutsikou, T.; Briana, D.D.; Lantzouraki, D.Z.; Paliatsiou, S.; Volaki, P.; Bratakos, S.; Malamitsi-Puchner, A.; Zoumpoulakis, P. Factors affecting human colostrum fatty acid profile: A case study. *PLoS ONE* **2017**, *12*, e0175817. [CrossRef] [PubMed]
33. Much, D.; Brunner, S.; Vollhardt, C.; Schmid, D.; Sedlmeier, E.M.; Brüderl, M.; Heimberg, E.; Bartke, N.; Boehm, G.; Bader, B.L.; et al. Breast milk fatty acid profile in relation to infant growth and body composition: Results from the INFAT study. *Pediatr. Res.* **2013**, *74*, 230–237. [CrossRef] [PubMed]
34. Berglund, S.K.; García-Valdés, L.; Torres-Espinola, F.J.; Segura, M.T.; Martínez-Zaldívar, C.; Aguilar, M.J.; Agil, A.; Lorente, J.A.; Florido, J.; Padilla, C.; et al. Maternal, fetal and perinatal alterations associated with obesity, overweight and gestational diabetes: An observational cohort study (PREOBE). *BMC Public Health* **2016**, *16*, 207. [CrossRef] [PubMed]
35. Chisaguano, A.M.; Lozano, B.; Moltó-Puigmartí, C.; Castellote, A.I.; Rafecas, M.; López-Sabater, M.C. Elaidic acid, vaccenic acid and rumenic acid (c9,t11-CLA) determination in human plasma phospholipids and human milk by fast gas chromatography. *Anal. Methods* **2013**, *5*, 1264. [CrossRef]
36. Borghi, E.; de Onis, M.; Garza, C.; Van den Broeck, J.; Frongillo, E.A.; Grummer-Strawn, L.; Van Buuren, S.; Pan, H.; Molinari, L.; Martorell, R.; et al. Construction of the World Health Organization child growth standards: Selection of methods for attained growth curves. *Stat. Med.* **2006**, *25*, 247–265. [CrossRef] [PubMed]
37. Duggan, M.B. Anthropometry as a tool for measuring malnutrition: Impact of the new WHO growth standards and reference. *Ann. Trop. Paediatr.* **2010**, *30*, 1–17. [CrossRef]
38. Goldstein, S.; Naglieri, J.A. *Encyclopedia of Child Behavior and Development*; Springer: Berlin/Heidelberg, Germany, 2011; ISBN 9780387775791.
39. Faucher, M.A.; Barger, M.K. Gestational weight gain in obese women by class of obesity and select maternal/newborn outcomes: A systematic review. *Women Birth* **2015**, *28*, e70–e79. [CrossRef] [PubMed]

40. Durie, D.E.; Thornburg, L.L.; Glantz, J.C. Effect of second-trimester and third-trimester rate of gestational weight gain on maternal and neonatal outcomes. *Obstet. Gynecol.* **2011**, *118*, 569–575. [CrossRef]

41. Hinkle, S.N.; Sharma, A.J.; Dietz, P.M. Gestational weight gain in obese mothers and associations with fetal growth. *Am. J. Clin. Nutr.* **2010**, *92*, 644–651. [CrossRef]

42. Patterson, E.; Wall, R.; Fitzgerald, G.F.; Ross, R.P.; Stanton, C. Health implications of high dietary omega-6 polyunsaturated Fatty acids. *J. Nutr. Metab.* **2012**, *2012*, 539426. [CrossRef]

43. Alberico, S.; Montico, M.; Barresi, V.; Monasta, L.; Businelli, C.; Soini, V.; Erenbourg, A.; Ronfani, L.; Maso, G.; Multicentre Study Group on Mode of Delivery in Friuli Venezia Giulia. The role of gestational diabetes, pre-pregnancy body mass index and gestational weight gain on the risk of newborn macrosomia: Results from a prospective multicentre study. *BMC Pregnancy Childbirth* **2014**, *14*, 23. [CrossRef] [PubMed]

44. Olsen, I.E.; Groveman, S.A.; Lawson, M.L.; Clark, R.H.; Zemel, B.S. New intrauterine growth curves based on United States data. *Pediatrics* **2010**, *125*, e214–e224. [CrossRef] [PubMed]

45. Moltó-Puigmartí, C.; Castellote, A.I.; Carbonell-Estrany, X.; López-Sabater, M.C. Differences in fat content and fatty acid proportions among colostrum, transitional, and mature milk from women delivering very preterm, preterm, and term infants. *Clin. Nutr.* **2011**, *30*, 116–123. [CrossRef] [PubMed]

46. Haddad, I.; Mozzon, M.; Frega, N.G. Trends in fatty acids positional distribution in human colostrum, transitional, and mature milk. *Eur. Food Res. Technol.* **2012**, *235*, 325–332. [CrossRef]

47. Lawn, J.E.; Blencowe, H.; Oza, S.; You, D.; Lee, A.C.C.; Waiswa, P.; Lalli, M.; Bhutta, Z.; Barros, A.J.D.; Christian, P.; et al. Every Newborn: Progress, priorities, and potential beyond survival. *Lancet* **2014**, *384*, 189–205. [CrossRef]

48. Morales, E.; Bustamante, M.; Gonzalez, J.R.; Guxens, M.; Torrent, M.; Mendez, M.; Garcia-Esteban, R.; Julvez, J.; Forns, J.; Vrijheid, M.; et al. Genetic Variants of the FADS Gene Cluster and ELOVL Gene Family, Colostrums LC-PUFA Levels, Breastfeeding, and Child Cognition. *PLoS ONE* **2011**, *6*, e17181. [CrossRef] [PubMed]

49. Shivappa, N.; Steck, S.E.; Hurley, T.G.; Hussey, J.R.; Hébert, J.R. Designing and developing a literature-derived, population-based dietary inflammatory index. *Public Health Nutr.* **2014**, *17*, 1689–1696. [CrossRef] [PubMed]

50. Yang, L.G.; Song, Z.X.; Yin, H.; Wang, Y.Y.; Shu, G.F.; Lu, H.X.; Wang, S.K.; Sun, G.J. Low n-6/n-3 PUFA Ratio Improves Lipid Metabolism, Inflammation, Oxidative Stress and Endothelial Function in Rats Using Plant Oils as n-3 Fatty Acid Source. *Lipids* **2016**, *51*, 49–59. [CrossRef]

51. Nishimura, R.Y.; Barbieiri, P.; de Castro, G.S.F.; Jordão, A.A.; da Silva Castro Perdoná, G.; Sartorelli, D.S. Dietary polyunsaturated fatty acid intake during late pregnancy affects fatty acid composition of mature breast milk. *Nutrition* **2014**, *30*, 685–689. [CrossRef]

52. Hadley, K.B.; Ryan, A.S.; Forsyth, S.; Gautier, S.; Salem, N., Jr. The Essentiality of Arachidonic Acid in Infant Development. *Nutrients* **2016**, *8*, 216. [CrossRef]

53. Lassek, W.D.; Gaulin, S.J.C. Maternal milk DHA content predicts cognitive performance in a sample of 28 nations. *Matern. Child Nutr.* **2015**, *11*, 773–779. [CrossRef] [PubMed]

54. Isanaka, S.; Villamor, E.; Shepherd, S.; Grais, R.F. Assessing the impact of the introduction of the World Health Organization growth standards and weight-for-height z-score criterion on the response to treatment of severe acute malnutrition in children: Secondary data analysis. *Pediatrics* **2009**, *123*, e54–e59. [CrossRef] [PubMed]

55. Rombaldi Bernardi, J.; de Souza Escobar, R.; Ferreira, C.F.; Pelufo Silveira, P. Fetal and neonatal levels of omega-3: Effects on neurodevelopment, nutrition, and growth. *Sci. World J.* **2012**, *2012*, 202473.

56. Pedersen, L.; Lauritzen, L.; Brasholt, M.; Buhl, T.; Bisgaard, H. Polyunsaturated fatty acid content of mother's milk is associated with childhood body composition. *Pediatr. Res.* **2012**, *72*, 631–636. [CrossRef] [PubMed]

57. Buss, J. Limitations of Body Mass Index to Assess Body Fat. *Workplace Health Saf.* **2014**, *62*, 264. [CrossRef] [PubMed]

58. Vanderwall, C.; Randall Clark, R.; Eickhoff, J.; Carrel, A.L. BMI is a poor predictor of adiposity in young overweight and obese children. *BMC Pediatr.* **2017**, *17*, 135. [CrossRef]

59. Macé, K.; Shahkhalili, Y.; Aprikian, O.; Stan, S. Dietary fat and fat types as early determinants of childhood obesity: A reappraisal. *Int. J. Obes.* **2006**, *30*, S50–S57. [CrossRef]

60. Innis, S.M. Impact of maternal diet on human milk composition and neurological development of infants. *Am. J. Clin. Nutr.* **2014**, *99*, 734S–741S. [CrossRef]

61. Bernard, J.Y.; Armand, M.; Garcia, C.; Forhan, A.; De Agostini, M.; Charles, M.A.; Heude, B. The association between linoleic acid levels in colostrum and child cognition at 2 and 3 y in the EDEN cohort. *Pediatr. Res.* **2015**, *77*, 829–835. [CrossRef]

62. Guxens, M.; Mendez, M.A.; Molto-Puigmarti, C.; Julvez, J.; Garcia-Esteban, R.; Forns, J.; Ferrer, M.; Vrijheid, M.; Lopez-Sabater, M.C.; Sunyer, J. Breastfeeding, Long-Chain Polyunsaturated Fatty Acids in Colostrum, and Infant Mental Development. *Pediatrics* **2011**, *128*, e880–e889. [CrossRef]

63. Bernard, J.Y.; Armand, M.; Peyre, H.; Garcia, C.; Forhan, A.; De Agostini, M.; Charles, M.A.; Heude, B.; EDEN Mother-Child Cohort Study Group (Etude des Déterminants pré- et postnatals précoces du développement et de la santé de l'Enfant). Breastfeeding, Polyunsaturated Fatty Acid Levels in Colostrum and Child Intelligence Quotient at Age 5–6 Years. *J. Pediatr.* **2017**, *183*, 43–50. [CrossRef] [PubMed]

64. Horta, B.L.; Loret de Mola, C.; Victora, C.G. Breastfeeding and intelligence: A systematic review and meta-analysis. *Acta Paediatr.* **2015**, *104*, 14–19. [CrossRef] [PubMed]

65. Jedrychowski, W.; Perera, F.; Jankowski, J.; Butscher, M.; Mroz, E.; Flak, E.; Kaim, I.; Lisowska-Miszczyk, I.; Skarupa, A.; Sowa, A. Effect of exclusive breastfeeding on the development of children's cognitive function in the Krakow prospective birth cohort study. *Eur. J. Pediatr.* **2012**, *171*, 151–158. [CrossRef] [PubMed]

66. WHO. *Breastfeeding*; WHO: Geneva, Switzerland, 2018.

67. Nyaradi, A.; Li, J.; Hickling, S.; Foster, J.; Oddy, W.H. The role of nutrition in children's neurocognitive development, from pregnancy through childhood. *Front. Hum. Neurosci.* **2013**, *7*, 97. [CrossRef] [PubMed]

68. Carson, V.; Hunter, S.; Kuzik, N.; Wiebe, S.A.; Spence, J.C.; Friedman, A.; Tremblay, M.S.; Slater, L.; Hinkley, T. Systematic review of physical activity and cognitive development in early childhood. *J. Sci. Med. Sport* **2016**, *19*, 573–578. [CrossRef] [PubMed]

69. Worobey, J. Physical activity in infancy: Developmental aspects, measurement, and importance. *Am. J. Clin. Nutr.* **2014**, *99*, 729S–733S. [CrossRef]

7

The Clinical Frailty Scale: Do Staff Agree?

Rebekah L. Young [1,*] **and David G. Smithard** [2,3]

[1] Newham University Hospital, Bart's Health NHS Trust, London E13 8SL, UK
[2] Queen Elizabeth Hospital, Lewisham and Greenwich NHS Trust, London SE18 4QH, UK; david.smithard@nhs.net
[3] Department of Sports Science, University of Greenwich, London SE10 9BD, UK
* Correspondence: rebekah.young5@nhs.net

Abstract: The term frailty is being increasingly used by clinicians, however there is no strict consensus on the best screening method. The expectation in England is that all older patients should have the Clinical Frailty Scale (CFS) completed on admission. This will frequently rely on junior medical staff and nurses, raising the question as to whether there is consistency. We asked 124 members of a multidisciplinary team (consultants, junior doctors, nurses, and allied health professionals; physiotherapists, occupational therapists, dietitians, speech and language therapists) to complete the CFS for seven case scenarios. The majority of the participants, 91/124 (72%), were trainee medical staff, 16 were senior medical staff, 12 were allied health professions, and 6 were nurses. There was broad agreement both between the professions and within the professions, with median CFS scores varying by a maximum of only one point, except in case scenario G, where there was a two-point difference between the most junior trainees (FY1) and the nursing staff. No difference (using the Mann–Whitney U test) was found between the different staff groups, with the median scores and range of scores being similar. This study has confirmed there is agreement between different staff members when calculating the CFS with no specific preceding training.

Keywords: frailty; clinical frailty score

1. Introduction

Frailty can be described as a clinical state in which the ability of older people to cope with every-day or acute stressors is compromised by increased vulnerability due to age-associated declines in physiological reserve and function across multiple organ systems [1]. It is estimated that around 10% of people aged over 65 years are frail, which increases to 25–50% of those aged over 85 [2]. Frailty can also be used to describe certain physical changes, such as muscle wasting and weakness, leading to reduced walking ability. The identification of these patients allows us to start a care pathway to address the issues contributing to frailty and avoid adverse outcomes.

All older people admitted to hospital should undergo a comprehensive geriatric assessment (CGA). It is recommended that this should commence on the day of admission [3]. An assessment of frailty is one component of the CGA, and similarly should be completed at the earliest opportunity. Assessments of frailty (frailty scales) are numerous [4] and rely on the recall of information, either by the patient or carer. The term frailty is being increasingly used by clinicians, however there is no strict consensus on the most appropriate screening scale [4].

The Clinical Frailty Scale, first described by Rockwood et al. in 2005 [5], is a nine-point scale where the assessor makes a judgement about the degree of a person's frailty based upon clinical assessment and has been adopted by the Acute Frailty Network in the UK. The advantage the CFS has over other scales is that it offers a pictorial representation with a small description and is quick and simple to administer.

As the various frailty scores measure slightly different things, it is possible to score as severely frail on one and moderately frail on another. It is therefore important that the same scale is used throughout any one service.

The expectation in England is that all older patients should have the Clinical Frailty Scale completed at the time of admission or soon after [6]. This will frequently rely on the junior trainee medical staff and nurses. This raises the question as to whether there is consistency in completing the assessments.

2. Methodology

The participants (consultants, junior doctors, nurses, and allied health professionals; physiotherapists, occupational therapists, dietitians, speech and language therapists) were approached on the ward and at time of clinical education sessions/conferences. A total of 124 people agreed to take part (Table 1). They were provided with seven clinical case scenarios (Table 2) based on actual clinical scenarios and asked to provide a frailty score by referring to the Clinical Frailty Scale (1–9) (Figure 1). The results were completed anonymously; participants were requested to provide their profession and grade where appropriate. The participants had no or limited experience using the CFS, nor was any training provided on how to use it. The nurses and allied health professionals were of varying levels of qualification, from newly qualified to senior staff.

Clinical Frailty Scale*

1 Very Fit – People who are robust, active, energetic and motivated. These people commonly exercise regularly. They are among the fittest for their age.

2 Well – People who have **no active disease symptoms** but are less fit than category 1. Often, they exercise or are very **active occasionally**, e.g. seasonally.

3 Managing Well – People whose **medical problems are well controlled**, but are **not regularly active** beyond routine walking.

4 Vulnerable – While **not dependent** on others for daily help, often **symptoms limit activities**. A common complaint is being "slowed up", and/or being tired during the day.

5 Mildly Frail – These people often have **more evident slowing**, and need help in **high order IADLs** (finances, transportation, heavy housework, medications). Typically, mild frailty progressively impairs shopping and walking outside alone, meal preparation and housework.

6 Moderately Frail – People need help with **all outside activities** and with **keeping house**. Inside, they often have problems with stairs and need **help with bathing** and might need minimal assistance (cuing, standby) with dressing.

7 Severely Frail – Completely dependent for personal care, from whatever cause (physical or cognitive). Even so, they seem stable and not at high risk of dying (within ~ 6 months).

8 Very Severely Frail – Completely dependent, approaching the end of life. Typically, they could not recover even from a minor illness.

9. Terminally Ill - Approaching the end of life. This category applies to people with **a life expectancy <6 months**, who are **not otherwise evidently frail**.

Scoring frailty in people with dementia

The degree of frailty corresponds to the degree of dementia. Common **symptoms in mild dementia** include forgetting the details of a recent event, though still remembering the event itself, repeating the same question/story and social withdrawal.

In **moderate dementia**, recent memory is very impaired, even though they seemingly can remember their past life events well. They can do personal care with prompting.

In **severe dementia**, they cannot do personal care without help.

 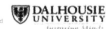 **DALHOUSIE UNIVERSITY** *Inspiring Minds*

Figure 1. The Clinical Frailty Scale (CFS) [5].

Table 1. Description of staff groups and previous experience with the CFS.

Staff Grade	Years Qualified	Experience with CFS
FY1	Immediately post qualification	None
SHO	Second year post training (may be longer depending on the individual)	None
Registrar	Min 4 years after undergraduate training	A few may have used the CFS
Consultant	At least nine years post graduate training	Depending on Specialty. Geriatricians would have experience other specialties not
Nursing/ AHP	Mixed 1–20	No exposure to CFS

Table 2. Clinical case scenarios.

	Case History
A.	84-year-old male. Admitted with a fall. Lives alone. Independent washing and dressing. Uses a walking stick in the house, housebound. Problems with urinary incontinence and wears pads. Has a BD care package when son away.
B.	81-year-old female. Walks with a Zimmer frame. Single level living. Undertakes a strip wash. Needs help with dressing, cooking, cleaning, shopping. Housebound. Carers 4 times a day. Unable to manage finances.
C.	91-year-old male. Independent with transfers from bed to chair but help otherwise to transfer chair to commode. Walks with a Zimmer frame but needs assistance. Help with personal activities of daily living (ADLs) (washing, dressing, shaving). Continence is an issue. Short term memory problems. Housebound. Unable to manage finances.
D.	74-year-old female. Working in an office, independent and self-caring. Drives a car. No care issues.
E.	89-year-old female. Walks with a stick and uses a 4-wheel shopper. Beginning to struggle with transfers (out of chair, off toilet) and lower half dressing. No package of care.
F.	84-year-old female. Recurrent falls and troubles with medication. Housebound, carers three times a day. Continent. Help with cooking, shopping and dressing. Requires help with medication. Cannot manage finances.
G.	82-year-old female. Falls, dementia. Independently mobile. Out shopping. Walks with a stick. Independent with personal and extended ADLS.

3. Results

The majority of participants—91/124 (72%)—were trainee medical staff, 16 were senior medical staff, 12 were allied health professions, and 6 were nurses (Figure 2).

There was broad agreement both between the professions and within the professions, with median CFS scores varying by a maximum of only one point, except in case scenario G, where there was a two-point difference between the most junior trainees (FY1) and the nursing staff (Figure 3). No difference (using multiple Mann–Whitney U) was found between different staff groups (basis between any two groups), with the median scores and range of scores all being very similar.

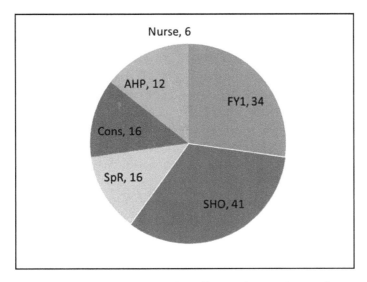

Figure 2. Distribution of staff completing the study.

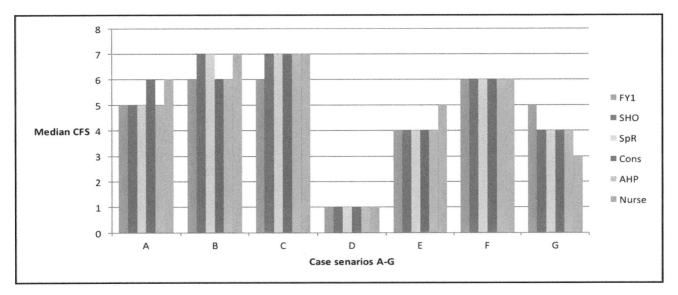

Figure 3. Chart to show the median CFS score calculated for each case scenario, divided by the member of the multidisciplinary team completing the score.

4. Discussion

The severity of prior frailty at the time of admission is a prognostic indicator of outcome (length of stay, institutionalisation, and mortality) from acute medical and surgical illness [7–10]. Holistic medical management uses information from many sources, one of which is a frailty scale. For any tool to be adopted into clinical practice, it needs to be simple and quick to use. The CFS meets both criteria (Figure 1) and is used widely used in many geriatric services in England; however, the CFS, like any other assessment tool, needs to be consistent in identifying and grading frailty between clinical staff and between clinical services.

In a study conducted by a university-associated tertiary hospital in Melbourne, Australia, all patients aged 65 and over admitted to the general medical unit during August and September 2013 had their baseline CFS score documented by a member of the treating medical team [11]. Despite the lack of prior training for medical staff on the use of the CFS, increasing frailty was correlated with functional decline and mortality, supporting the validity of the CFS as a frailty screening tool for clinicians. This study, however, did not compare the scores between staff groups.

In a retrospective note review by a medical student, a CFS was completed and then compared to one completed by a nurse specialist during a comprehensive geriatric assessment. The agreement between the two assessments, using Cohen's Kappa, was 0.63 [12]. An ICU-based study compared medical students with ICU doctors completing the CFS during patients' stays and again found an agreement of 0.64 [13]. Rolfson et al. found a good interrater reliability with the Edmonton Frailty Scale completed by Geriatric specialist nurses [14].

In this study, the largest disagreement was with case scenario G, where there was a two-point difference between the most junior trainees (FY1) and the nursing staff. This could be explained by the fact the patient was independent with activities of daily living, but also suffering from falls, indicating that she may need more help. Overall, there was broad agreement, and therefore the CFS can be documented on patient admission and we can be reassured of the score's consistency, despite it being used by different staff groups. The routine identification of frailty is good practice, as the identification of these patients allows us to start a care pathway to address the issues contributing to frailty and avoid adverse outcomes.

5. Conclusions

This study has confirmed that there is agreement between different staff members when conducting the CFS with no specific preceding training.

Author Contributions: Both authors contributed to the design and implementation of the research, D.G.S. performed data analysis, and both authors assisted in writing the manuscript. All authors have read and agreed to the published version of the manuscript.

References

1. WHO Clinical Consortium on Healthy Ageing: Topic Focus: Frailty and Intrinsic Capacity: Report of Consortium Meeting, 2016 in Geneva, Switzerland. Available online: https://www.who.int/ageing/health-systems/first-CCHA-meeting-report.pdf?ua=1 (accessed on 24 June 2020).

2. Romero-Ortuno, R.; O'Shea, D. Fitness and frailty: opposite ends of a challenging continuum! Will the end of age discrimination make frailty assessments an imperative? *Age Ageing* **2013**, *42*, 279–280. [CrossRef] [PubMed]

3. British Geriatrics Society, Fit for frailty guideline. Available online: https://www.bgs.org.uk/sites/default/files/content/resources/files/2018-05-23/fff_full.pdf (accessed on 24 June 2020).

4. Wou, F.; Gladman, J.; Bradshaw, L.; Franklin, M.; Edmans, J.; Conroy, S. The predictive properties of frailty-rating scales in the acute medical unit. *Eur. Geriatr. Med.* **2013**, *4*, S74. [CrossRef]

5. Rockwood, K.; Song, X.; Macknight, C.; Bergman, H.; Hogan, D.B.; McDowell, I.; Mitnitski, A. A global clinical measure of fitness and frailty in elderly people. *Can. Med Assoc. J.* **2005**, *173*, 489–495. [CrossRef] [PubMed]

6. Specialised Clinical Frailty Network, the Clinical Frailty Scale. Available online: https://www.scfn.org.uk/clinical-frailty-scale (accessed on 24 June 2020).

7. Darvall, J.N.; Bellomo, R.; Paul, E.; Subramaniam, A.; Santamaria, J.D.; Bagshaw, S.M.; Rai, S.; E Hubbard, R.; Pilcher, D. Frailty in very old critically ill patients in Australia and New Zealand: a population-based cohort study. *Med J. Aust.* **2019**, *211*, 318–323. [CrossRef] [PubMed]

8. O'Caoimh, R.; Costello, M.; Small, C.; Spooner, L.; Flannery, A.; O'Reilly, L.; Heffernan, L.; Mannion, E.; Maughan, A.; Joyce, A.; et al. Comparison of Frailty Screening Instruments in the Emergency Department. *Int. J. Environ. Res. Public Heal.* **2019**, *16*, 3626. [CrossRef] [PubMed]

9. Kahlon, S.; Pederson, J.; Majumdar, S.R.; Belga, S.; Lau, D.; Fradette, M.; Boyko, D.; Bakal, J.A.; Johnston, C.; Padwal, R.; et al. Association between frailty and 30-day outcomes after discharge from hospital. *Can. Med Assoc. J.* **2015**, *187*, 799–804. [CrossRef] [PubMed]

10. Patel, K.V.; Brennan, K.L.; Brennan, M.L.; Jupiter, D.C.; Shar, A.; Davis, M.L. Association of a Modified Frailty Index With Mortality After Femoral Neck Fracture in Patients Aged 60 Years and Older. *Clin. Orthop. Relat. Res.* **2013**, *472*, 1010–1017. [CrossRef] [PubMed]

11. Gregorevic, K.J.; E Hubbard, R.; Lim, W.K.; Katz, B. The clinical frailty scale predicts functional decline and mortality when used by junior medical staff: a prospective cohort study. *BMC Geriatr.* **2016**, *16*, 117. [CrossRef] [PubMed]
12. Davies, J.; Whitlock, J.; Gutmanis, I.; Kane, S.-L. Inter-Rater Reliability of the Retrospectively Assigned Clinical Frailty Scale Score in a Geriatric Outreach Population. *Can. Geriatr. J.* **2018**, *21*, 1–5. [CrossRef] [PubMed]
13. Pugh, R.; Ellison, A.; Pye, K.; Subbe, C.P.; Thorpe, C.M.; Lone, N.; Clegg, A. Feasibility and reliability of frailty assessment in the critically ill: a systematic review. *Crit. Care* **2018**, *22*, 49. [CrossRef] [PubMed]
14. Rolfson, D.B.; Majumdar, S.R.; Tsuyuki, R.T.; Tahir, A.; Rockwood, K. Validity and reliability of the Edmonton frailty score. *Age and Ageing* **2006**, *35*, 526–529. [CrossRef] [PubMed]

8

Considerations for the Development of Innovative Foods to Improve Nutrition in Older Adults

Mariane Lutz [1,2,*], **Guillermo Petzold** [1,3] **and Cecilia Albala** [1,4]

1. Thematic Task Force on Healthy Aging, CUECH Research Network, Viña del Mar 2520000, Chile; gpetzold@ubiobio.cl (G.P.); calbala@uchile.cl (C.A.)
2. Interdisciplinary Center for Health Studies, CIESAL, Faculty of Medicine, Universidad de Valparaíso, Angamos 655, Reñaca, Viña del Mar 2520000, Chile
3. Department of Food Engineering, Universidad del Bio-Bio, Andrés Bello 720, Casilla 447, Chillán 3780000, Chile
4. Institute of Nutrition and Food Technology, INTA, Universidad de Chile, El Líbano 5524, Macul, Santiago 7810000, Chile
*   Correspondence: mariane.lutz@uv.cl

Abstract: The population of older adults is growing globally. This increase has led to an accumulation of chronic illnesses, so-called age-related diseases. Diet and nutrition are considered the main drivers of the global burden of diseases, and this situation applies especially to this population segment. It relates directly to the development of coronary heart disease, hypertension, some types of cancer, and type 2 diabetes, among other diseases, while age-associated changes in body composition (bone and muscle mass, fat, sarcopenia) constitute risk factors for functional limitations affecting health status and the quality of life. Older adults present eating and swallowing problems, dry mouth, taste loss, and anorexia among other problems causing "anorexia of aging" that affects their nutritional status. The strategies to overcome these situations are described in this study. The impact of oral food processing on nutrition is discussed, as well as approaches to improve food acceptance through the design of innovative foods. These foods should supply a growing demand as this group represents an increasing segment of the consumer market globally, whose needs must be fulfilled.

Keywords: older adults; aging; food; nutrition; acceptability

1. Introduction

The increasing life expectancy of the world population, along with decreased mortality, has led to a rapid aging of the population in many countries [1]. The success in improving survival does not necessarily mean that the additional years are healthy or endured with a good quality of life. In fact, as mortality decreases and life expectancy increases, the question about the quality of the years gained, in the different regions of the world, arises. The rapid increase of the population over 60 years old, or older adults (OA), has led to an accumulation of chronic illnesses, the so-called age-related diseases (ARDs). This, together with the decrease in the function of organs and systems, increases vulnerability to a variety of stressors, augmenting functional limitations, disability, and dependency. The situation, however, is not inevitable or irreversible. Although the prevention of chronic diseases and the promotion of health should optimally be carried out throughout the life cycle, many disability-adjusted life years (DALYs) lost can be avoided through proper action initiated in OA [2]. Consequently, the current challenge is to decrease the gap between health expectancy and healthy life expectancy, as expressed by independence, autonomy, and functionality.

Nutrition and physical activity are among the main determinants of health. Diet and nutrition are considered the main drivers of the global burden of diseases [3]. Their global impact is huge, and their association to ARDs such as coronary heart disease, hypertension, some types of cancer, and type 2 diabetes, is well established. On the other hand, age-associated changes in body composition, including a decrease in bone and muscle mass, and a redistribution and increase of body fat, can lead, among others, to impaired immunity, metabolic disorders, frailty, sarcopenia, and osteoporosis, all of which constitute risk factors for functional limitations, falls, fractures, disability, dependency, institutionalization and mortality, affecting health status and the quality of life.

Although the importance of nutrition in OA is well established, undernutrition has not been given sufficient importance. A review of studies carried out mainly in European countries using the Mini Nutritional Assessment (MNA) screening tool found a prevalence of undernutrition of 5.8% in community dwelling, 38.7% in hospitalized patients, 50.5% in rehabilitation care, and 13.8% in institutionalized OA [4]. The Survey on Health, Well-Being, and Aging (SABE) survey, carried out in the capital cities of Latin America and the Caribbean in 1999–2000, revealed that, according to MNA, the prevalence of undernutrition among community-dwelling OA fluctuated between 1% and 8.3% and the risk of malnutrition ranged from 9.1% to 41.8% [5].

Other important physiological changes in OA include eating and swallowing impairment, such as chewing difficulty, dry mouth, taste loss, and loss of appetite, among others. These problems decrease the oral processing capability, which has attracted the attention of the food industry and researchers to provide technological solutions of foods with nutritive properties and attractive sensory attributes [6].

The aim of this publication is to describe some major physiological changes associated with aging and how these changes impact the nutritional status of OA, facts that should be taken into account to prevent the negative impact of aging on their quality of life. Accordingly, the need for innovative foods that consider rheological or texture properties especially directed towards OA is described, as a strategy to improve their acceptability and, consequently, the nutritional status of this increasing population group.

2. Nutritional Status in Aging

Along with the increasing prevalence of certain diseases, the changes in body composition associated to aging influence the nutritional status of OA [7]. Roubenoff [8] distinguishes three interrelated types of changes associated with undernutrition that may occur either as a consequence of the aging process, concomitant diseases, or both—wasting (an unintentional loss of weight, primarily caused by a deficient dietary intake, affecting fat and fat free mass); cachexia (the loss of fat free mass or body cell mass and no initial weight loss, characterized by hypercatabolism and sarcopenia); and loss of muscle mass (which seems to be a condition inherently related to aging, usually with pre-existing cachexia or sarcopenia, with low muscle mass, muscle strength, and physical performance, caused by mechanisms that involve, among others, protein synthesis, proteolysis, neuromuscular integrity and muscle fat content). In many OA the etiology is multi-factorial [9].

The physiological changes that lead to these situations include the loss of appetite [10], mainly due to decreased chemosensory functions and decreased secretions of the hormones that regulate appetite. Cox et al. [11] assessed nine interventional treatment strategies for the anorexia of aging, which aimed to improve appetite, of which food flavor enhancement, oral nutritional supplements, amino acid precursors, fortified foods, and megestrol acetate medication proved to be effective.

Chewing difficulties, swallowing problems, thirst, hunger, and diminished smell and taste are detrimental for the psychological satisfaction and pleasure associated with eating, resulting in a decrease in energy intake. Anorexia may also lead to wasting and sarcopenia (defined as "a syndrome characterized by progressive and generalized loss of skeletal muscle mass and strength with a risk of adverse outcomes such as physical disability, poor quality of life, and death" [9,12–14]), poor endurance, and decreased mobility [15]. Consequently, there are multiple causes of weight loss in the elderly, including the decline of chemosensory function (smell and taste), reduced efficiency of chewing, slowed gastric emptying, and alterations to the neuroendocrine axis (changes in the levels of leptin, cholecystokinin, neuropeptide Y, and other hormones and peptides), which contribute to anorexia [16,17].

3. Anorexia and Malnutrition in OA

Poor nutritional status is one of the main risk factors for frailty, a condition characterized by the inability to respond to stress and preserve homeostasis [18], and associated with both macro- and micronutrients deficiencies [19]. Frail persons are at a high risk of disability, dependency, cognitive impairment, and mortality [20]. In fact, frailty is considered as a state of pre-disability, and has been described as a situation between normal aging and disability (or even death) [21]. Tsutsumimoto et al. [22] investigated whether the anorexia of aging had a significant impact on incident disability and a possible direct association with future disability, or an indirect association with this condition via frailty. The authors showed that OA with anorexia had a higher proportion of frailty and a higher prevalence of disability compared to those without it. In addition, anorexia indirectly affected incident disability via frailty status. The pathophysiology of frailty is complex and multi-factorial, and nutrition is an important factor in its onset and a specific target for treatment [23]. Frailty involves a decrease in dietary intake, coupled with a decline in physical exercise, which leads to a loss of muscle mass, thus making OA more vulnerable to develop complications such as sarcopenia, comorbidities, or disability [18].

Chronic undernutrition (insufficient protein and energy intake) leads to weight loss and sarcopenia (which may, in turn, cause low muscle strength and feelings of exhaustion), while frailty itself may have a negative effect on eating and, consequently, on the nutritional status [24]. When lean body mass is lost, while fat mass is preserved or even increased, the state is called sarcopenic obesity [25]. In this situation, the relationship between age-related reduction of muscle mass and strength is often independent of body mass. It had long been thought that the loss of weight, along with the loss of muscle mass, were major factors affecting muscle weakness in OA [26]. However, changes in muscle composition are also important, e.g., fat infiltration into muscle lowers work performance [27].

Undernutrition involving protein-energy wasting in OA has been extensively described [28,29]. Inadequate food intake, reduced capacity to use available proteins, and a higher need for proteins due to a cumulative physical decline [30] contribute to the alteration of the nutritional state. Efforts have been made to improve protein intake through various strategies, including the use of nutritional supplements [31] and dietary enrichment or food and meal fortification, in which protein intake is increased by augmenting protein density [32]. In a systematic review of clinical studies determining the effects of dietary enrichment with conventional foods on energy and protein intake in OA, Trabal and Farran-Codina [33] concluded that any intervention that increases energy and nutrient density while holding constant or reducing portion sizes, constitutes a desired approach—having observed that low-volume, energy-dense foods increase energy intake without affecting appetite. However, the authors could not get conclusive results, mainly due to the lack of large-scale clinical trials with long-term interventions that allow the establishment of the effects of the treatments reported to address malnutrition in OA. Besides, OA usually exhibit both short- and long-term satiety signals (mostly peripheral) which contrast energy balance and contribute to malnutrition.

4. Protein Needs in OA

OA need more protein due to a series of physiological changes, including a declining anabolic response to protein intake. In fact, OA develop resistance to the positive effects of dietary protein on protein synthesis, limiting muscle accretion and maintenance, in a situation described as "anabolic resistance" [34]. Besides, there is a need to offset the catabolic conditions associated with the multiple chronic and acute diseases that commonly occur in OA, among other situations. Many of these relate to modifications of hormone production and sensitivity, which involves growth hormones (GH), insulin-like growth factor (IGF-I), corticosteroids, androgens, estrogens, and insulin, which affect the anabolic/catabolic state of muscle protein metabolism [35–37]. Metabolic changes associated with aging also include increased splanchnic sequestration and decreased postprandial availability of amino acids (AA), a lower postprandial perfusion of muscle, decreased muscle uptake of dietary AA, reduced anabolic signaling for protein synthesis, a reduced ability to use available protein (insulin resistance, protein anabolic resistance, high splanchnic extraction, immobility), and a reduced digestive capacity [30,38]. On the other hand, the main factors that influence protein use in OA include inadequate intake of protein (anorexia or appetite loss, gastrointestinal disturbances) or a greater need for protein (inflammatory disease, increased oxidative modification of proteins), all of which indicate that protein needs are augmented. A high proportion of inadequate protein intake has been observed in OA [39] and some studies had estimated that 15% to 38% of older men and 27% to 41% of older women consume less protein than recommended [40]. The AA composition of dietary proteins impacts anabolic potency at a muscular level. Leucine is the main regulator of protein turnover in muscle, through the activation of mTOR signaling. Although aged muscle has a reduced anabolic response to small doses of essential AA, 2.5–3 g of leucine are able to reverse this anabolic resistance [41].

The PROT-AGE Study Group established that, in order to maintain and regain muscle, OA should consume an average daily intake in the range of 1.0 to 1.2 g/kg body weight/day. In case of acute or chronic disease, the need of dietary protein increases to 1.2 to 1.5 g/kg body weight/day; and people with severe illness, injury, or marked malnutrition may need 2.0 g/kg body weight/day [30]. In OA, dietary protein or AA supplementation promote protein synthesis and can enhance recovery of physical function [42], improving muscle strength and function more readily than muscle mass [41,43,44]. Observational studies have supported an association between protein intake and muscle strength and mass [45,46], and the ingestion of ~20 g whey protein has been shown to increase muscle protein synthesis rates in healthy OA [47,48]. In fact, it has been recommended that due to the blunted sensitivity of OA muscles to low doses of AA, dietary protein should be distributed to at least 25 to 30 g of high quality protein per meal, containing approximately 2.5 to 2.8 g of leucine, to stimulate muscle protein synthesis [30,49].

An additional approach regarding the sources of proteins to supply the needs of OA takes into consideration their sustainability. A sustainable diet should increase plant protein sources and reduce animal protein intake. The impacts of these more environmentally-friendly diets on the nutritional state of OA are just beginning to be addressed, considering that plant foods are also sources of dietary fiber and a variety of phytochemicals, and may eventually reduce the bioavailability of some nutrients [50]. The recommendations for increased high-quality protein intake in OA should also take into consideration an adequate supply of calcium for preserving bone and muscle mass and, additionally, it is also relevant to reach an adequate energy supply to achieve the optimal protein utilization, with a high P% (proportion of dietary energy derived from proteins) [51].

5. Strategies to Contrast Anorexia and Malnutrition

The most commonly described dietary strategies to deliver proteins and other nutrients to OA include fractioning food intake in small digestible meals, improving taste and flavor, and/or limiting the intake of cholecystokinin (CCK)-stimulating foods such as fats and proteins [10], although in this case the energy and protein densities may be reduced. A strategy that can be used for OA who require increased energy and nutrient intakes is to offer frequent, small servings of food with high energy and nutrient density [52], such as frozen ready-to-eat meals [53]. Besides changes in the amount of food and type of food intake, OA eat fewer snacks between meals [54], experience less cravings for food [55], and feel less hungry and more satiated than younger individuals [56]. Another factor affecting low energy intake and low body weight in OA is small dietary variety, since energy intake is greater when a variety of foods is provided [57,58]. Finally, as highlighted by de Boer et al. [59], the effects of non-physiological anorexia of aging should be considered, including socio-economic factors such as depression, alcoholism, poverty, widowhood, environment changes, social isolation, and loneliness.

6. Foods for OA: The Importance of Texture and Other Sensory Attributes

Good nutrition may help prevent, modulate, or ameliorate age related diseases [60]. However, the physiological changes and dysfunctions in OA cause a series of eating and swallowing problems, considering that the oral food processing (the first step of food consumption) includes not only the intake of food, digestion and absorption of nutrients, and conditioning their bioavailability, but also comprises important sensory attributes. Various approaches have been proposed to improve food acceptance through intelligent design or modifications of the food matrix. Among these, in case of the chewing difficulty of OA due to the lack of functional teeth, an efficient reduction of food size is suggested; while in most of the OA with eating difficulties it is necessary to modify the texture of food as an efficient solution to improve food intake [6].

The development of innovative foods is important to counteract the deficiencies of macro- and micronutrients intake in OA, fortifying the food products with selected ingredients, vitamins, and minerals [61]. In this context, the need of OA for food products with adequate sensory values and optimal nutritional quality is of crucial importance [62]. As mentioned above, an important nutritional concern is to provide OA with sufficiently high-quality proteins [50], while the decline of food chemosensory perception in OA forces the food industry to develop more palatable foods, improving attractive properties such as taste, smell, temperature, color, and texture that positively influence food intake [63]. Accordingly, several strategies have been proposed to make foods for OA more palatable and stimulate their appetite. For example, van der Meij et al. [64] highlight the importance of providing a variety of adapted meals and snacks of different colors. In a similar strategy, Griep et al. [65] showed that intensely flavored products such as a meat substitute (Quorn) and yoghurt increase food intake in OA. On the other hand, an increase in food intake has been observed via flavored additives such as monosodium glutamate [66,67], or the natural flavoring of roast beef, bacon, cheese, citrus or pomegranate byproducts and spices such as rosemary, garlic, paprika, and onion [68,69]. The effect of natural food flavors on food intake in hospitalized OA patients in Hong Kong showed that total energy and protein intakes were increased by 13–26% and 15–28%, respectively, with flavor enhancement [70].

The food industry needs to develop and offer innovative food products with modified texture or rheology, palatable, and nutritious [63] to help overcome aging related anorexia [71]. Texture modified foods are processed products with a soft texture or a reduced particle size, as well as thickened liquids (drinks) oriented towards the market segment of OA with eating dysfunctions [72]. Food textures for the OA population should be soft and moist, while sticky and adhesive textures should be avoided as well as fibrous structures that are not easily disintegrated [73]. Soft texture foods are preferred, because they are easily disintegrated and mixed in the mouth, avoiding mastication [74]. Additionally, OA usually have difficulties forming the food bolus, which in some cases leads to a very long time of chewing before swallowing, which negatively affects the sensory experience associated with that food. Accordingly, Laguna et al. [75] tested the oral processing of foods in OA using gels of different textures (varying in hardness), and reported that not only the texture or consistency (hardness) is important, but also the heterogeneity of the food matrix. The physical characteristics of foods influence their oral processing, affecting mainly the number of chews and time spent in the mouth—major considerations in the design of foods for OA. Moreover, the flow and properties of saliva normally change with age, which can result in dry mouth conditions and taste aberrations [76]. Limited salivation is an important physiological dysfunction, with a 38% drop of the salivary flow in OA and the consequent problems forming the food bolus [77]. Salivation is very important to food processing, involving lubrication and food bolus formation in the mouth, and is consequently also related to the textural experience and overall sensory experience [76]. In this context, Assad-Bustillos et al. [78] reported that soft aerated cereal foods stimulate the salivary flow rate, the food bolus properties and the perception of oral comfort (the oral sensations perceived when eating a food) in OA, priming over the dental status. In addition, Lorieau et al. [79] demonstrated that soft model cheeses tested by OA led to a softer bolus that was more easily formed, the soft cheeses being more comfortable than dryer cheeses as their textures were perceived as soft, fatty and melting.

Another alternative to offering innovative acceptable foods for OA is to modify the culinary processes used to improve oral comfort when they eat. Among these, blade tenderization is an effective technique for improving meat texture. It involves meat perforation with sharp edged blades that are closely spaced to cut muscle fibers and ensure tenderness. Vandenberghe-Descamps et al. [80] demonstrated that easy-to-do culinary processes improve oral comfort, facilitate the formation of a food bolus and ameliorate food texture while eating meat. Regarding roast beef, the cumulative effect of blade tenderization, marinade and low-temperature cooking were the optimal conditions to obtain meat that is easy to chew, humidifies well with saliva, and can be smoothly swallowed, as well as any tender and juicy product.

The food industry should consider the fact that foods for the OA represent an interesting segment of the world consumer market. In the US, this segment holds more than a third of the country's wealth. In Europe, consumption by adults over 50 years old has increased three times as fast as those under this age. Clearly, the stereotype of an OA who is conservatively spending on food and beverages in the face of very limited income is increasingly out of date. In addition, OA constitute the largest percentage of television audiences (>50%) and the largest consumers of printed material, representing an audience prone to receive information about new food products that leverage innovations in the food science and technology area [81].

7. Conclusions

OA experience a series of age-related physiological changes that lead to detrimental nutritional impacts. In order to improve their food intake to accomplish their nutritional needs, overcome changes in their appetite, improve their oral processing of foods, and to increase sensory attributes, the food industry needs to develop intelligent foods through novel design. Among the current alternatives directed towards the growing OA population group, new texture-modified foods represent an efficient, nutritious, and palatable solution to overcome their eating and swallowing difficulties. Innovative foods should supply a growing demand as OA represent an interesting and increasing segment of the consumer market globally, whose needs must be fulfilled (Figure 1).

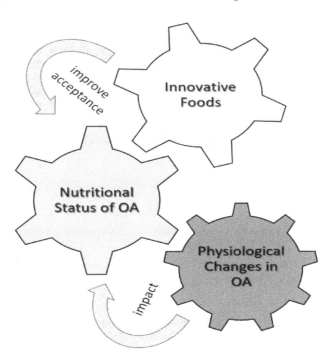

Figure 1. The physiological changes in older adults (OA) impact their nutritional status. Innovative foods with high acceptability must be developed to improve their nutritional status.

Author Contributions: M.L. conceived the subject and aim of the review and wrote the paper; G.P. provided information on sensory and texture aspects of foods; C.A. provided information on physiological changes of aging that affect nutritional status.

References

1.   World Health Organization. Global Health Observatory Data Repository. Mortality and Global Health Estimates. Available online: http://apps.who.int/gho/data/node.home (accessed on 3 April 2019).

2.   Prince, M.J.; Wu, F.; Guo, Y.; Gutierrez Robledo, L.M.; O'Donnell, M.; Sullivan, R.; Yusuf, S. The burden of disease in older people and implications for health policy and practice. *Lancet* **2015**, *385*, 549–562. [CrossRef]

3.   Global Nutrition Report. From Promise to Impact: Ending Malnutrition by 2030 Independent Expert Group, Washington, DC, USA. Available online: http://www.ifpri.org/publication/global-nutrition-report-2016-promise-impact-ending-malnutrition-2030 (accessed on 30 March 2019).

4.   Kaiser, M.J.; Bauer, J.M.; Rämsch, C.; Uter, W.; Guigoz, Y.; Cederholm, T.; Thomas, D.R.; Anthony, P.S.; Charlton, K.E.; Maggio, M.; et al. Mini Nutritional Assessment International Group. Frequency of malnutrition in older adults: A multinational perspective using the mini nutritional assessment. *J. Am. Geriatr. Soc.* **2010**, *58*, 1734–1738. [CrossRef] [PubMed]

5.   Lera, L.; Sánchez, H.; Ángel, B.; Albala, C. Mini Nutritional Assessment short-form: Validation in five Latin American cities. SABE Study. *J. Nutr. Health Aging* **2016**, *20*, 797–805. [CrossRef] [PubMed]

6.   Wang, X.; Chen, J. Food oral processing: Recent developments and challenges. *Curr. Opin. Colloid Interface Sci.* **2017**, *28*, 22–30. [CrossRef]

7.   Hickson, M.; Frost, G. An investigation into the relationships between quality of life, nutritional status and physical function. *Clin. Nutr.* **2004**, *23*, 213–221. [CrossRef]

8.   Roubenoff, R. The pathophysiology of wasting in the elderly. *J. Nutr.* **1999**, *129*, 256S–259S. [CrossRef] [PubMed]

9.   Cruz-Jentoft, A.J.; Bahat, G.; Bauer, J.; Boirie, Y.; Bruyère, O.; Cederholm, T.; Cooper, C.; Landi, F.; Rolland, Y.; Sayer, A.A.; et al. Sarcopenia: Revised European consensus on definition and diagnosis. *Age Ageing* **2018**, *48*, 16–31. [CrossRef] [PubMed]

10. Di Francesco, V.; Fantin, F.; Omizzolo, F.; Residori, L.; Bissoli, L.; Bissoli, L.; Bosello, O.; Zamboni, M. The anorexia of aging. *Dig. Dis.* **2007**, *25*, 129–137. [CrossRef]

11. Cox, N.J.; Ibrahim, K.I.; Sayer, A.A.; Robinson, S.M.; Roberts, H.C. Assessment and treatment of the anorexia of aging: A systematic review. *Nutrients* **2019**, *11*, 144. [CrossRef]

12. Fielding, R.A.; Vellas, B.; Evans, W.J.; Bhasin, S.; Morley, J.E.; Newman, A.B.; Abellan van Kan, G.; Andrieu, S.; Bauer, J.; Breuille, D.; et al. Sarcopenia: An undiagnosed condition in older adults. Current consensus definition: Prevalence, etiology, and consequences. International Working Group on Sarcopenia. *J. Am. Med. Dir. Assoc.* **2011**, *12*, 249–256. [CrossRef]

13. Cruz-Jentoft, A.J.; Baeyens, J.P.; Bauer, J.M.; Boirie, Y.; Cederholm, T.; Landi, F.; Martin, F.C.; Michel, J.P.; Rolland, Y.; Schneider, S.M.; et al. Sarcopenia: European consensus on definition and diagnosis. *Age Ageing* **2010**, *39*, 412–423. [CrossRef] [PubMed]

14. Cruz-Jentoft, A.J.; Landi, F.; Schneider, S.M.; Zuñiga, C.; Arai, H.; Boirie, Y.; Chen, L.K.; Fielding, R.A.; Martin, F.C.; Michel, J.P.; et al. Prevalence of and interventions for sarcopenia in ageing adults: A systematic review. Report of the International Sarcopenia Initiative (EWGSOP and IWGS). *Age Ageing* **2014**, *43*, 748–759. [CrossRef] [PubMed]

15. Morley, J.E. Anorexia, sarcopenia, and aging. *Nutrition* **2001**, *17*, 660–663. [CrossRef]

16. Alibhai, S.M.; Greenwood, C.; Payette, H. An approach to the management of unintentional weight loss in elderly people. *Can. Med. Assoc. J.* **2005**, *172*, 773–780. [CrossRef] [PubMed]

17. Wernette, C.M.; White, D.; Zizza, C.A. Signaling proteins that influence energy intake may affect unintentional weight loss in elderly persons. *J. Am. Diet. Assoc.* **2011**, *111*, 864–873. [CrossRef] [PubMed]

18. Fried, L.P.; Tangen, C.M.; Walston, J.; Newman, A.B.; Hirsch, C.; Gottdiener, J.; Seeman, T.; Tracy, R.; Kop, W.J.; Burke, G.; et al. Frailty in older adults: Evidence for a phenotype. *J. Gerontol. A Biol. Sci. Med. Sci.* **2001**, *56*, M146–M156. [CrossRef] [PubMed]

19. Bonnefoy, M.; Berrut, G.; Lesourd, B.; Ferry, M.; Gilbert, T.; Guérin, O.; Hanon, O.; Jeandel, C.; Paillaud, E.; Raynaud-Simon, A.; et al. Frailty and nutrition: Searching for evidence. *J. Nutr. Health Aging* **2015**, *19*, 250–257. [CrossRef] [PubMed]

20. Walston, J.; Hadley, E.C.; Ferrucci, L.; Guralnik, J.M.; Newman, A.B.; Studenski, S.A.; Ershler, W.B.; Harris, T.; Fried, L.P. Research Agenda for Frailty in Older Adults: Toward a better understanding of physiology and etiology: Summary from the American Geriatrics Society/National Institute on Aging Research Conference on Frailty in Older Adults. *J. Am. Geriatrics Soc.* **2006**, *54*, 991–1001. [CrossRef] [PubMed]

21. Van Kan, G.A.; Rolland, Y.M.; Morley, J.E.; Vellas, B. Frailty: Toward a clinical definition. *J. Am. Med. Dir. Assoc.* **2007**, *9*, 71–72. [CrossRef]

22. Tsutsumimoto, K.; Doi, T.; Makizako, H.; Hotta, R.; Nakakubo, S.; Makino, K.; Suzuki, T.; Shimada, H. Aging-related anorexia and its association with disability and frailty. *J. Cachexia Sarcop. Muscle* **2018**, *9*, 834–843. [CrossRef]

23. Clegg, A.; Young, J.; Iliffe, S.; Rikkert, M.O.; Rockwood, K. Frailty in elderly people. *Lancet* **2013**, *381*, 752–762. [CrossRef]

24. Yannakoulia, M.; Ntanasi, E.; Anastasiou, C.A.; Scarmeas, M. Frailty and nutrition: From epidemiological and clinical evidence to potential mechanisms. *Metab. Clin. Exper.* **2017**, *68*, 64–76. [CrossRef]

25. Prado, C.M.; Lieffers, J.R.; McCargar, L.J.; Reiman, T.; Sawyer, M.B.; Sawyer, M.B.; Martin, L.; Baracos, V.E. Prevalence and clinical implications of sarcopenic obesity in patients with solid tumours of the respiratory and gastrointestinal tracts: A population-based study. *Lancet Oncol.* **2008**, *9*, 629–635. [CrossRef]

26. Stenholm, S.; Harris, T.B.; Rantanen, T.; Visser, M.; Kritchevsky, S.B.; Ferrucci, L. Sarcopenic obesity: Definition, cause and consequences. *Curr. Opin. Clin. Nutr. Metab. Care* **2008**, *11*, 693–700. [CrossRef] [PubMed]

27. Visser, M.; Kritchevsky, S.B.; Goodpaster, B.H.; Newman, A.B.; Nevitt, M.; Stamm, E.; Harris, T.B. Leg muscle mass and composition in relation to lower extremity performance in men and women aged 70 to 79: The health, aging and body composition study. *J. Am. Geriatr. Soc.* **2002**, *50*, 897–904. [CrossRef] [PubMed]

28. DiMaria-Ghalili, R.; Amella, E. Nutrition in older adults: Intervention and assessment can help curb the growing threat of malnutrition. *Am. J. Nurs.* **2005**, *105*, 40–50. [CrossRef] [PubMed]

29. Morley, J.E. Undernutrition in older adults. *Fam. Pract.* **2012**, *29*, i89–i93. [CrossRef]

30. Bauer, J.; Biolo, G.; Cederholm, T.; Cesari, M.; Cruz-Jentoft, J.; Morley, J.E.; Phillips, S.; Sieber, C.; Stehle, P.; Teta, D.; et al. Evidence-based recommendations for optimal dietary protein intake in older people: A position paper from the PROT-AGE study group. *J. Am. Med. Dir. Assoc.* **2013**, *14*, 542–559. [CrossRef]

31. Silver, H.J. Oral strategies to supplement older adults' dietary intakes: Comparing the evidence. *Nutr. Rev.* **2009**, *67*, 21–31. [CrossRef]

32. Milne, A.C.; Potter, J.; Vivanti, A.; Avenell, A. Protein and energy supplementation in elderly people at risk from malnutrition. *Cochrane Database Syst. Rev.* **2009**, *2*, CD003288. [CrossRef]

33. Trabal, J.; Farran-Codina, A. Effects of dietary enrichment with conventional foods on energy and protein intake in older adults: A systematic review. *Nutr. Rev.* **2015**, *73*, 624–633. [CrossRef] [PubMed]

34. Burd, N.A.; Gorissen, S.H.; van Loon, L.J. Anabolic resistance of muscle protein synthesis with aging. *Exerc. Sport Sci. Rev.* **2013**, *41*, 169–173. [CrossRef] [PubMed]

35. Chernoff, R. Protein and older adults. *J. Am. Coll. Nutr.* **2004**, *23*, 627S–630S. [CrossRef] [PubMed]

36. Adamo, M.L.; Farrar, R.P. Resistance training, and IGF involvement in the maintenance of muscle mass during the aging process. *Ageing Res. Rev.* **2006**, *5*, 310–331. [CrossRef] [PubMed]

37. Walrand, S.; Guillet, C.; Salles, J.; Cano, N.; Boirie, Y. Physiopathological mechanism of sarcopenia. *Clin. Geriatr. Med.* **2011**, *27*, 365–385. [CrossRef] [PubMed]

38. Deutz, N.E.P.; Bauer, J.M.; Barazzoni, R.; Biolo, G.; Boirie, Y.; Bosy-Westphal, A.; Cederholm, T.; Cruz-Jentoft, A.; Krznariç, Z.; Nair, K.S.; et al. Protein intake and exercise for optimal muscle function with aging: Recommendations from the ESPEN Expert Group. *Clin. Nutr.* **2014**, *33*, 929–936. [CrossRef] [PubMed]

39. Fulgoni, V.L. Current protein intake in America: Analysis of the National Health and Nutrition Examination Survey, 2003–2004. *Am. J. Clin. Nutr.* **2008**, *87*, 1554S–1557S. [CrossRef]

40. Kerstetter, J.E.; O'Brien, K.O.; Insogna, K.L. Low protein intake: The impact on calcium and bone homeostasis in humans. *J. Nutr.* **2003**, *133*, 855S–861S. [CrossRef]

41. Tieland, M.; van de Rest, O.; Dirks, M.L.; van der Zwaluw, N.; Mensink, M.; van Loon, L.J.; de Groot, L.C. Protein supplementation improves physical performance in frail elderly people: A randomized, double-blind, placebo-controlled trial. *J. Am. Med. Dir. Assoc.* **2012**, *13*, 720–726. [CrossRef]

42. Paddon-Jones, D.; Sheffield-Moore, M.; Zhang, X.J.; Volpi, E.; Wolf, S.E.; Aarsland, A.; Ferrando, A.A.; Wolfe, R.R. Amino acid ingestion improves muscle protein synthesis in the young and elderly. *Am. J. Physiol. Endocrinol. Metab.* **2004**, *286*, E321–E328. [CrossRef]

43. Pohlhausen, S.; Uhlig, K.; Kiesswetter, E.; Diekmann, R.; Heseker, H.; Volkert, D.; Stehle, P.; Lesser, S. Energy and protein intake, anthropometrics, and disease burden in elderly home-care receivers—A cross-sectional study in Germany (ErnSIPP Study). *J. Nutr. Health Aging* **2016**, *20*, 361–368. [CrossRef] [PubMed]

44. Kramer, I.F.; Verdijk, L.V.; Hamer, H.M.; Verlaan, S.; Luiking, Y.C.; Kouw, I.W.K.; Senden, J.M.; van Kranenburg, J.; Gijsen, A.P.; Bierau, J.; et al. Both basal and post-prandial muscle protein synthesis rates, following the ingestion of a leucine-enriched whey protein supplement, are not impaired in sarcopenic older males. *Clin. Nutr.* **2017**, *36*, 1440–1449. [CrossRef] [PubMed]

45. Isanejad, M.; Mursu, J.; Sirola, J.; Kröger, H.; Rikkonen, T.; Tuppurainen, M.; Erkkilä, A.T. Dietary protein intake is associated with better physical function and muscle strength among elderly women. *Br. J. Nutr.* **2016**, *115*, 1281–1291. [CrossRef] [PubMed]

46. Landi, F.; Calvani, R.; Tosato, M.; Martone, A.M.; Picca, A.; Ortolani, E.; Savera, G.; Salini, S.; Ramaschi, M.; Bernabei, R.; et al. Animal-derived protein is associated with muscle mass and strength in community-dwellers: Results from the Milan EXPO Survey. *J. Nutr. Health Aging* **2017**, *21*, 1050–1056. [CrossRef] [PubMed]

47. Paddon-Jones, D.; Sheffield-Moore, M.; Katsanos, C.S.; Zhang, X.J.; Wolfe, R.R. Differential stimulation of muscle protein synthesis in elderly humans following isocaloric ingestion of amino acids or whey protein. *Exp. Gerontol.* **2006**, *41*, 215–219. [CrossRef]

48. Kramer, I.F.; Verdijk, L.B.; Hamer, H.M.; Verlaan, S.; Luiking, Y.; Kouw, I.W.; Senden, J.M.; van Kranenburg, J.; Gijsen, A.P.; Poeze, M.; et al. Impact of the macronutrient composition of a nutritional supplement on muscle protein synthesis rates in older men: A randomized, double blind, controlled trial. *J. Clin. Endocrinol. Metab.* **2015**, *100*, 4124–4132.

49. Bauer, J.; Verlaan, S.; Bautmans, I.; Brandt, K.; Donini, L.M.; Maggio, M.; McMurdo, M.E.; Mets, T.; Seal, C.; Wijers, S.L.; et al. Effects of a vitamin D and leucine-enriched whey protein nutritional supplement on measures of sarcopenia in older adults, the PROVIDE Study: A randomized, double-blind, placebo-controlled trial. *J. Am. Med. Dir. Assoc.* **2015**, *16*, 740–747. [CrossRef]

50. Lonnie, M.; Hooker, E.; Brunstrom, J.M.; Corfe, B.M.; Green, M.A.; Watson, A.W.; Williams, E.A.; Stevenson, E.J.; Penson, S.; Johnstone, A.M.; et al. Protein for Life: Review of optimal protein intake, sustainable dietary sources and the effect on appetite in ageing adults. *Nutrients* **2018**, *10*, 360. [CrossRef]

51. De Souza Genaro, P.; Araujo Martini, L. Effect of protein intake on bone and muscle mass in the elderly. *Nutr. Rev.* **2010**, *68*, 616–623. [CrossRef]

52. Nieuwenhuizen, W.F.; Weenen, H.; Rigby, P.; Hetherington, M.M. Older adults and patients in need of nutritional support: Review of current treatment options and factors influencing nutritional intake. *Clin. Nutr.* **2010**, *29*, 160–169. [CrossRef]

53. Höglund, E.; Ekman, S.; Stuhr-Olsson, G.; Lundgren, C.; Albinsson, M.S.; Signäs, M.; Karlsson, C.; Rothenberg, E.; Wendin, K. A meal concept designed for older adults—Small, enriched meals including dessert. *Food Nutr. Res.* **2018**, *62*, 1572–1579. [CrossRef] [PubMed]

54. De Castro, J.M. Age-related changes in spontaneous food intake and hunger in humans. *Appetite* **1993**, *21*, 255–272. [CrossRef] [PubMed]

55. Pelchat, M.L.; Schaefer, S. Dietary monotony and food cravings in young and elderly adults. *Physiol. Behav.* **2000**, *68*, 353–359. [CrossRef]

56. Clarkson, W.K.; Pantano, M.M.; Morley, J.E.; Horowitz, M.; Littlefield, J.M.; Burton, F.R. Evidence for the anorexia of aging: Gastrointestinal transit and hunger in healthy elderly versus young adults. *Am. J. Physiol.* **1997**, *272*, R243–R248.

57. Roberts, S.B.; Hajduk, C.L.; Howarth, N.C.; Russell, R.; McCrory, M.A. Dietary variety predicts low body mass index and inadequate macronutrient and micronutrient intakes in community-dwelling older adults. *J. Gerontol. A Biol. Sci. Med. Sci.* **2005**, *60A*, 613–621. [CrossRef] [PubMed]

58. Hays, N.P.; Roberts, S.B. The anorexia of aging in humans. *Physiol. Behav.* **2006**, *88*, 257–266. [CrossRef] [PubMed]

59. De Boer, A.; Ter Horst, G.J.; Lorist, M.M. Physiological and psychosocial age-related changes associated with reduced food intake in older persons. *Ageing Res. Rev.* **2013**, *12*, 316–328. [CrossRef] [PubMed]

60. Clegg, M.E.; Williams, E.A. Optimizing nutrition in older people. *Maturitas* **2018**, *112*, 34–38. [CrossRef] [PubMed]

61. Baugreet, S.; Hamill, R.M.; Kerry, J.P.; McCarthy, S.N. Mitigating nutrition and health deficiencies in older adults: A role for food innovation? *J. Food Sci.* **2017**, *82*, 848–855. [CrossRef]

62. Schwartz, C.; Vandenberghe-Descamps, M.; Sulmont-Rossé, C.; Tournier, C.; Feron, G. Behavioral and physiological determinants of food choice and consumption at sensitive periods of the life span, a focus on infants and elderly. *Innov. Food Sci. Emerg. Technol.* **2018**, *46*, 91–106. [CrossRef]

63. Aguilera, J.M.; Park, D.J. Texture-modified foods for the elderly: Status, technology and opportunities. *Trends Food Sci. Technol.* **2016**, *57*, 156–164. [CrossRef]

64. Van der Meij, B.S.; Wijnhoven, H.A.; Finlayson, G.S.; Oosten, B.S.; Visser, M. Specific food preferences of older adults with a poor appetite. A forced-choice test conducted in various care settings. *Appetite* **2015**, *90*, 168–175. [CrossRef] [PubMed]

65. Griep, M.I.; Mets, T.F.; Massart, D.L. Effects of flavour amplification of Quorn (R) and yoghurt on food preference and consumption in relation to age, BMI and odour perception. *Br. J. Nutr.* **2000**, *83*, 105–113. [CrossRef]

66. Schiffman, S.S. Intensification of sensory properties of foods for the elderly. *J. Nutr.* **2000**, *130* (Suppl. 4S), 927s–930s. [CrossRef]

67. Dermiki, M.; Prescott, J.; Sargent, L.J.; Willway, J.; Gosney, M.A.; Methven, L. Novel flavours paired with glutamate condition increased intake in older adults in the absence of changes in liking. *Appetite* **2015**, *90*, 108–113. [CrossRef] [PubMed]

68. Smith, J.S.; Ameri, F.; Gadgil, P. Effect of marinades on the formation of heterocyclic amines in grilled beef steaks. *J. Food Sci.* **2008**, *73*, T100–T105. [CrossRef] [PubMed]

69. Best, R.L.; Appleton, K.M. Comparable increases in energy, protein and fat intakes following the addition of seasonings and sauces to an older person's meal. *Appetite* **2011**, *56*, 179–182. [CrossRef]

70. Di Francesco, V.; Zamboni, M.; Dioli, A.; Zoico, E.; Mazzali, G.; Omizzolo, F.; Bissoli, L.; Solerte, S.B.; Benini, L.; Bosello, O. Delayed postprandial gastric emptying and impaired gallbladder contraction together with elevated cholecystokinin and peptide YY serum levels sustain satiety and inhibit hunger in healthy elderly persons. *J. Gerontol.* **2005**, *60*, 1581–1585. [CrossRef] [PubMed]

71. Wysokiński, A.; Sobów, T.; Kłoszewska, I.; Kostka, T. Mechanisms of the anorexia of aging—A review. *Age (Dordr)* **2015**, *37*, 9821. [CrossRef]

72. Cichero, J.A.Y. Texture-modified meals for hospital patients. In *Modifying Food Texture*; Chen, J., Rosenthal, A., Eds.; Woodhead Publishing: Cambridge, UK, 2015; Volume 2, p. 135e162.

73. Cichero, J.A.Y. Adjustment of food textural properties for elderly patients. *J. Text. Stud.* **2016**, *47*, 277–283. [CrossRef]

74. Ishihara, S.; Nakao, S.; Nakauma, M.; Funami, T.; Hori, K.; Ono, T.; Kohyama, K.; Nishinariet, K. Compression test of food gels on artificial tongue and its comparison with human test. *J. Text. Stud.* **2013**, *44*, 104–114. [CrossRef]

75. Laguna, L.; Hetherington, M.M.; Chen, J.; Artigas, G.; Sarkar, A. Measuring eating capability, liking and difficulty perception of older adults: A textural consideration. *Food Qual. Prefer.* **2016**, *53*, 47–56. [CrossRef]

76. Xu, F.; Laguna, L.; Sarkar, A. Aging-related changes in quantity and quality of saliva: Where do we stand in our understanding? *J. Text. Stud.* **2019**, *50*, 27–35. [CrossRef] [PubMed]

77. Vandenberghe-Descamps, M.; Labouré, H.; Prot, A.; Septier, C.; Tournier, C.; Feron, G. Salivary flow decreases in healthy elderly people independently of dental status and drug intake. *J. Text. Stud.* **2016**, *47*, 353–360. [CrossRef]

78. Assad-Bustillos, M.; Tournier, C.; Feron, G.; Guessasma, S.; Reguerre, A.L.; Della Valle, G. Fragmentation of two soft cereal products during oral processing in the elderly: Impact of product properties and oral health status. *Food Hydrocoll.* **2019**, *91*, 153–165. [CrossRef]

79.   Lorieau, L.; Septier, C.; Laguerre, A.; Le Roux, L.; Hazart, E.; Ligneul, A.; Famelart, M.H.; Dupont, D.;
      Floury, J.; Feron, G.; et al. Bolus quality and food comfortability of model cheeses for the elderly as influenced
      by their texture. *Food Res. Internat.* **2018**, *111*, 31–38. [CrossRef] [PubMed]

80.   Vandenberghe-Descamps, M.; Sulmont-Rossé, C.; Septier, C.; Follot, C.; Feron, G.; Labouré, H. Impact of
      blade tenderization, marinade and cooking temperature on oral comfort when eating meat in an elderly
      population. *Meat Sci.* **2018**, *145*, 86–93. [CrossRef] [PubMed]

81.   Murphy, C.; Vertrees, R. Sensory functioning in older adults: Relevance for food preference. *Curr. Opin.
      Food Sci.* **2017**, *15*, 56–60. [CrossRef]

9

Prevalence of Medication-Dietary Supplement Combined use and Associated Factors

Ignacio Aznar-Lou [1,2,*], Cristina Carbonell-Duacastella [1], Ana Rodriguez [3], Inés Mera [3] and Maria Rubio-Valera [1,2,4]

[1] Teaching, Research & Innovation Unit, Institut de Recerca Sant Joan de Déu, Esplugues de Llobregat, Parc Sanitari Sant Joan de Déu, 08830 Sant Boi de Llobregat (Barcelona), Spain
[2] Centro de Investigación Biomédica en Red en Epidemiología y Salud Pública, CIBERESP, 28029 Madrid, Spain
[3] Spanish Society of Community and Family Pharmacy (SEFAC), 28045 Madrid, Spain
[4] School of Pharmacy, University of Barcelona, 08028 Barcelona, Spain
[*] Correspondence: i.aznar@pssjd.org

Abstract: Introduction: The use of medication has increased in recent years in the US while the use of dietary supplements has remained stable but high. Interactions between these two kinds of products may have important consequences, especially in the case of widely used medications such as antihypertensives and antibiotics. The aim of this paper is to estimate the prevalence of potentially serious drug–dietary supplement interactions among tetracyclines, thiazides, and angiotensin II receptor blocker users by means of the NHANES 2013–2014 dataset. Methods: Data from 2013–2014 NHANES were obtained. Potential interactions analysed were tetracyclines with calcium, magnesium, and zinc, thiazides with vitamin D, and angiotensin II receptors blockers with potassium. Prevalence was calculated for each potential interaction. Logistic regression was used to assess associated factors. Results: 864 prescriptions issued to 820 patients were analysed. Overall prevalence of potential interaction was 49%. Older age and higher educational level were strongly associated with being at risk of a potential interaction. Factors such as age, race, civil status, citizenship, country of birth, BMI, and physical activity did not show notable associations. Conclusions: Healthcare professionals should be aware of other medical products when they prescribe or dispense a medication or a dietary supplement, especially to the older population and people with a higher educational level.

Keywords: prevalence; interactions; dietary supplements; antibiotics; antihypertensive medication

1. Introduction

The use of prescription medicines has increased recently in the United States (US) [1]. This general increase is not homogenous across all drug classes. While important increases are noted in the consumption of some prescription drugs such as anti-hypertensive agents (i.e., angiotensin II receptor blockers and thiazides), consumption of other drug classes, for instance oral antibiotics, has decreased. The use of dietary supplements is high and has remained stable over recent years in the general population in the US. The latest figures point to a prevalence in the use of dietary supplements of around 50% [2]. This use is higher in the older population, and among females, non-Hispanic whites, and people with a higher level of education.

One of the main health concerns related to the use of prescription medicines is the potential risk of adverse events and interactions. Interactions may occur between medications but also between medications and dietary supplements [3]. Qato et al. reported a range of prevalences of concomitant use of medication prescription and dietary supplements of between 0.2% and 2% of the general population [4]. Drug–drug interactions are usually checked by prescription and dispensing systems, which will prompt a warning message to the physician or pharmacist if a drug–drug interaction is detected. However, these systems have no information on patients' use of dietary supplements, as most of these supplements are obtained over the counter [3].

Interactions between prescription medication and dietary supplements may occur with widely used medications, such as antihypertensive agents and antibiotics [5,6]. The consequences of these interactions may vary between drugs and dietary supplements. Certain minerals including calcium, magnesium, and zinc may interact with tetracycline. The effects of these interactions could cause a reduction in tetracycline absorption (decreasing or eliminating the therapeutic effect) [3,5]. Other minerals, such as potassium, can cause interactions with anti-hypertensive drugs, including angiotensin II receptor blockers, provoking hyperkalaemia [5]. The use of thiazides has to be especially controlled in patients with osteoporosis because they could also interact with vitamin D and/or calcium causing hypercalcaemia and a potential metabolic alkalosis [5].

Since consumption of dietary supplements is rarely supervised by healthcare professionals, this information may help these professionals in their prescription and medication-counselling practice [3]. Specifically, although studies regarding consequences of prescription medication and dietary supplement interaction do exist, only a few of them have focused on American populations [4], revealing the lack of information. Thus, the aim of this paper is to estimate the prevalence of potentially serious drug–dietary supplement interactions among tetracyclines, thiazides, and angiotensin II receptor blocker users by means of the NHANES 2013–2014 dataset. The secondary aim of this paper is to outline the profile of a patient at risk of interactions between medication and dietary supplements. The NHANES survey is among the few large population-based nationally representative health and nutrition studies to apply standard design, and it includes the most detailed information regarding dietary habits and dietary supplement intake, as well as medication prescription. Due to the potential consequences of prescription medication and dietary supplement interaction, it is important to discern what patient profile is at the greatest risk of consuming dietary supplements that cause serious interactions. Thus, the information derived from our study will be important for effective US and international public health planning.

2. Methods

2.1. Study Design

We obtained data from the 2013–2014 National Health and Nutrition Examination Survey (NHANES). NHNAES is a nationally representative cross-sectional survey conducted by the National Center for Health Statistics (NCHS) and Centers for Disease Control and Prevention. NHANES includes information about the non-institutionalised US population. This database is used worldwide and has produced satisfactory results [6,7].

2.2. Ethics

The NCHS Research Ethics Review Board (ERB) approved the 2013–2014 study protocol (protocol 2011-17). NHANES and all participants provided written informed consent.

2.3. Interactions under Study

Table 1 shows the drug–dietary supplement interactions studied. We considered medication groups if they represented a prevalence of use higher than 2% of the population included in the database.

Table 1. Drug–dietary supplement interactions and their consequences.

Prescription Medicine	Dietary Supplement	Potential Clinical Consequences of the Interaction	Prevalence of Potential Interactions
Tetracyclines	Calcium	Decreased therapeutic effect as a consequence of a reduction in the absorption of tetracycline [3].	44.3%
	Magnesium	Decreased therapeutic effect as a consequence of a reduction in the absorption of tetracycline [3,5].	26.9%
	Zinc	Decreased therapeutic effect as a consequence of a reduction in the absorption of tetracycline [3,5].	37.4%
Thiazides	Calcium	Hypercalcemia and metabolic alkalosis. Thiazides reduce the urinary excretion of calcium. Vitamin D increases the absorption of calcium [5].	53.5%
	Vitamin D		52.1%
Angiotensin II receptor blockers	Potassium	Higher risk of hyperkalaemia, especially in patients with decreased renal function, heart failure, or diabetes [5].	28.8%

Tetracycline interacts with divalent ions such as calcium, magnesium, and zinc, forming a relatively stable and poorly absorbed chelate, preventing absorption of the antibiotic due to a lower amount of calcium in the gut available to be absorbed. This interaction may reduce or even abolish the therapeutic effect of the antibiotic, thereby diminishing anti-infectious efficiency. For this reason, tetracycline should be taken one hour before or two hours after meals [3,5].

Thiazide diuretics can cause increased calcium reabsorption in distal tubules of the kidneys, which contributes to hypercalcemia. Another cause of hypercalcemia is the excess of vitamin D, for example, through high doses of oral supplements, which increases the absorption of calcium in the gut. Due to the retention of calcium in the body, metabolic alkalosis may be developed [5].

Finally, angiotensin II receptor blockers are potassium-sparing and can, therefore, have additional hyperkalaemic effects if combined with potassium supplements or salt substitutes containing potassium. The use of potassium supplements is the main risk factor for developing hyperkalaemia, as this causes a rapid rate of increase in serum potassium levels. Other contributory risk factors such as poor renal function, heart failure, and diabetes should also be considered, as they are associated with a faster rate of hyperkalaemia progress [5,8].

3. Population and Prescription Medication Information

The sample was composed of tetracyclines, thiazides, and/or angiotensin II receptor blocker users. These drugs were chosen due to the potential severity of their interactions and their high prevalence of use in the American population. Prescription medication information was obtained through the Prescription Medication subsection included in The Dietary Supplement and Prescription Medication section of the Sample Person Questionnaire. This section provides personal information on the use of prescription medication in the month prior to the participant's interview. The name of the medication was provided by the participant to the interviewer, who entered it into the computer where it was automatically matched to a generic drug name and code. Medication is presented following the WHO Drug Statistics Methodology of ATC index [9].

Tetracyclines: We considered a patient to be a tetracycline consumer if he/she reported having taken a medication with a generic drug name included in the ATC group J01AA.

Thiazides: We considered a patient to be a thiazide consumer if he/she reported having taken a medication with a generic drug name included in the ATC group C03AA.

Angiotensin II receptor blockers: We considered a patient to be an angiotensin II receptor blocker consumer if he/she reported having taken a medication with a generic drug name included in the ATC group C09CA.

4. Dietary Supplement Information

Dietary supplement information was obtained through the dietary supplement subsection also included in The Dietary Supplement and Prescription Medication section of the Sample Person Questionnaire. This subsection allows for collection of personal data on the use of dietary supplements in the month prior to the participant's interview. Interviewers reported the supplement product name, which was automatically disaggregated to up to 34 nutrients.

We considered a participant to be a nutrient supplement consumer if he/she had taken any supplement containing at least one of the nutrients under study (Table 1).

5. Other Covariates

Demographic covariates were sex, age, race/ethnicity (Hispanic origin: Mexican-American, other Hispanic, non-Hispanic white, non-Hispanic black, other race), educational level (primary, secondary, university), civil status (married/with partner, widow/er, divorced, single), citizenship (American/non-American), and country of birth (U.S./Other country).

We also considered body mass index (BMI) and physical activity. BMI was determined from height and weight measured by health technicians previously trained by an expert anthropometrist. We categorised this variable as follows: underweight (<18.5), normal weight (18.5–24.9), overweight (25.0–29.9), and obesity type I (30.0–34.9) and obesity type II and type III (≥35.0).

Physical activity was self-reported and measured through a question asking if participants did any moderate-intensity sports in a typical week. The answer was dichotomic (yes/no).

6. Statistical Analysis

Prevalence rates were calculated for each potential interaction described in Table 1. The reference population consisted of those who reported having taken one of the medications under study.

A multivariate logistic regression analysis was conducted to determine the factors associated with a higher probability of having a potential interaction using the presence/absence of the interaction as the dependent variable and demographic and clinical variables as independent variables. The regression model provided odds ratios (OR) and 95% confidence intervals for the associations between the dependent variable and each of the independent variables. Crude associations obtained from bivariate logistic regressions were also presented.

To test potential interactions between demographic and clinical variables, such as age and physical exercise or gender and BMI, we tested the association between the probability of having a potential interaction and the interacting term of the dependent variables. The interacting terms were not statistically significant and, therefore, were not included in the final model.

All analyses were performed taking into account the appropriate weights. This procedure was developed with the goal of obtaining nationally representative estimates and accounting for unequal probability of selection derived from study design and non-response.

STATA 13.1MP was used to perform the statistical analyses.

7. Results

7.1. Sample Demographic Characteristics

The total sample was made up of 864 prescriptions issued to 820 individuals. Five per cent of those prescriptions involved tetracyclines, 61% involved thiazides, and 46% angiotensin II receptor blockers. Some of these prescriptions consisted of a combination of a thiazide and an angiotensin II inhibitor.

Sociodemographic characteristics are shown in Table 2. The proportion of women was 57%. The majority of the sample was non-Hispanic white (70%) and had secondary-level education (57%). Regarding civil status, 66% of the sample was defined as married or with a partner. Some 88% had been born in the U.S. and a higher percentage (97%) had American citizenship. The main BMI category was type II or III obesity (32%). Only 30% of the sample did moderate-intensity sport.

Table 2. Sociodemographic characteristics of the sample (n = 820).

	% or Mean	95% CI
Gender,% (n)		
Men	42.6 (350)	38.7; 46.7
Women	57.3 (470)	53.3; 61.3
Age, mean (range)	61.4 (20–80)	60.3; 62.6
Age group,% (n)		
20–39	6.4 (41)	4.6; 8.8
40–59	34.1 (249)	29.4; 39.2
60–79	50.0 (470)	45.6; 54.4
≥80	9.5 (104)	7.6; 11.9
Race,% (n)		
Mexican-American	3.9 (63)	2.0; 7.7
Other Hispanic	3.5 (62)	2.3; 5.5
Non-Hispanic white	70.4 (357)	65.5; 75.0
Non-Hispanic black	15.6 (237)	11.4; 21.0
Other race	6.4 (101)	4.4; 9.2
Education,% (n)		
Primary	15.7 (191)	11.9; 20.5
Secondary	57.4 (450)	53.6; 61.1
University	26.9 (179)	22.7; 31.7
Civil status *,% (n)		
Married/with partner	65.5 (482)	62.0; 68.9
Widow/er	12.9 (131)	10.4; 15.8
Divorced	14.4 (131)	12.3; 16.9
Single	7.1 (75)	5.2; 9.5
Citizenship *,% (n)		
American	88.3 (633)	84.4; 91.3
Non-American	11.7 (186)	8.7; 15.6
Country of birth *,% (n)		
U.S.	97.7 (779)	96.1; 98.6
Other country	2.3 (40)	1.4; 3.9
Body mass index (categories),% (n)		
Underweight	0.5 (5)	0.1; 2.2
Normal weight	10.6 (109)	7.6; 14.5
Overweight	30.7 (247)	26.4; 35.3
Obesity type I	26.5 (206)	22.2; 31.4
Obesity types II and III	31.6 (253)	28.3; 35.2
Physical activity in a typical week,% (n)		
Yes	40.4 (313)	35.9; 45.0
No	59.6 (507)	55.0; 64.1

* The following variables contain one missing value: civil status, citizenship and country of birth.

7.2. Prevalence of Potential Interactions

Table 1 shows the prevalence of potential interactions among the sample. Forty-four percent of the people using tetracyclines were consuming calcium and 26% and 37% of them were consuming magnesium and zinc, respectively. Among the users of thiazides, 54% and 52% used calcium and vitamin D, respectively. Finally, 26% of consumers of antagonist II receptor blockers presented a potential interaction due to the concomitant use of potassium. Overall, 49% of the participants were at risk of at least one of the studied interactions.

7.3. Factors Associated with Potential Interactions

Table 3 shows the factors associated with suffering a potential interaction between medications and dietary supplements. According to the adjusted analysis, age and educational level were strongly associated with the probability of a potential interaction. Also, compared to the non-Hispanic white population, the non-Hispanic black population presented a lower probability of a potential interaction.

The remaining variables (sex, civil status, citizenship, country of birth, BMI category, and physical activity) showed no statistically significant association with the risk of a potential interaction.

Table 3. Factors associated with potential interactions based on the multivariate weighted logistic regression model $^\$$.

	Bivariate Analysis		Multivariate Analysis	
	OR	95% CI	OR	95% CI
Gender				
Men	ref		ref	-
Women	1.08	0.79; 1.49	1.23	0.87; 1.75
Age (1 year increase)	1.02	1.01; 1.03	1.02	1.01; 1.03
Race				
Non-Hispanic white	ref		ref	-
Other Hispanic	0.42	0.17; 1.03	0.44	0.14; 1.33
Mexican-American	0.44	0.24; 0.80	0.55	0.25; 1.20
Non-Hispanic black	0.42	0.29; 0.60	0.45	0.30; 0.66
Other race	0.58	0.83; 1.78	0.60	0.29; 1.26
Education				
Primary	ref		ref	-
Secondary	2.10	1.31; 3.40	1.95	1.18; 3.23
University	2.03	1.24; 3.31	1.63	1.01; 2.63
Civil status *				
Married/with partner	ref		ref	-
Widow/er	0.98	0.66; 1.46	0.84	0.50; 1.43
Divorced	0.92	0.65; 1.32	1.05	0.71; 1.56
Single	0.56	0.25; 1.26	0.95	0.39; 2.34
Citizenship *				
American	ref		ref	-
Non-American	0.40	0.16; 0.99	0.86	0.27; 2.72
Country of birth *				
U.S.	ref		ref	-
Other country	0.65	0.41; 1.02	1.12	0.57; 2.20
Body mass index (categories)				
Underweight *				
Normal weight	ref		ref	-
Overweight	0.90	0.53; 1.51	0.77	0.45; 1.29
Obesity type I	1.23	0.77; 1.97	1.00	0.59; 1.71
Obesity types II and III	1.17	0.83; 1.67	1.04	0.74; 1.48
Physical activity in a typical week				
Yes	ref		ref	-
No	0.69	0.41; 1.17	0.71	0.41; 1.24

$^\$$ Potential interactions include the interaction of tetracyclines with calcium, magnesium or zinc, thiazides with vitamin D and Angiotensin II receptor blockers with potassium; * Few values to be considered. CI = Confidence interval; OR = Odds ratio.

Older people had a higher risk of using a prescription medication and a dietary product with a potential interaction effect (OR = 1.02 (95% CI 1.01, 1.03)) per year, i.e., OR is 1.22 in patients 10 years older). People with a higher educational level (secondary or university) showed a higher risk of using a dietary product with a potential interaction with one prescription medicine (OR = 2.0 (95%CI 1.18; 3.23) and OR = 1.6 (95% CI 1.01; 2.63), respectively).

8. Discussion

One in every two people who take one of the considered medications is at risk of a potential interaction. Specifically, older people and the population with a higher educational level represent a profile at risk of a potential interaction between medications and nutritional supplements. Older people are also more likely to use both drugs and supplements because of a higher potential to get sick [10]. This is an important issue from a public health perspective, as there are population groups, such as the older population, who are high consumers of these two kinds of health products. This study is one of the first to examine factors associated with specific medication-dietary supplement interactions [11,12].

Qato et al. already showed that more than two-thirds of older adults used prescription medication with OTC medication or dietary supplements [4]. This is in line with our results indicating that the older population has greater probability of suffering a potential interaction. According to Kantor et al. supplement use in the US showed a downward trend among young adults aged 20 to 39 years, stable use among middle-aged adults aged 40–64 years, and an increase among adults over 65 years of age; this last population has a greater probability of being under pharmacotherapeutic treatment due to their clinical status [2]. In this population, the intake of both products is essential. Polypharmacy is a well-known phenomenon that is mainly observed in older populations [13]. The appropriateness of these medications is questioned in some cases [14]; however, in other situations such as antihypertensive or diuretic medication, the need is beyond doubt as cardiovascular illnesses are among the most important causes of death and disability in the US [15]. A similar scenario is observed with dietary supplements, where the effect of the supplementation may reduce the risk of several chronic diseases [16,17].

People with a primary level of education showed lower likelihood of being at risk of a potential interaction. This group also has a lower likelihood of taking dietary supplements. An explanation for this might be that people with a higher educational level might be over-concerned due to a flood of health information about health, and they might be taking dietary supplements when they do not need them. However, this result may also indicate a higher concern regarding the health of people with a higher education; higher education mediates the impact on health outcomes through health literacy [18]. Furthermore, people with a higher education level, which are likely to have a higher socioeconomic status, may have more resources to access dietary products.

These results are especially important for healthcare professionals. Determining whether patients at risk of suffering a potential interaction are taking a dietary supplement that might interact with their prescribed medication is important. In the case of tetracyclines, the effect of the drug may be decreased and the patient may be uncovered for a potential infection; in the case of thiazides, patients may suffer metabolic alkalosis; and in the case of angiotensin II receptor blockers, cardiac function may be affected. This information should be considered at the time of prescription or dispensation. A secondary assessment could be made to analyze whether this supplement is really needed, and if so, to try to adapt it to the pharmacologic treatment. In addition, the assistance of a specialist, such as a nutritionist, is recommendable.

In this line, public policies designed to inform healthcare professionals how to detect potential interactions and tools to help them identify them are highly recommended. These tools could be incorporated in the respective electronic tools of prescription and dispensing, and they might not only remind healthcare professionals to ask about the use of those dietary supplements that may generate an interaction, but also offer alternatives to avoid the interaction in the event that the supplement is recommended. In addition, it is important to inform citizens that, before taking a supplement, it is desirable to consult their doctors to verify that the supplement is necessary and safe taking into account their prescription drugs.

This study has several strengths. It is among the first to evaluate medication use with specific dietary supplements in a representative sample of the American population, providing useful information for targeted public health planning. In the NHANES, medication and dietary supplement use were assessed through in-home interviews, and boxes were seen by the interviewers in most participants. This reduces the recall bias, which is especially notable in medication [1]. However, the present study also has several limitations. First, there is no certainty that the interactions detected occurred. Furthermore, some of these interactions were dose-dependent, and information on dose was not available. Second, information only showed self-reported recent consumption, so it was impossible to discern whether the consumption was concurrent. Finally, other important medication groups that might generate serious interactions, such as quinolones, were not assessed due to their limited representation in the sample. These limitations are not restricted to the present study, as the methodology and analysis strategy followed were similar to those of previous studies based on the NHANES database [4].

9. Conclusions

There are two main population groups at risk of potential interactions: older people and the population with a higher educational level. With respect to other races, non-Hispanic whites present a higher risk of potential interactions. These results add important information about ways of approaching patients when they receive a prescription or ask for a medication. Health policy should take this information into account so as to inform healthcare professionals, and electronic tools should be developed or adapted to help in the re-assessment of their pharmacotherapeutic planning.

Author Contributions: Conceptualization, I.A.-L. and M.R.-V.; methodology, I.A.-L. and M.R.-V.; formal analysis, I.A.-L., M.R.-V. and C.C.-D. investigation; investigation, C.C.-D., I.M. and A.R.; writing-original draft, I.A.-L. and C.C.-D.; writing—review and editing, I.M., A.R., supervision M.R.-V.

Acknowledgments: I.A.-L. and M.R.-V. have a research contract with the CIBERESP (CB16/02/00429) funded by the Instituto de Salud Carlos III, and CCD has a research contract with the Instituto de Salud Carlos III (PI15/00114). Both contracts are co-funded by the European regional development fund (ERDF). We are grateful to Stephen Kelly and Tom Yohannan for their contribution to editing the English of the article.

References

1.   Kantor, E.D.; Rehm, C.D.; Haas, J.S.; Chan, A.T.; Giovannucci, E.L. Trends in prescription drug use among adults in the United States from 1999–2012. *JAMA* **2015**, *314*, 1818–1830. [CrossRef] [PubMed]

2.   Kantor, E.D.; Rehm, C.D.; Du, M.; White, E.; Giovannucci, E.L. Trends in dietary supplement use among US adults from 1999–2012. *JAMA* **2016**, *316*, 1464–1474. [CrossRef] [PubMed]

3.   Bushra, R.; Aslam, N.; Khan, A.Y. Food-drug interactions. *Oman Med. J.* **2011**, *26*, 77–83. [CrossRef] [PubMed]

4.   Qato, D.M.; Wilder, J.; Schumm, L.P.; Gillet, V.; Alexander, G.C. Changes in prescription and over-the-counter medication and dietary supplement use among older adults in the United States, 2005 vs. 2011. *JAMA Intern. Med.* **2016**, *176*, 473–482. [CrossRef] [PubMed]

5.   Baxter, K. *Stockley Interacciones Farmacológicas (Stockley's Drug Interactions)*, 3rd ed.; Pharma, E., Ed.; Pharmaceutical Press: London, UK, 2009.

6.   Tyrovolas, S.; Koyanagi, A.; Kotsakis, G.A.; Panagiotakos, D.; Shivappa, N.; Wirth, M.D.; Hébert, J.R.; Haro, J.M. Dietary inflammatory potential is linked to cardiovascular disease risk burden in the US adult population. *Int. J. Cardiol.* **2017**, *240*, 409–413. [CrossRef] [PubMed]

7.   Malek, A.M.; Newman, J.C.; Hunt, K.J.; Marriott, B.P. Race/Ethnicity, Enrichment/Fortification, and Dietary Supplementation in the U.S. Population, NHANES 2009–2012. *Nutrients* **2019**, *11*, 1005. [CrossRef] [PubMed]

8.   Indermitte, J.; Burkolter, S.; Drewe, J.; Krähenbühl, S.; Hersberger, K.E. Risk factors associated with a high velocity of the development of hyperkalaemia in hospitalised patients. *Drug Saf.* **2007**, *30*, 71–80. [CrossRef] [PubMed]

9.   Norwegian Insitute of Public Health WHO Collaborating Centre for Drug Statistics Methodology. International Language for Drug Utilization Research. Available online: https://www.whocc.no/ (accessed on 27 August 2019).

10. Kuerbis, A.; Sacco, P.; Blazer, D.G.; Moore, A.A. Substance abuse among older adults. *Clin. Geriatr. Med.* **2014**, *30*, 629–654. [CrossRef] [PubMed]

11. Nahin, R.L.; Pecha, M.; Welmerink, D.B.; Sink, K.; Dekosky, S.T.; Fitzpatrick, A.L. Concomitant use of prescription drugs and dietary supplements in ambulatory elderly people: Clinical investigations. *J. Am. Geriatr. Soc.* **2009**, *57*, 1197–1205. [CrossRef] [PubMed]

12. Qato, D.M.; Alexander, G.C.; Conti, R.M.; Johnson, M.; Schumm, P.; Lindau, S.T. Use of prescription and over-the-counter medications and dietary supplements among older adults in the United States. *JAMA J. Am. Med. Assoc.* **2008**, *300*, 2867–2878.

13. Oktora, M.P.; Denig, P.; Bos, J.H.J.; Schuiling-Veninga, C.C.M.; Hak, E. Trends in polypharmacy and dispensed drugs among adults in the Netherlands as compared to the United States. *PLoS ONE* **2019**, *14*, e0214240. [CrossRef] [PubMed]

14. Vozoris, N.T. Benzodiazepine and opioid co-usage in the US population, 1999–2014: An exploratory analysis. *Sleep* **2019**, *42*, zsy264. [CrossRef] [PubMed]

15. Dwyer-Lindgren, L.; Bertozzi-Villa, A.; Stubbs, R.W.; Morozoff, C.; Kutz, M.J.; Huynh, C.; Barber, R.M.; Shackelford, K.A.; Mackenbach, J.P.; van Lenthe, F.J.; et al. US county-level trends in mortality rates for major causes of death, 1980–2014. *JAMA J. Am. Med. Assoc.* **2016**, *316*, 2385–2401. [CrossRef] [PubMed]

16. Parva, N.R.; Tadepalli, S.; Singh, P.; Qian, A.; Joshi, R.; Kandala, H.; Nookala, V.K.; Cheriyath, P. Prevalence of Vitamin D Deficiency and Associated Risk Factors in the US Population (2011–2012). *Cureus* **2018**, *10*, e2741. [CrossRef] [PubMed]

17. McKay, D.L.; Perrone, G.; Rasmussen, H.; Dallal, G.; Hartman, W.; Cao, G.; Prior, R.L.; Roubenoff, R.; Blumberg, J.B. The Effects of a Multivitamin/Mineral Supplement on Micronutrient Status, Antioxidant Capacity and Cytokine Production in Healthy Older Adults Consuming a Fortified Diet. *J. Am. Coll. Nutr.* **2000**, *19*, 613–621. [CrossRef] [PubMed]

18. Van Der Heide, I.; Wang, J.; Droomers, M.; Spreeuwenberg, P.; Rademakers, J.; Uiters, E. The relationship between health, education, and health literacy: Results from the dutch adult literacy and life skills survey. *J. Health Commun.* **2013**, *18*, 172–184. [CrossRef] [PubMed]

10

The Relationship of Balance Disorders with Falling, the Effect of Health Problems and Social Life on Postural Balance in the Elderly Living in a District in Turkey

Tahsin Barış Değer [1,*], Zeliha Fulden Saraç [2], Emine Sumru Savaş [2] and Selahattin Fehmi Akçiçek [2]

[1]   Directorate of Health Affairs, Söke Municipality, Söke, Aydın 09200, Turkey
[2]   Geriatrics Section, Faculty of Medicine, Ege University, Bornova, Izmir 35100, Turkey;
      fulden.sarac@ege.edu.tr (Z.F.S.); emine.sumru.savas@ege.edu.tr (E.S.S.); fehmi.akcicek@gmail.com (S.F.A.)
*   Correspondence: baris.deger@soke.bel.tr

Abstract: The aim of this study was to determine the prevalence of balance disorders; the effects of sociodemographic, medical, and social conditions on postural balance; and the relationship between balance and falls in elderly individuals. The study design was cross-sectional. A total of 607 community-dwelling elderly individuals with a mean age of 73.99 ± 6.6 years were enrolled after being selected by stratified random sampling. The study was performed as a face-to-face survey in the homes of elderly individuals. Sociodemographic and medical data were obtained from elderly individuals using the Elderly Identification Form. Balance disorders were determined using the Berg Balance Scale (BBS). In this study, the prevalence of balance disorders was found to be 34.3% in the community-dwelling elderly. Older age, physical disability, having four or more chronic illnesses, the presence of incontinence, having a history of falls, not walking regularly, absence of free time activity, and obesity were found to be associated with an increased prevalence of balance disorders. Balance disorders are commonly seen in the elderly and may be triggered by a variety of biological and social factors. It is crucial to develop and implement national health and social policies to eliminate the causes of this problem, as well as to prioritize preventive health services in the ever-increasing elderly population.

Keywords: balance disorder; prevalence; elderly; fall; medical conditions; social mobility

1. Introduction

Balance is the ability to collect sensory and proprioceptive signals related to a person's position in space and to produce the appropriate motor responses to control body movement [1]. When this ability deteriorates, due to both disease and the normal aging process, the risk of falling increases in the elderly [2]. Balance disorders are one of the most important reasons leading to falls [3]. Falling increases the possibility of death and disability; furthermore, it may cause the loss of independence [4]. In 2014, an estimated 29 million falls were reported in the US. Twenty-seven thousand older adults died, and 7 million were injured because of falls [5]. Approximately 68% of hospitalizations of injured elderly individuals were reported to be because of falls, and this rate reached 86% in individuals aged ≥85 years [6]. Falls in the elderly population cause long-term immobilization and related complications. Therefore, balance disorders in elderly individuals are a symptom that leads to functional insufficiency. As a result of dynamic postural control, appropriate rehabilitation following the early detection of balance disorders and environmental modifications could prevent falls and increase an individual's quality of life [7].

Balance disorders generate a significant healthcare burden due to the rise in hospitalization, morbidities, and mortalities in the elderly population [8]. Most of the patients who present to emergency services complain of balance disorders. In otology and neurology clinics, in which patients commonly present with balance disorders and dizziness, the rate of balance disorder is about 20% [9]. Thirteen percent of community-dwelling individuals aged 65–69 years and 46% of those aged ≥85 years have balance disorders [10]. There are many factors that lead to balance disorders, including cardiovascular diseases, metabolic diseases, musculoskeletal disorders, neurological disorders, visual and hearing disturbance, fear of falling, surgical operations, and specific medications [11].

Factors related to the risk of falling were taken into consideration in a report published by the World Health Organization (WHO) on the elderly in 2007. It was reported that balance disorders contribute to the occurrence of falls, and that balance exercises are a useful way to protect from falls. [12]. Goal number three of the Turkey Healthy Aging Implementation Program in the Healthy Aging Action Plan and Implementation Program published by the Ministry of Health for 2015–2020 includes a statement on the development of preventive and rehabilitative approaches to determine and decrease the risk factors leading to balance disorders, falling, and fear of falling in old age [13].

This study was conducted to determine the prevalence of balance disorders in the elderly population, identify the health (chronic illnesses, drug use) and social (leisure time activities) causes of balance disorders, and determine the role of balance disorders in falls.

2. Materials and Methods

2.1. Subjects

This was a cross-sectional study involving community-dwelling elderly individuals aged >65 years in a center in the Söke district of Aydın. A total of 607 elderly individuals with a mean age of 73.99 ± 6.6 (65–102) years were selected by the stratified random sampling method. The 65–74-year age group was stratified as the first group, the 75–84-year age group was the second group, and the ≥85-year age group was the third group. The study was performed as face-to-face surveys at the homes of elderly individuals. A total of 668 elderly individuals were asked to participate in the study, but those individuals who were bedridden, who were diagnosed with dementia, and who did not pass the Mini Mental State Examination (MMSE; cut-off score of 23) were not included in the study [14]. Eventually, 607 elderly individuals who agreed to voluntarily participate in the study formed the sample used for our study. Informed consent was given by all participants.

2.2. Evaluation Parameters

Elderly Identification Form: This form recorded information about the participants, including their age, gender, marital status, number of people in their household, economic level, education level, presence of illnesses, disability status, fall history, fear of falling, drugs used, presence of incontinence, nocturia, walking habits, leisure time activities, and body mass index. This form was created by the investigators.

Berg Balance Scale (BBS): This test, which was developed to measure balance performance in elderly individuals, consists of 14 instructions. Participants are given 0–4 points for each instruction according to their ability to perform the task; the maximum total score for the test is 56. It is a practical test that can be conducted in 15–20 min in the homes of the community-dwelling elderly individuals. The cut-off score for the test is 45. A score of 45–56 is an indication of an acceptable functional level. A score below 45 point is considered to indicate a balance disorder [15–17]. The Turkish translation and the transcultural adaptation of the BBS were previously studied in 60 elderly individuals with various comorbidities aged >65 years, and the validity and reliability have been reported [18].

2.3. Methods

The study started with the selection of Address-Based Population Registration System data with a stratified random sampling method for individuals over 65 years of age. The elders who were selected by this method represented elderly people living in the district center. Thus, the sample used was representative of the group of universe of elderly people in the district center. Four different teams were formed in the study, and these teams visited the elderly in their homes. The MMSE was applied to elderly people who participated voluntarily, who were not bedridden, and who had not been diagnosed with dementia. The Elderly Identification Form was given to participants to determine their socio-demographic and health characteristics, as well as to gather information about their free life activities. Sociodemographic, social, and health data were recorded on the form. Participants' health reports were reviewed. The drugs they used were noted. The participants completed the BBS assessment, and their BBS scores were noted. The weights and heights of the participants were measured, and BMI values were calculated.

The present study was submitted to and approved by the Clinical Research Ethics Committee of the Ege University Faculty of Medicine (Decision Number: 16–3.2/7, Date: April 7, 2016). The study was conducted in accordance with the Declaration of Helsinki. All participants provided informed consent before being included in the study as a participant.

2.4. Statistics

Analysis of the data was done using SPSS (Version 18.0, SPSS Inc., Chicago, IL, USA). Chi-square tests were used to analyze balance disorders and fall variables. Univariate binary logistic regression analysis and multiple binary logistic regression analyses were conducted on all variables. For the results of the statistical analysis, p-values of <0.05 were considered significant.

3. Results

3.1. The Prevalence of Balance Disorders (Mean Value of BBS)

The BBS was used to measure the prevalence of balance disorders in the participants. In elderly individuals, the cut-off (sorter) value for balance disorders is 45 points [19,20]. The prevalence of a balance disorder in the elderly individuals in our study was 34.3%. The average BBS score was 43.49 ± 14.2.

3.2. The Relationship between Balance and Falls

For individuals with a balance disorder, 58.1% had fallen in the past year, and 90.3% had a fear of falling; in those without a balance disorder, 29.8% had fallen, and 60.3% had a fear of falling (Table 1).

Table 1. The relationship between balance and falling.

	Fell Last Year			**Fear of Falling**		
	Yes (n = 237)	No (n = 370)	Chi-square (p-value)	Yes (n = 427)	No (n = 178)	Chi-square (p-value)
Balance disorder (n = 208)	121 (58.1%)	87 (41.8%)	$X^2 = (p < 0.001)$	187 (90.3%)	20 (9.7%)	$X^2 = (p < 0.001)$
No balance disorder (n = 389)	116 (29.8%)	283 (72.7%)		240 (60.3%)	158 (39.7%)	

Chi-square test, $p < 0.05$: statistically significant.

3.3. Multiple Logistic Regression Analysis and the Effects of Sociodemographic, Medical, and Social Data on Balance Disorders

The sample of 607 participants was composed of 347 people aged 65–74 (first group), 214 aged 75–84 (second group), and 46 aged over 85 years old (third group). The association of age with balance disorders was statistically significant according to the multiple logistic regression analysis ($p = 0.002$).

The prevalence of balance disorders increased as age increased. Balance disorders were 1.97 times higher in the second group ($p = 0.006$, OR = 1.97, 95% CI = 1.21–3.20) and 3.63 times higher in the third group ($p = 0.003$, OR = 3.63, 95% CI = 1.54–8.55), compared with the first group.

Three hundred and sixty-one of the 607 participants (59.47%) were females.

Participants included non-literate individuals, primary school quitters, primary school graduates (n = 276), secondary school graduates, high school graduates, and university graduates.

Participants included widows (divorced or had lost their husband/wife) and married individuals.

Participants included those living alone, with their spouses, with their spouses and children, only with their children, and with relatives/carers.

Considering economic situations, there were people without incomes, those receiving the elderly/widow/disabled wage, those receiving the retirement wage, and those using wages earned by their spouse.

The variables gender, education level, marital status, living status, and economic situation were not found to be statistically significant in our study, according to the multiple logistic regression analysis.

Our study included elderly participants without any obstacles, elderly participants with a visual impairment, elderly participants with a hearing impairment, and elderly participants with disabilities. When the relationship between the disability status of elderly people and balance disorders was examined, with the group without obstacles taken as the reference group, participants with walking disabilities had a balance disorder 2.80 times higher than the reference group ($p = 0.013$, OR = 2.80, 95% CI = 1.24–6.33). The disability variable was found to be statistically significant (Table 2).

Two hundred and thirty-seven participants had fallen at least once in the past year. Fall history was statistically associated with the presence of a balance disorder in our study, according to the multiple logistic regression analysis. The prevalence of balance disorders among those who had fallen in the past year was 2.25 times higher than in those who had not fallen ($p < 0.001$, OR = 2.25, 95% CI = 1.46–3.46).

The prevalence of chronic disease was determined. Only 10.7% (n = 65) of the participants did not have any chronic illnesses. The number of chronic diseases was not statistically significantly associated with the prevalence of balance disorders in our study, according to multiple logistic regression analysis, but a significant association was shown in elderly people with four or more diseases ($p = 0.047$, OR = 3.54, 95% CI = 1.01–12.32).

Daily medication use was recorded for each participant. Hundreds of medications were classified according to their indications to determine which drugs can alter balance. For example, a participant using three medications (amlodipine [a selective calcium channel blocker], silazapril and hydrochlorothiazide [an angiotensin-converting enzyme inhibitor combination], and acetylsalicylic acid [an antithrombotic agent]) was categorized into a group of participants "using only one group of medications" (cardiovascular drug group). Medications were determined by group number instead of individual drugs. Our study included participants using neurological disease drugs, cardiovascular group drugs, diabetes medications, vertigo medications, thyroid medications, rheumatic disease drugs, pain killers, and depression group drugs. 12.8% of the participants (n = 78) did not use any medication (Table 2). The drug group use variable was not shown to be significantly associated with balance disorders in our study.

One hundred and seventy-seven of the participants stated that they could not hold urine during the day. In addition, 87 of the participants stated that they could not hold urine sometimes. Urinary incontinence was found to be statistically significantly associated with balance disorders ($p = 0.002$). Compared with the participants who had no difficulty with urinary incontinence, balance disorders were 2.4 times more prevalent in the participants who had urinary incontinence ($p = 0.001$, OR = 2.4, 95%CI = 1.46–3.95).

Table 2. Univariate logistic regression analysis and multiple logistic regression analysis.

Variant	Reference Group (n)	Other Groups (n)	Univariate Logistic Regression			** Multiple Logistic Regression		
			P	OR	95% C.I.	P	OR	95% C.I.
Age						0.002 *		
	6574 years (n = 347)	7584 (n = 214)	<0.001	2.34	1.623.36	0.006 *	1.97	1.213.20
		≥85 (n = 46)	<0.001	4.24	2.258.01	0.003 *	3.63	1.548.55
Gender	male (n = 246)	female (n = 361)	<0.001	2.30	1.603.30	0.211	0.65	0.34–1.26
Education						0.162		
	university-high (n = 54)	non-literate (n = 160)	<0.001	8.20	3.3220.24	0.071	2.72	0.918.08
		quit prim. s. (n = 90)	0.001	5.09	1.9713.14	0.082	2.69	0.888.20
		primary s. (n = 276)	0.011	3.15	1.297.66	0.259	1.80	0.645.00
		secondary s. (n = 27)	0.044	3.36	1.0311.01	0.061	3.85	0.9315.84
Marital status	married (n = 407)	widow (n = 200)	<0.001	2.95	2.074.21	0.494	1.65	0.397.04
Living						0.946		
	with spouse (n = 291)	living alone (n = 115)	<0.001	3.20	2.035.03	0.466	1.76	0.388.06
		spouse-child (n = 113)	0.359	1.25	0.772.03	0.584	1.18	0.642.15
		children (n = 75)	<0.001	3.29	1.945.57	0.582	1.52	0.336.92
		relative/carer (n = 13)	0.273	1.90	0.605.99	0.665	1.48	0.248.93
Economic						0.123		
	retired (n = 298)	no income (n = 140)	0.003	1.91	1.242.94	0.105	1.82	0.883.78
		aged wage (n = 53)	<0.001	3.51	1.926.41	0.544	1.29	0.562.95
		wage spouse(n = 116)	<0.001	2.83	1.804.44	0.397	0.72	0.351.51
Disability						0.027 *		
	no (n = 463)	blind (n = 42)	0.005	2.48	1.314.69	0.082	2.03	0.914.51
		hearing imp. (n = 57)	0.126	1.56	0.882.75	0.776	0.89	0.421.90
		walking imp. (n = 45)	<0.001	6.10	3.1011.99	0.013 *	2.80	1.246.33
Fall history	no (n = 370)	yes (n = 237)	<0.001	3.39	2.394.81	<0.001 *	2.25	1.463.46
Number CD						0.205		
	no (n = 65)	1 (n = 117)	0.326	1.52	0.653.52	0.390	1.70	0.505.74
		2 (n = 160)	0.004	3.17	1.456.89	0.152	2.43	0.728.24
		3 (n = 109)	0.001	3.90	1.748.70	0.090	2.98	0.8410.55
		≥4 (n = 156)	<0.001	6.55	3.0314.15	0.047 *	3.54	1.0112.32
Number MG						0.831		
	no (n = 78)	1 (n = 160)	0.265	1.47	0.742.91	0.450	0.65	0.221.95
		2 (n = 164)	0.011	2.37	1.224.59	0.524	0.70	0.232.09
		≥3 (n = 205)	<0.001	4.27	2.258.09	0.697	0.80	0.262.44
Incontinence						0.002 *		
	no (n = 343)	yes (n = 177)	<0.001	5.30	3.567.89	0.001 *	2.40	1.463.95
		sometimes (n = 87)	<0.001	2.75	1.664.54	0.057	1.81	0.983.35
Nocturia	no (n = 280)	yes (n = 327)	<0.001	2.83	1.984.05	0.577	1.14	0.711.81
Walking	yes (n = 384)	no (n = 223)	<0.001	4.18	2.935.97	0.001 *	2.21	1.413.48
LTA						0.079		
	3+ (n = 77)	no (n = 60)	<0.001	9.88	4.1723.40	0.024 *	3.40	1.179.88
		1+2 (n = 470)	<0.001	4.08	1.988.40	0.097	2.04	0.874.77
BMI						0.093		
	<25 (n = 114)	2529.9 (n = 217)	0.340	1.29	0.762.19	0.206	1.54	0.783.03
		3034.9 (n = 170)	0.002	2.36	1.394.04	0.044 *	2.09	1.024.28
		≥35 (n = 106)	<0.001	3.25	1.825.82	0.019 *	2.53	1.165.50

* Statistically significant ($p < 0.05$), OR: Odds ratio, C.I.: Confidence interval, CD: Chronic disease, MG: Medication group, LTA: Leisure time activities, BMI: Body Mass Index, prim. s.: Primary school, s.: School, imp.: Impairment, ** Multiple logistic regression analysis with enter method.

The study included elderly participants who did not urinate while sleeping at night and those who got up and went to urinate two or more times at night. Nocturia was not statistically significantly associated with balance disorders.

A total of 63.2% of the participants (n = 384) stated that they went out of the house and walked to go to the market, street market, mosque, coffee shop, or park. A lack of walking was statistically significantly associated with balance disorders. Balance disorders were 2.21 times more prevalent in the participants who did not walk than in those who walked to the market or those who took walks in the park ($p = 0.001$, OR = 2.21, 95% CI = 1.41–3.48).

Participants were asked about hobbies and interests to learn about leisure time activities. Participants reported eight types of hobby activities. These activities included reading activities; artistic activities, such as painting, music, and poetry; sports activities, such as swimming, fishing, and hunting; gardening and field work; making handcrafts; using the computer, foundation memberships; and mental games like chess and puzzles. Participation in leisure time activities was not statistically significantly associated with balance disorders, but, compared with the elderly who participated in three or more leisure time activities, the prevalence of balance disorders in participants who did not participate in activities was 3.4 times higher ($p = 0.024$, OR = 3.4, 95% CI = 1.17–9.88).

The BMI values of participants were measured. Individuals were classified as normal weight (<25), overweight (25–29.9), obese (30–34.9), or overly obese (≥35). BMI was not statistically significantly associated with balance disorders, but, compared with the participants with BMI < 25, balance disorders were approximately two times more common in obese ($p = 0.044$, OR = 2.09, 95% CI = 1.02–4.28) and overly obese participants ($p = 0.019$, OR = 2.53, 95% CI = 1.16–5.50).

4. Discussion

In this study, the prevalence of balance disorders was found to be 34.3% in the community-dwelling elderly. Older age, physical disability, the presence of incontinence, having a history of falls, having four or more chronic illnesses, not walking regularly, absence of free time activity, and obesity were found to be associated with an increased prevalence of balance disorders.

International studies have investigated balance disorders in elderly individuals living in the community. In a study conducted in the UK in 2008, the prevalence of balance disorders was found to be 21.5% among elderly individuals living in the community [21]. In a study conducted in the United States that was published in 2012 including participants aged ≥65 years with an average age of 74.4 years, the prevalence of balance disorders was approximately 20% [22]. In a study conducted in Scotland published in 1994, the prevalence of balance disorders was found to be 30% [23]. In another BBS-based study published in the US in 2006 including 101 community-dwelling volunteers aged >65 years, the prevalence of balance disorders was found to be 32% [24]. In our study, we found the prevalence of balance disorders to be 34.3%, which is in good agreement with the literature.

Şahin and colleagues performed a Turkish validity and reliability study of the BBS in 2008 including 60 healthy individuals aged >65 years. The average BBS score in that study was 47.63 ± 9.88 [18]. In a study conducted by Soyuer et al. using the BBS, the average BBS score was 45.42 ± 12.11 in nursing home residents [25]. In another study, the average BBS score was 41.3 ± 9 [26]. We found an average score of 43.49 ± 14.23 in our study.

In a study about the effect of age on balance disorders, a decrease in BBS scores with age was reported [27]. In another study, increased age was associated with decreasing BBS scores [28]. In our study, we also found that balance disorders were significantly more common in those aged 75–84 years and in those aged >85 years than in those aged 65–74 years.

In a study published in 2012, in which the effect of gender on the prevalence of balance disorders was examined, the prevalence of balance disorders was reported to be higher in females than in males [22]. In another study published in 2013, BBS scores were lower for female participants [27]. However, gender was not found to be a meaningful variable in our study.

Regarding the relationship between visual disturbance, balance, and falls, visual disturbance was found to be associated with the prevalence of falling [29]. In another study, elderly patients with visual disorders were found to have lower balance scores than a control group [30]. In another study, peripheral visual loss was reported to have a negative effect on balance control [31]. In our study, although overall disability status was significantly associated with balance disorders, visual disability had no effect on balance. At the same time, walking impairment was associated with balance.

In a study published in 2012, one-third of participants with balance disorders participated in no exercise-related activities or social activities [22]. In our study, participants who did not walk and who did not participate in any free time activities had a high likelihood of having a balance disorder. Our data match those reported by others. In a study published in 2019, the effect of exercise on falls was reported. Sherrington et al. found that participation in exercise mainly involving balance and functional exercises, plus resistance exercise, was associated with a reduction in falls. However, Sherrington et al. did not find enough evidence to determine the effect of walking programs on falls [32]. In contrast, in our study, we found a lower prevalence of balance disorders in those who walked regularly than in those who did not walk.

We think that the causes of balance disorders in elderly people with a walking disability and those who do not walk regularly may be sarcopenia and demineralization. It is known that the most important muscle for balance is the quadriceps femoris. We think that the loss of this muscle has a negative effect on balance in elderly people who do not walk regularly. In addition, loss of minerals from bone and decreased signal frequency from the proprioceptive receptors may have negative effects. As a result, we advise elderly people to walk regularly.

When we look at the relationship between postural balance and falls, posturographic vestibular rehabilitation has been reported to improve balance in elderly individuals and to reduce the number of falls [33]. Impaired balance has been reported as one of the long term risk factors for falls in men [34]. In another study, participants were classified into the non-fall group, one-time fall group, and repeated fall group. Both the dynamic balance and static balance scores were found to be higher in the non-fall group than in the one-time fall group and repeated fall group [35]. In our study, the prevalence of balance disorders was found to be significantly higher in people with a fall history.

In a study that was conducted to show the relationship between balance disorders and a fear of falling, the presence of balance, gait, and cognitive disorders was reported to be significantly higher in elderly individuals with a fear of falling [36]. In another study that used the Berg Balance Scale, lower BBS scores were found in the group with a fear of falling compared to those in the group without a fear of falling [27]. In our study, the presence of balance disorders was found to be significantly higher in those who had a fear of falling than in those who did not have a fear of falling ($p < 0.001$) (Table 1)

In a study on obesity in the elderly, an increased Body Mass Index (BMI) was associated with decreases in both dynamic stability and balance in the elderly [37]. In a study published in 2018, older participants were classified into obese, normal weight, and weak groups according to Body Mass Index scores. The one-leg standing time test was applied to determine balance scores. In the obese group, the one-leg standing time was much shorter than in the normal weight group of community-dwelling elderly women [38]. In our study, the prevalence of balance disorders was found to be higher in obese (BMI = 30–34.9) and overly obese (BMI ≥ 35) elderly individuals ($p = 0.044$ and $p = 0.019$, respectively) than in individuals of normal weight.

Balance disorders, incontinence, fall history, and age have been associated with each other in many studies published in this area [39,40]. These variables were found to be significant in the multiple logistic regression analysis in our study, too.

Our study had both limitations and significant contributions. In terms of limitations, some of the survey data were determined from the statements of elderly individuals—fall history, for example. In addition, the participants in our study consisted of elderly people living in a district center, and different socio-demographic data could be obtained from elderly people living in other parts of the country. In terms of contributions, to our knowledge, no previous study in this area has been conducted in Turkey using the stratified random sampling method to interview a large sample of community-dwelling elderly individuals face-to-face at their homes. We were able to get the right data because we applied the BBS test. In addition to academic data, our study also guided a local government social project. Walking support materials (walking stick, walker, wheelchair) were given to the elderly who were identified as having a balance disorder. Our work has created awareness in the community (see Appendix A).

Our research data may be used as reference for other academic studies in this area. The identification of the relationship between equilibrium and falling in the elderly and the emergence of many health and social causes of balance disorders are very valuable. More work is needed to determine the mechanisms behind each of these reasons. Awareness of these causes is needed for both individual and social preventive health practices. Following the collection of these data, people have learned that they need to change their lifestyles to protect their health. The local government has launched projects to support elderly people after obtaining these data. It has opened courses where seniors can spend their leisure time, with picture, music, craft, and folklore courses. Using the sociodemographic data of the elderly collected in this study, a journal called "Old Age Atlas of Söke" was published in the district. Söke Municipality published this journal to district people. This journal increased the awareness of people in the district about old age and old age problems. The social contributions of the study were appreciated by people in the district in addition to the academic contributions.

Balance disorders, which are considered to have several biological and social etiologies, are a major geriatric problem which lead leading to falling and increased morbidity and mortality rates. The development of national health and social policies that address the underlying causes of this problem and the introduction of preventive health care services should be the primary steps towards helping today's increasingly elderly population. The concept of "age-friendly" should be widespread in all segments of the society, including the private sector and public services.

Author Contributions: Conceptualization, T.B.D., S.F.A., and E.S.S.; methodology, T.B.D. and S.F.A.; validation, T.B.D.; investigation, T.B.D.; writing—original draft preparation, T.B.D.; writing—review and editing, T.B.D., Z.F.S., and E.S.S.; supervision, T.B.D. and Z.F.S.; project administration, Z.F.S. and S.F.A.; funding acquisition, Z.F.S. and E.S.S.

Acknowledgments: This manuscript was prepared as part of the PhD thesis of the corresponding author. It was also partially summarized at the International Academic Geriatrics Congress 2017 as an oral presentation. We would like to thank Timur KÖSE and retired Oktay TEKEŞİN for their support with this study.

Appendix A.

In addition to the academic content of our study, a social aspect was also included. Walking support materials (walking stick, walker, wheelchair) were given to the elderly people who were identified as having a balance disorder. These support materials were gifted to the elderly by Söke Municipality to allow them to participate in a social life and to protect them from falls. The data from our study allowed us to implement a project called "age-friendly municipality."

References

1. Sturnieks, D.L.; St George, R.; Lord, S.R. Balance disorders in the elderly. *Neurophysiol. Clin.* **2008**, *38*, 467–478. [CrossRef] [PubMed]
2. Nnodim, J.O.; Yung, R.L. Balance and its clinical assessment in older adults—A review. *J. Geriatr. Med. Gerontol.* **2015**, *1*, 003. [CrossRef]
3. Perera, T.; Tan, J.L.; Cole, M.H.; Yohanandan, S.A.C.; Silberstein, P.; Cook, R.; Peppard, R.; Aziz, T.; Coyne, T.; Brown, P.; et al. Balance control systems in Parkinson's disease and the impact of pedunculopontine area stimulation. *Brain* **2018**, *141*, 3009–3022. [CrossRef]
4. Cameron, I.D.; Dyer, S.M.; Panagoda, C.E.; Murray, G.R.; Hill, K.D.; Cumming, R.G.; Kerse, N. Interventions for preventing falls in older people in care facilities and hospitals. *Cochrane Database Syst. Rev.* **2018**, *9*. [CrossRef]
5. Bergen, G.; Stevens, M.R.; Burns, E.R. Falls and fall injuries among adults aged ≥65 years—United States, 2014. *MMWR Morb. Mortal. Wkly. Rep.* **2016**, *65*, 993–998. [CrossRef]
6. Covington, D.L.; Maxwell, J.G.; Clancy, T.V. Hospital resources used to treat the injured elderly at North Carolina trauma centers. *J. Am. Geriatr. Soc.* **1993**, *41*, 847–852. [CrossRef]
7. Onat, Ş.Ş.; Delialioğlu, S.Ü.; Özel, S. The relationship of balance between functional status and quality of life in the geriatric population. *Turk. J. Phys. Med. Rehabil.* **2014**, *60*, 147–154. [CrossRef]
8. Nguyen, T.Q.; Young, J.H.; Rodriguez, A.; Zupancic, S.; Lie, D.Y.C. Differentiation of patients with balance insufficiency (vestibular hypofunction) versus normal subjects using a low-cost small wireless wearable gait sensor. *Biosensors* **2019**, *9*, 29. [CrossRef] [PubMed]

9.   Von Brevern, M.; Radtke, A.; Lezius, F.; Feldmann, M.; Ziese, T.; Lempert, T.; Neuhauser, H. Epidemiology of benign paroxysmal positional vertigo: A population based study. *J. Neurol Neurosurg. Psychiatr.* **2007**, *78*, 710–715. [CrossRef] [PubMed]

10. Felsenthal, G.; Ference, T.S.; Young, M.A. Aging of organ systems. In *Downey and Darling's Physiological Basis of Rehabilitation Medicine*, 3th ed.; Gonzales, E.G., Myers, S.A., Edelstein, J.E., Lieberman, J.S., Downey, J.A., Eds.; Butterwoth Heinemann: Boston, MA, USA, 2001; pp. 561–577.

11. Salzman, B. Gait and balance disorders in older adults. *Am. Fam. Physician* **2010**, *82*, 61–68.

12. World Health Organization. WHO global report on falls prevention in older age. 2007, pp. 15–18. Available online: https://www.who.int/ageing/publications/Falls_prevention7March.pdf (accessed on 23 February 2019).

13. Turkey Healthy Aging Action Plan and Implementation Programme 2015–2020, Ankara. 2015; p. 33. Available online: https://sbu.saglik.gov.tr/Ekutuphane/kitaplar/Sağl\T1\ikl\T1\i%20Yaş.%202015--2020%20Pdf.pdf (accessed on 24 February 2019). (In Turkish)

14. Güngen, C.; Ertan, T.; Eker, E.; Yaşar, R.; Engin, F. Reliability and Validity of The Standardized Mini Mental State Examination in The Diagnosis of Mild Dementia in Turkish Population. *Turk. J. Psychiatry* **2002**, *13*, 273–281.

15. Berg, K.O.; Maki, B.E.; Williams, J.I.; Holliday, P.J.; Wood-Dauphinee, S.L. Clinical and laboratory measures of postural balance in an elderly population. *Arch. Phys. Med. Rehabil.* **1992**, *73*, 1073–1080.

16. Berg, K.; Wood-Dauphinee, S.; Williams, J.I.; Maki, B. Measuring balance in the elderly: Validation of an instrument. *Can. J. Pub. Health* **1992**, *2*, 7–11.

17. Berg, K.; Wood-Dauphinee, S.; Williams, J.I. The Balance Scale: Reliability assessment with elderly residents and patients with an acute stroke. *Scand. J. Rehabil. Med.* **1995**, *27*, 27–36. [PubMed]

18. Sahin, F.; Yilmaz, F.; Ozmaden, A.; Kotevolu, N.; Sahin, T.; Kuran, B. Reliability and validity of the Turkish version of the Berg Balance Scale. *J. Geriatr. Phys. Ther.* **2008**, *31*, 32–37. [CrossRef]

19. Kornetti, D.L.; Fritz, S.L.; Chiu, Y.P.; Light, K.E.; Velozo, C.A. Rating scale analysis of the Berg Balance Scale. *Arch. Phys. Med. Rehabil.* **2004**, *85*, 1128–1135. [CrossRef] [PubMed]

20. Dogan, A.; Mengulluoglu, M.; Ozgırgın, N. Evaluation of the effect of ankle-foot orthosis use on balance and mobility in hemiparetic stroke patients. *Disabil. Rehabil.* **2011**, *33*, 1433–1439. [CrossRef]

21. Stevens, K.N.; Lang, I.A.; Guralnik, J.M.; Melzer, D. Epidemiology of balance and dizziness in a national population: Findings from the English Longitudinal Study of Ageing. *Age Ageing* **2008**, *37*, 300–305. [CrossRef]

22. Lin, H.W.; Bhattacharyya, N. Balance Disorders in the elderly: Epidemiology and functional impact. *Laryngoscope* **2012**, *122*, 1858–1861. [CrossRef]

23. Colledge, N.R.; Wilson, J.A.; Macintyre, C.C.; Mac Lennan, W.J. The prevalence and characteristics of dizziness in an elderly community. *Age Ageing* **1994**, *23*, 117–120. [CrossRef]

24. Hawk, C.; Hyland, J.K.; Rupert, R.; Colonvega, M.; Hall, S. Assessment of balance and risk for falls in a sample of community-dwelling adults aged 65 and older. *Chiropr. Osteopat.* **2006**, *14*, 3. [CrossRef]

25. Soyuer, F.; Şenol, V.; Elmalı, F. Physical activity, balance and mobility functions of individuals over 65 years of age in the nursing homes. *Van Med. J.* **2012**, *19*, 116–121. (In Turkish). Available online: https://www.journalagent.com/vtd/pdfs/VTD_19_3_116_121.pdf. (accessed on 5 February 2019).

26. Holbein-Jenny, M.A.; Billek-Sawhney, B.; Beckman, E.; Smith, T. Balance in personal care home residents: A comparison of the Berg Balance Scale, the Multi-Directional Reach Test, and the Activities-Specific Balance Confidence Scale. *J. Geriatr. Phys. Ther.* **2005**, *28*, 48–53. [CrossRef]

27. Ulus, Y.; Akyol, Y.; Tander, B.; Durmuş, D.; Bilgici, A.; Kuru, Ö. The relationship between fear of falling and balance in community-dwelling older people. *Turk. J. Geriatr.* **2013**, *16*, 260–265. Available online: http://geriatri.dergisi.org/uploads/pdf/pdf_TJG_745.pdf. (accessed on 11 February 2019).

28. Steffen, T.M.; Hacker, T.A.; Mollinger, L. Age and gender related test performance in community-dwelling elderly people: Six-minute walk test, Berg Balance Scale, timed up-go test and gait speeds. *Physical. Ther.* **2002**, *82*, 128–137. [CrossRef]

29. Guimarâes, J.M.N.; Farinatti, P.T.V. Descriptive analysis of variables theoretically associated to the risk of falls in elder women. *Rev. Bras. Med. Esport.* **2005**, *11*, 280–286. Available online: http://www.scielo.br/pdf/rbme/v11n5/en_27593.pdf. (accessed on 11 February 2019).

30. Popescu, M.L.; Boisjoly, H.; Schmaltz, H.; Kergoat, M.J.; Rousseau, J.; Moghadaszadeh, S.; Djafari, F.; Freeman, E.E. Age-related eye disease and mobility limitations in older adults. *Invest. Ophthalmol. Vis. Sci.* **2011**, *9*, 7168–7174. [CrossRef]

31. Kotecha, A.; Chopra, R.; Fahy, R.T.; Rubin, G.S. Dual tasking and balance in those with central and peripheral vision loss. *Invest. Ophthalmol Vis. Sci.* **2013**, *54*, 5408–5415. [CrossRef] [PubMed]

32. Sherrington, C.; Fairhall, N.J.; Wallbank, G.K.; Tiedemann, A.; Michaleff, Z.A.; Howard, K.; Clemson, L.; Hopewell, S.; Lamb, S.E. Exercise for preventing falls in older people living in the community. *Cochrane Database Syst. Rev.* **2019**, *31*. [CrossRef]

33. Soto-Varela, A.; Gayoso-Diz, P.; Faraldo-García, A.; Rossi-Izquierdo, M.; Vaamonde-Sánchez-Andrade, I.; Del-Río-Valeiras, M.; Lirola-Delgado, A.; Santos-Pérez, S. Optimising costs in reducing rate of falls in older people with the improvement of balance by means of vestibular rehabilitation (ReFOVeRe study): A randomized controlled trial comparing computerised dynamic posturography vs. mobile vibrotactile posturography system. *BMC Geriatr.* **2019**, *19*, 1. [CrossRef]

34. Ek, S.; Rizzuto, D.; Fratiglioni, L.; Calderón-Larrañaga, A.; Johnell, K.; Sjöberg, L.; Xu, W.; Welmer, A.K. Risk factors for injurious falls in older adults: The role of sex and length of follow-up. *J. Am. Geriatr Soc.* **2019**, *67*, 246–253. [CrossRef]

35. Jeon, M.; Gu, M.O.; Yim, J. Comparison of Walking, Muscle Strength, Balance, and Fear of Falling Between Repeated Fall Group, One-time Fall Group, and Nonfall Group of the ElderlyReceiving Home Care Service. *Asian Nurs. Res. (Korean Soc. Nurs. Sci).* **2017**, *11*, 290–296. [CrossRef]

36. Vellas, B.J.; Wayne, S.J.; Romero, L.J.; Baumgartner, R.N.; Garry, P.J. Fear of falling and restriction of mobility in elderly fallers. *Age Ageing* **1997**, *26*, 189–193. [CrossRef]

37. Gao, X.; Wang, L.; Shen, F.; Ma, Y.; Fan, Y.; Niu, H. Dynamic walking stability of elderly people with various BMIs. *Gait Posture* **2019**, *68*, 168–173. [CrossRef]

38. Nonaka, K.; Murata, S.; Shiraiwa, K.; Abiko, T.; Nakano, H.; Iwase, H.; Naito, K.; Horie, J. Physical characteristics vary according to body mass index in Japanese community-dwelling elderly women. *Geriatrics* **2018**, *3*, 87. [CrossRef]

39. Tkacheva, O.N.; Runikhina, N.K.; Ostapenko, V.S.; Sharashkina, N.V.; Mkhitaryan, E.A.; Onuchina, J.S.; Lysenkov, S.N.; Yakhno, N.N.; Press, Y. Prevalence of geriatric syndromes among people aged 65 years and older at four community clinics in Moscow. *Clin. Interv. Aging.* **2018**, *13*, 251–259. [CrossRef]

40. Almeida Abreu, H.C.; Oliveira Reiners, A.A.; Souza Azevedo, R.C.; Silva, A.M.C.; Oliveira Moura Abreu, D.R.; Oliveira, A.D. Incidence and predicting factors of falls of older inpatients. *Rev. Saude Publica* **2015**, *49*. [CrossRef]

11

The Effect of an Infant Formula Supplemented with AA and DHA on Fatty Acid Levels of Infants with Different FADS Genotypes: The COGNIS Study

Isabel Salas Lorenzo [1,2], Aida M. Chisaguano Tonato [3], Andrea de la Garza Puentes [1,2,4,*], Ana Nieto [5,6], Florian Herrmann [5,6], Estefanía Dieguez [5,6], Ana I. Castellote [1,2,7], M. Carmen López-Sabater [1,2,7,*], Maria Rodríguez-Palmero [8] and Cristina Campoy [5,6,9]

[1] Department of Nutrition, Food Sciences and Gastronomy, Faculty of Pharmacy and Food Sciences, University of Barcelona, Av. Joan XXIII 27-31, E-08028 Barcelona, Spain; salas.lorenzo.i@gmail.com (I.S.L.); aicastellote@ub.edu (A.I.C.)

[2] Institut de Recerca en Nutrició i Seguretat Alimentària de la UB (INSA-UB), 08921 Barcelona, Spain

[3] Nutrition, Faculty of Health Sciences, University of San Francisco de Quito, Quito 170157, Ecuador; achisaguano@usfq.edu.ec

[4] Parc Sanitari Sant Joan de Déu, Fundació Sant Joan de Déu, Institut de Recerca Sant Joan de Déu, 08830 Sant Boi de Llobregat, Spain

[5] Centre of Excellence for Paediatric Research EURISTIKOS, University of Granada, 18071 Granada, Spain; ananietoruiz@gmail.com (A.N.); herrmann@florian-herrmann.de (F.H.); estefaniadieguez@ugr.es (E.D.); ccampoy@ugr.es (C.C.)

[6] Department of Paediatrics, University of Granada, 18071 Granada, Spain

[7] CIBER Physiopathology of Obesity and Nutrition CIBERobn, Institute of Health Carlos III, 28029 Madrid, Spain

[8] Basic Research Department. Ordesa Laboratories, 08830 Barcelona, Spain; Maria.Rodriguez@ordesa.es

[9] CIBER Epidemiology and Public Health CIBEResp, Institute of Health Carlos III, 28029 Madrid, Spain

[*] Correspondence: adelagarza@ub.edu (A.d.l.G.P.); mclopez@ub.edu (M.C.L.-S.)

Abstract: Polymorphisms in the fatty acid desaturase (FADS) genes influence the arachidonic (AA) and docosahexaenoic (DHA) acid concentrations (crucial in early life). Infants with specific genotypes may require different amounts of these fatty acids (FAs) to maintain an adequate status. The aim of this study was to determine the effect of an infant formula supplemented with AA and DHA on FAs of infants with different FADS genotypes. In total, 176 infants from the COGNIS study were randomly allocated to the Standard Formula (SF; n = 61) or the Experimental Formula (EF; n = 70) group, the latter supplemented with AA and DHA. Breastfed infants were added as a reference group (BF; n = 45). FAs and FADS polymorphisms were analyzed from cheek cells collected at 3 months of age. FADS minor allele carriership in formula fed infants, especially those supplemented, was associated with a declined desaturase activity and lower AA and DHA levels. Breastfed infants were not affected, possibly to the high content of AA and DHA in breast milk. The supplementation increased AA and DHA levels, but mostly in major allele carriers. In conclusion, infant FADS genotype could contribute to narrow the gap of AA and DHA concentrations between breastfed and formula fed infants.

Keywords: fatty acids; omega 6; omega 3; breast milk; infant formula; fatty acid desaturases; early life nutrition; control formula; intervention formula; exclusive breastfeeding

---

1. Introduction

Long chain polyunsaturated fatty acids (LCPUFA) have an important role in the immune system regulation, blood clots, neurotransmitters, cholesterol metabolism, and in the structure of membrane phospholipids in the brain and the retina [1]. Attention has been devoted especially to arachidonic acid (AA) and docosahexaenoic acid (DHA), due to their key role for optimal health, cognition and development during fetal and early postnatal life [2]. Breastmilk is usually the only external source of AA and DHA for infants during the first months of life [3,4]. When breastfeeding is not possible, infants require breast milk substitutes [5], which are usually supplemented with nutrients to match the breast milk content [6]. However, there is still debate and different opinions in regards of DHA and AA supplementation in infant formulas. The European Food Safety Authority (EFSA) [7] and the Commission Delegated Regulation (EU) 2016/127 [8] have proposed DHA supplementation as mandatory for infant formulas, while no minimum amount of AA was determined to be necessary, setting AA supplementation as an optional ingredient. However, it has been observed that when infants receive both AA and DHA supplementation they have better outcomes in cognitive performance than receiving DHA alone [9]. Other authors have even found that DHA alone did not influenced cognitive development at all [10]. Therefore, whether DHA should be supplemented alone or with AA remains controversial. Additionally, there is no agreed specific dose for supplementation, and there is little evidence of the long-term effect.

LCPUFAs can also be endogenously synthesized from the essential fatty acids (FAs): linoleic acid (LA) and alpha-linolenic acid (ALA). LCPUFA synthesis requires desaturation and elongation reactions. D6 and D5 desaturases (D6D and D5D) are two key enzymes that catalyze the synthesis by introducing *cis* double bonds at specific positions. Fatty acid desaturase genes FADS1 and FADS2 encode D5D and D6D, respectively, making them a rate limiting factor in LCPUFA conversion [11]. However, the endogenous synthesis of AA and DHA from their precursors is limited in humans as Demmelmair et al. observed in women that only 1.2% of the AA is directly derived from LA intake [12]. Likewise, both blood and tissue levels of PUFAs are influenced to a large extent by genetic heritability [13]. There are many studies showing the major impact of gene variants of the FADS gene cluster on the FA composition of blood, tissues and human milk [14–16]. For instance, single nucleotide polymorphisms (SNPs) in the FADS gene modulate the capacity for endogenous synthesis of LCPUFAs by compromising the desaturase activity of the involved enzymes [17–21]. It has been observed that up to 28% of variation of AA blood levels is due to FADS genetic variants, while LA is affected in 9% [13]. Furthermore, Baylin et al. observed that an impaired desaturase activity may induce an unbalanced proportion of n3 (e.g., the FADS2 deletion could prevent the conversion of the precursor ALA into LCPUFAs) [22]. Likewise, Schaeffer et al. observed that variants in the FADS1 and FADS2 genes showed strong associations with levels of n6 (e.g., LA, gamma-linolenic acid (GLA), dihomo-gamma-linolenic acid (DGLA), AA, and adrenic acid (AdA)), and n3 FAs (ALA, eicosapentaenoic acid (EPA), docosapentaenoic acid (DPA) [13], and DHA [23]). It has also been observed that variants in the FADS cluster can also influence total LDL, and DHL cholesterol, triglycerides, phospholipids, C-reactive protein, proinflamatory eicosanoids and cardiovascular disease endpoints [24,25].

Even though there is wide evidence of the effect of FADS genetic variants in FA concentrations of different biological tissues, there is little evidence for infants during their first year of life [19,26–28], which is a critical period of early life programming in which LCPUFAs play an important role [29]. Studying this could identify vulnerable groups in the pediatric population and contribute to the refinement of current recommendations and legislations in regards to infant AA and DHA supplementation. Given the low rates of exclusive breastfeeding in Europe, and while efforts are still being made to promote it, it is important to secure an appropriate source of LCPUFAs for infants who are not breastfed to promote their development. Therefore, the aim of this study was to determine the effect of an infant formula supplemented with AA and DHA on fatty acid levels of three-month-old infants with different FADS genotypes.

2. Materials and Methods

2.1. Ethics Statement

This study was carried out in accordance with the ethical standards established by the Declaration of Helsinki (2004), the Good Clinical Practice recommendations of the EEC (document 111/3976/88 July 1990) and the current Spanish legislation governing clinical research in humans (Royal Decree 561/1993 on clinical trials). In addition, the study was approved by the San Cecilio University Hospital Ethics Committee and the Faculty of Medicine at the University of Granada.

2.2. Study Population and Design

We analyzed 176 infants from the total of 220 participants in the COGNIS study (A Neurocognitive and Immunological Study of a New Formula for Healthy Infants), which is an interventional, randomized, and double-blinded study registered at www.ClinicalTrials.gov (NCT02094547). Full-term infants were recruited at the University Hospitals (Clinical San Cecilio and Mother-Infant Hospital) in the city of Granada (Spain), where samples and data were also collected. Each parent or legal guardian signed a written informed consent before the recruitment. To be eligible for enrolment of COGNIS study, infants had to meet the following inclusion criteria: 0–2 month old full-term infants, adequate birth weight for gestational age, normal Apgar score, umbilical pH $\geq$ 7.10 (normal range), availability to continue throughout the entire study period, signed informed consent, and for infants in the SF and EF groups, a maximum of 30 days of exclusive breastfeeding was considered and a minimum of 70% of infant formula consumption was required afterwards. Participants were excluded if they were participating in other studies, if they had nervous system or gastrointestinal disorders, and if the mother had a disease history or had received harmful drug treatment during pregnancy. Questionnaires and medical records were used to obtain maternal characteristics, including maternal age, gestational age, pre-pregnancy BMI, pre-pregnancy weight, smoking status during pregnancy, educational level, and Edinburgh scale. Likewise, infant characteristics such as gender, birth weight, birth length, and birth head circumference were obtained. The study design and information of the COGNIS participants are given in Figure 1.

After inclusion, infants were randomly allocated to the Standard Formula (SF) or the Experimental Formula (EF) group. Later, a third group was added with infants who were Exclusively Breastfed (BF) for at least 2 months to function as the control group.

After infant randomization, the research team decided to withdraw from the trial those infants who met the following criteria: Infants fed with infant formulas unrelated to COGNIS study, breastfed infants with formula intake >25% before 6 months, formula fed infants with human milk intakes higher than 25% beyond the 3rd month of life, any adverse event that could interfere with study follow-up, cow's milk protein allergy/intolerance or lactose intolerance, infant formula intake rejection or neurological disorder.

All infants from COGNIS study were followed up at 2, 3, 6, 12, 18 months of life and 2.5 years of age. During the follow-up visits, and depending on the subject age, different assessment procedures and data collection were carried out; however, those will be explored elsewhere. Nevertheless, for the purpose to obtain a better control of records avoiding possible twists on data due to factors that involved other time lines, such as mixed feeding in the 1st month of life or initiation of complementary feeding at 6 months, this study only takes into account infants from the second visit (3 months of age).

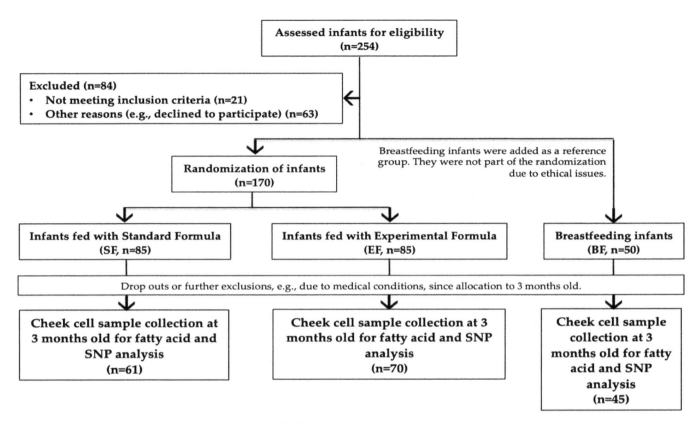

Figure 1. Participants in the COGNIS study and classification following type of feeding.

2.3. Formulas

Infant formulas from SF and EF were based on cow's milk and were provided by ORDESA Laboratories, S.L., Barcelona, Spain. The experimental formula was characterized by the presence of LCPUFAs AA (*Mortierella alpine*) and DHA (fish oil), milk fat globule membrane (MFGM) components {10% of total protein content (wt:wt}, symbiotics, gangliosides, nucleotides and sialic acid (Nutriexpert® factor). Fat blend, OMEGA FATS (palm, palm-kemel, rapeseed, sunflower, oleic sunflower fatty acids) and BETAPOL (Palm, palm-kemel, sunflower and rapeseed oils) were present in both formulas. For more information regarding the lipid profile, consult the Supplementary Materials (Table S2). Additionally, both formulas followed the guidelines of the Committee on Nutrition of the European Society for Pediatric Gastroenterology, Hepatology and Nutrition (ESPGHAN), and the international and national recommendations for the composition of infant formulas. Nutritional composition of infant formulas is shown in Table 1.

Table 1. Standard and Experimental Infant Formula Nutrition Facts per 100 mL.

	Standard Formula	Experimental Formula
	100 mL (13.5%)	100 mL (13.5%)
Energy (kcal/kJ)	69/288	68/285
Proteins * (g)	1.35	1.35
Casein/whey (%)	40/60	40/60
Carbohydrates (g)	7.97	7.56
Lactose (g)	7.17	6.82
Maltodextrin (g)	0.8	0.7
Fat # (g)	3.5	3.5
Linoleic acid (LA, mg)	579	569
α-Linolenic acid (ALA, mg)	49	49
Arachidonic acid (AA, mg)	-	15.8
Docosahexaenoic acid (DHA, mg)	-	11.2

Powder diluted in water (13.5%) * With alpha-lactoalbumin (15% of total protein) and with Immunoglobulins. # With 22% of palmitic acid in beta position.

2.4. Cheek Cell Sample Collection

Cheek cell samples were collected at 3 months of age to analyze FAs and genotype FADS SNPs. Samples were collected 1 h after feeding by scraping the inside of the cheeks with a Rovers® EndoCervex-Brush®. The tip of the brush was transferred and jolted in a cryotube with distilled water, shaking the tip before removing the brush. After centrifugation, the supernatant was carefully discarded. The cell pellets were stored at −80 °C until analysis.

2.5. Cheek Cell Fatty Acid Analysis

A modified version of the method described by de la Garza et al. [30] was used to analyze FAs from the glycerophospholipid fraction. Methanol with butylated hydroxytoluene (BHT) was used for lipid extraction. FA reactions with sodium methylate in methanol (25 wt% in methanol) and boron trifluoride methanol solution (14% v/v) were used to obtain FA methyl esters (FAMEs). Next, the FAs were separated by rapid gas chromatography following the method developed by Bondia et al. [31]. The system consisted of a Shimadzu GC-2010 gas chromatograph (Kyoto, Japan) equipped with a "split-splitless" injector, an automatic injector with AOC-20i-AOC-20s sampler and a flame ionization detector (FID). The separation of the methyl esters from the FAs was carried out with a fast capillary column of fused silica VF-23ms (10 m × 0,10 mm internal diameter, 0,10 μm film thickness) coated with a stationary phase 100% cyanopropyl-phenyl-methyl-polysiloxane of varian (Palo Alto, CA, USA). The methyl esters of the FAs were identified by comparison with the retention times of standards, FAME-37 and PUFA-2 animal. Quantification was done by normalization, expressing the results in relative amounts (percentage). Enzyme activities were estimated as product:precursor indexes of individual FAs as follows: GLA:LA and DGLA:LA indexes for D6D enzyme activity, and the AA:DGLA index for D5D enzyme activity. Additionally, AA:LA and eicosapentaenoic acid (EPA):ALA indexes were analyzed.

2.6. SNP Selection and Genotyping

SNPs within the FADS gene were selected if they were documented in previous studies for comparison purposes [19,27,32–38] and if their minor allele frequency (MAF) was higher than 10%. DNA material was extracted from infant cheek cells. FADS1 (rs174537, rs174545, rs174546, rs174548, and rs174553) and FADS2 (rs1535, rs174570, and rs2072114) SNPs were genotyped from 2.5 μl of DNA mixed with 2.5 μL of 2X TaqMan® OpenArray® Genotyping Master Mix. Analysis was then performed with 4 μL of the mixture in a microplate using the TaqMan® OpenArray® genotyping technology. Analyses were carried out at the *Autonomous University of Barcelona* (UAB) using the QuantStudio 12 k Flex® instrument (ThermoFisher) and the corresponding OpenArray® SNP Genotyping Analysis software.

2.7. Statistical Analysis

SPSS statistical software package for Windows (version 20.0; SPSS Inc., Chicago, IL, USA) was used to perform the statistical analyses. Data were tested for normality using the Kolmogorov-Smirnov test and non-normal data were log transformed. This exploratory study evaluated the associations between SNPs and PUFAs within the study groups using a linear regression analysis. We decided to analyze each SNP individually to provide more evidence about their effects on LCPUFAs levels in the first stage of life, given the lack of literacy in this period of life. Heterozygotes and minor allele homozygotes were analyzed together as one group to improve sample size. However, this codification implies an additive and dominant model. SNPs were studied as a numeric variable by coding them according to the minor allele count; 0 for major homozygotes and 1 for heterozygotes and minor allele homozygotes. We also tested the analyses with the three allele groups and confirmed that the results showed the same tendency. The Hardy-Weinberg equilibrium and genotype distribution were analyzed with the x^2-test (Supplementary Materials Table S1). We used a multivariate general linear model (GLM) to compare FA levels (mean ± standard deviation) between the study groups and according to FADS genotype. FAs were expressed as the percentage of total FAs. The analyses were corrected for potential confounders such as maternal characteristics (pre-pregnancy body mass index, age, education and smoking status), and gender of the child. The p-value cut-off has been reconsidered and changed according to Bonferroni correction (0.05/8 SNPs × 3 groups = 24) and assuming a moderate correlation of 30% between SNPs. The significance cut-off values resulted at <0.005 and this has been applied to each trait.

3. Results

3.1. Sample Characteristics

The population has the characteristics shown in Table 2. Mothers from the BF group were more likely to have a higher level of education and were older than mothers from the EF group. The EF group had more male infants than the BF group. No differences were observed in infant anthropometric data.

Table 2. Characteristics of the population.

Characteristics	SF		EF		BF		p
	N	Mean ± SD	N	Mean ± SD	N	Mean ± SD	
Maternal characteristics							
Age (years)	61	30.31 [ab] ± 6.53	70	29.97 ± 6.22 [a]	45	33.24 ± 5.39 [b]	0.014
Gestational age (months)	61	39.52 ± 1.29	70	39.26 ± 1.44	45	39.4 ± 1.3	0.55
Pre-pregnancy weight (kg)	56	65.43 ± 12.92	63	64.26 ± 12.52	43	65.66 ± 10.4	0.81
Pre-pregnancy BMI (kg/m²) (%)							0.76
Underweight	3	5.45	8	12.7	5	11.63	
Normal weight	29	52.73	29	46.03	23	53.49	
Overweight	14	25.45	15	23.81	11	25.58	
Obesity	9	16.36	11	17.46	4	9.3	
Education (%)							<0.001
Primary	14	22.58	15	21.43	1	2.22	
Secondary	18	29.03	25	35.71	4	8.89	
Professional	12	19.35	16	22.86	13	28.89	
Bachelor degree	18	29.03	14	20	27	60	
Smoking during pregnancy (Yes, %)	10	20.83	10	15.87	2	5.13	0.11
Edinburgh Scale (%)							0.42
No depression	49	79.03	53	76.81	39	86.67	
Probable depression	13	20.97	16	23.19	6	13.33	
Infant characteristics							
Sex, male (%)	37	59.68 [ab]	44	62.86 [a]	18	40.00 [b]	0.042
Birth weight (kg)	61	3.34 ± 0.41	70	3.32 ± 0.5	45	3.35 ± 0.42	0.91
Birth length (cm)	61	50.67 ± 2.01	68	50.72 ± 2.1	45	50.62 ± 2.39	0.97
WAZ	61	0.04 ± 0.86	68	0.02 ± 0.97	44	0.13 ± 0.86	0.81
LAZ	61	0.58 ± 1.03	68	0.59 ± 1.08	44	0.71 ± 0.98	0.79
BMIZ	61	−0.39 ± 0.93	68	−0.39 ± 1.04	44	−0.37 ± 0.95	0.99

The presented values are means and proportions. Different superscript letters indicate differences among study groups according to ANOVA and Bonferroni post-hoc test. A chi-square test was applied to qualitative variables. Significance level was established at $p < 0.05$. SF, Standard Formula; EF, Experimental Formula; BF, Breastfeeding; WAZ, weight for age z-score; LAZ, length for age z-score; HAZ, height for age z-score.

3.2. Associations of FADS SNPs with Fatty Acids

Table 3 shows nominal and significant associations between PUFAs and FADS minor alleles after adjusting for maternal age, maternal education, maternal smoking habit, and sex of infant.

The most significant associations ($p < 0.005$) were found in the EF group, where minor allele carriership of rs174537 was negatively associated with LA, AA and DHA (βc −0.376, −0.440, and −0.415, respectively), and FADS minor allele carriership of rs2072114 was negatively associated with AA and the AA:LA index (βc −0.522 and −0.450, respectively).

Within the SF group, nominal negative associations were found after correcting for confounders, while the BF group showed none.

The complete analysis can be found in Supplementary Materials Table S3.

Table 3. Associations between FADS genes and fatty acids levels in infants.

Fatty Acids and Gene	SNP	M/m	Standard Formula (n = 46) (n = 46)				Experimental Formula (n = 56) (n = 56)				Breastfeeding (n = 33) (n = 33)			
			β	P	βc	Pc	β	P	βc	Pc	β	P	βc	Pc
C18:2n6 (LA)														
FADS1	rs174537	G/T	−0.035	0.818	−0.132	0.408	−0.361	**0.006**	−0.376	**0.005** *	−0.027	0.880	−0.094	0.687
FADS1	rs174545	C/G	−0.035	0.818	−0.132	0.408	−0.322	**0.015**	−0.351	**0.008**	0.026	0.888	−0.092	0.688
FADS1	rs174546	C/T	−0.035	0.818	−0.132	0.408	−0.322	**0.015**	−0.351	**0.008**	−0.027	0.880	−0.094	0.687
FADS1	rs174553	A/G	−0.035	0.818	−0.132	0.408	−0.322	**0.015**	−0.351	**0.008**	−0.027	0.880	−0.094	0.687
FADS2	rs1535	A/G	−0.035	0.818	−0.132	0.408	−0.346	**0.008**	−0.357	**0.008**	−0.027	0.880	−0.094	0.687
FADS2	rs174570	C/T	0.155	0.304	0.137	0.406	−0.272	**0.043**	−0.207	0.134	−0.106	0.558	−0.162	0.464
C20:3n6 (DGLA)														
FADS2	rs174570	C/T	−0.276	0.063	−0.230	0.167	−0.327	**0.014**	−0.288	**0.034**	−0.123	0.495	−0.046	0.815
FADS2	rs2072114	A/G	−0.056	0.709	−0.079	0.632	−0.368	**0.005** *	−0.342	**0.014**	−0.090	0.618	−0.145	0.446
C20:4n6 (AA)														
FADS1	rs174537	G/T	−0.297	**0.045**	−0.224	0.155	−0.396	**0.002** *	−0.440	**0.001** *	0.023	0.897	0.035	0.876
FADS1	rs174545	C/G	−0.297	**0.045**	−0.224	0.155	−0.351	**0.007**	−0.375	**0.006**	0.046	0.803	0.036	0.873
FADS1	rs174546	C/T	−0.297	**0.045**	−0.224	0.155	−0.351	**0.007**	−0.375	**0.006**	0.023	0.897	0.035	0.876
FADS1	rs174548	C/G	−0.118	0.436	−0.073	0.653	−0.360	**0.006**	−0.367	**0.007**	0.052	0.773	0.034	0.878
FADS1	rs174553	A/G	−0.297	**0.045**	−0.224	0.155	−0.351	**0.007**	−0.375	**0.006**	0.023	0.897	0.035	0.876
FADS2	rs1535	A/G	−0.297	**0.045**	−0.224	0.155	−0.340	**0.010**	−0.374	**0.007**	0.023	0.897	0.035	0.876
FADS2	rs174570	C/T	−0.412	**0.004** *	−0.347	**0.030**	−0.262	0.051	−0.237	0.096	−0.257	0.148	−0.187	0.379
FADS2	rs2072114	A/G	−0.077	0.613	−0.049	0.761	−0.502	**<0.001** *	−0.522	**<0.001** *	−0.059	0.746	−0.054	0.797
C22:4n6 (AdA)														
FADS1	rs174537	G/T	−0.350	**0.017**	−0.408	**0.010**	−0.346	**0.009**	−0.365	**0.006**	0.015	0.933	−0.042	0.855
FADS1	rs174545	C/G	−0.350	**0.017**	−0.408	**0.010**	−0.333	**0.011**	−0.330	**0.014**	0.005	0.979	−0.042	0.856
FADS1	rs174546	C/T	−0.350	**0.017**	−0.408	**0.010**	−0.333	**0.011**	−0.330	**0.014**	0.015	0.933	−0.042	0.855
FADS1	rs174548	C/G	−0.280	0.059	−0.372	**0.022**	−0.332	**0.012**	−0.317	**0.016**	−0.027	0.883	−0.140	0.542
FADS1	rs174553	A/G	−0.350	**0.017**	−0.408	**0.010**	−0.333	**0.011**	−0.330	**0.014**	0.015	0.933	−0.042	0.855
FADS2	rs1535	A/G	−0.350	**0.017**	−0.408	**0.010**	−0.348	**0.008**	−0.354	**0.009**	0.015	0.933	−0.042	0.855
FADS2	rs174570	C/T	−0.222	0.138	−0.244	0.147	−0.374	**0.004** *	−0.337	**0.013**	−0.046	0.799	0.029	0.897
FADS2	rs2072114	A/G	0.060	0.693	0.025	0.883	−0.362	**0.006**	−0.302	**0.032**	0.011	0.953	−0.019	0.931
C22:5n6 (DPAn6)														
FADS1	rs174545	C/G	−0.111	0.463	−0.054	0.739	−0.255	0.056	−0.288	**0.038**	0.102	0.577	0.068	0.742
FADS1	rs174546	C/T	−0.111	0.463	−0.054	0.739	−0.255	0.056	−0.288	**0.038**	0.100	0.578	0.068	0.741
FADS1	rs174553	A/G	−0.111	0.463	−0.054	0.739	−0.255	0.056	−0.288	**0.038**	0.100	0.578	0.068	0.741
C18:3n3 (ALA)														
FADS2	rs174570	C/T	0.303	**0.040**	0.279	0.079	−0.040	0.772	−0.042	0.765	−0.061	0.736	−0.089	0.665
C20:5n3 (EPA)														
FADS1	rs174537	G/T	−0.287	0.053	−0.315	0.057	−0.249	0.065	−0.331	**0.017**	0.113	0.530	0.269	0.243
FADS1	rs174545	C/G	−0.287	0.053	−0.315	0.057	−0.225	0.093	0.310	**0.025**	0.162	0.374	0.274	0.236
FADS1	rs174546	C/T	−0.287	0.053	−0.315	0.057	−0.225	0.093	0.310	**0.025**	0.113	0.530	0.269	0.243
FADS1	rs174548	C/G	−0.238	0.112	−0.284	0.093	−0.247	0.064	−0.303	**0.026**	0.158	0.380	0.296	0.198
FADS1	rs174553	A/G	−0.287	0.053	−0.315	0.057	−0.225	0.093	−0.310	**0.025**	0.113	0.530	0.269	0.243
GLA:LA (D6D)														
FADS2	rs174570	C/T	−0.394	**0.007**	−0.338	**0.037**	−0.049	0.722	−0.127	0.361	−0.078	0.670	0.007	0.973
DGLA:LA (D6D)														
FADS1	rs174537	G/T	−0.24	**0.010**	−0.17	0.28	0.06	0.62	−0.01	0.94	0.09	0.62	0.19	0.38
FADS1	rs174545	C/G	−0.24	**0.010**	−0.17	0.28	0.04	0.72	−0.03	0.81	0.07	0.71	0.19	0.40
FADS1	rs174546	C/T	−0.24	**0.010**	−0.17	0.28	0.04	0.72	−0.03	0.81	0.09	0.62	0.19	0.38
FADS1	rs174553	A/G	−0.24	**0.010**	−0.17	0.28	0.04	0.72	−0.03	0.81	0.09	0.62	0.19	0.38
FADS2	rs174570	C/T	−0.40	**0.006**	−0.34	**0.032**	−0.21	0.12	−0.20	0.15	−0.08	0.64	0.01	0.93
FADS2	rs2072114	A/G	−0.18	0.22	−0.14	0.36	−0.29	**0.026**	−0.26	0.06	−0.09	0.59	−0.14	0.47
AA:LA (D6D + D5D)														
FADS1	rs174537	G/T	−0.36	**0.013**	−0.28	0.06	−0.22	0.09	−0.26	0.06	0.04	0.81	0.09	0.66
FADS1	rs174545	C/G	−0.36	**0.013**	−0.28	0.06	−0.20	0.13	−0.21	0.13	0.04	0.83	0.09	0.67
FADS1	rs174546	C/T	−0.36	**0.013**	−0.28	0.06	−0.20	0.13	−0.21	0.13	0.04	0.81	0.09	0.66
FADS1	rs174548	C/G	−0.18	0.24	−0.15	0.36	−0.27	**0.045**	−0.26	0.06	−0.01	0.95	−0.05	0.83
FADS1	rs174553	A/G	−0.36	**0.013**	−0.28	0.06	−0.20	0.13	−0.21	0.13	0.04	0.81	0.09	0.66
FADS2	rs1535	A/G	−0.36	**0.013**	−0.28	0.06	−0.17	0.18	−0.20	0.14	0.04	0.81	0.09	0.66
FADS2	rs174570	C/T	−0.47	**0.001** *	−0.41	**0.007**	−0.13	0.32	−0.14	0.32	−0.24	0.16	−0.12	0.54
FADS2	rs2072114	A/G	−0.16	0.27	−0.12	0.43	−0.43	**0.001** *	−0.450	**0.001** *	−0.07	0.67	−0.05	0.79
AA:DGLA (D5D)														
FADS1	rs174548	C/G	−0.226	0.132	−0.160	0.333	−0.269	**0.043**	−0.285	**0.041**	−0.133	0.462	−0.108	0.636
FADS2	rs1535	A/G	−0.195	0.195	−0.141	0.386	−0.261	0.050	−0.283	**0.049**	−0.072	0.691	−0.071	0.757
C22:6n3 (DHA)														
FADS1	rs174537	G/T	−0.257	0.085	−0.303	0.054	−0.393	**0.003** *	−0.415	**0.002** *	0.057	0.753	0.176	0.432
FADS1	rs174545	C/G	−0.257	0.085	−0.303	0.054	−0.341	**0.010**	−0.339	**0.013**	0.089	0.629	0.177	0.429
FADS1	rs174546	C/T	−0.257	0.085	−0.303	0.054	−0.341	**0.010**	−0.339	**0.013**	0.057	0.753	0.176	0.432
FADS1	rs174548	C/G	−0.144	0.339	−0.211	0.192	−0.338	**0.010**	−0.328	**0.015**	0.101	0.577	0.164	0.463
FADS1	rs174553	A/G	−0.257	0.085	−0.303	0.054	−0.341	**0.010**	−0.339	**0.013**	0.057	0.753	0.176	0.432
FADS2	rs1535	A/G	−0.257	0.085	−0.303	0.054	−0.342	**0.009**	−0.354	**0.010**	0.057	0.753	0.176	0.432
FADS2	rs174570	C/T	−0.233	0.120	−0.258	0.114	−0.265	**0.048**	−0.238	0.092	−0.352	**0.045**	−0.274	0.196
FADS2	rs2072114	A/G	0.071	0.637	0.056	0.732	−0.289	**0.029**	−0.244	0.093	−0.081	0.654	−0.017	0.934

Table 3. *Cont.*

Fatty Acids and Gene	SNP	M/m	Standard Formula (n = 46) (n = 46)				Experimental Formula (n = 56) (n = 56)				Breastfeeding (n = 33) (n = 33)			
			β	P	βc	Pc	β	P	βc	Pc	β	P	βc	Pc
EPA:ALA (D6D + D5D)														
FADS1	rs174537	G/T	−0.37	**0.010**	−0.35	**0.022**	−0.13	0.32	−0.19	0.15	0.08	0.65	−0.04	0.83
FADS1	rs174545	C/G	−0.37	**0.010**	−0.35	**0.022**	−0.08	0.52	−0.14	0.30	0.06	0.71	−0.04	0.84
FADS1	rs174546	C/T	−0.37	**0.010**	−0.35	**0.022**	−0.08	0.52	−0.14	0.30	0.08	0.65	−0.04	0.83
FADS1	rs174553	A/G	−0.37	**0.010**	−0.35	**0.022**	−0.08	0.52	−0.14	0.30	0.08	0.65	−0.04	0.83
FADS2	rs1535	A/G	−0.37	**0.010**	−0.35	**0.022**	−0.07	0.61	−0.13	0.34	0.08	0.65	−0.04	0.83
FADS2	rs174570	C/T	−0.37	**0.010**	−0.37	**0.019**	−0.06	0.61	−0.07	0.58	−0.14	0.43	−0.09	0.65

Associations between SNPs and FAs were determined using linear regression analysis. βc and Pc are values corrected for potential confounders such as maternal age, maternal education, smoking and infant gender. SNPs were coded according to minor allele count and analyzed as a numeric variable. "β" = beta per minor allele standardized per the major allele. p-values < 0.05 are highlighted in bold and significant associations that persisted after Bonferroni corrections are additionally denoted by asterisks (* p < 0.005). M: Major allele; m: minor allele; SNP, single nucleotide polymorphism; LA: Linoleic Acid; GLA: gamma-linolenic acid; DGLA: dihomo-gamma-linolenic acid; AA: Arachidonic Acid; AdA: adrenic acid; DPA*n*6: docosapentaenoic acid *n*6; ALA: alpha-linolenic Acid; EPA: eicosapentaenoic acid; DHA: docosahexaenoic Acid.

3.3. Fatty Acid Comparison by FADS Genotype among Feeding Practice Groups

LCPUFA levels were statistically different among the feeding practice groups when classifying infants by FADS genotype (Table 4). Among major homozygotes, both the BF and EF groups had a higher AA level than the SF group, but when infants carried minor alleles, those with breastfeeding showed a higher AA level than both the EF and SF groups. DHA levels also exhibited differences. Among major homozygotes, infants in the BF and EF groups showed a higher DHA level than infants in the SF group. On the other hand, among minor allele carriers, the EF group presented a higher DHA level than the SF group, but the BF group had the highest DHA level of all. The complete analysis can be found in Supplementary Materials Table S4.

Table 4. Fatty acids according to infant SNPs and study group.

Fatty Acids and Gene	SNP	M/m	MM								MM	Mm + mm								
			Standard Formula		Experimental Formula		Breastfeeding		p	Standard Formula		Experimental Formula		Breastfeeding		p
			N	Mean ± SD	N	Mean ± SD	N	Mean ± SD		N	Mean ± SD	N	Mean ± SD	N	Mean ± SD	
C20:4n6 (AA)																
FADS1	rs174537	G/T	30	2.0000 ± 0.64 [a]	41	2.4900 ± 0.53 [b]	18	2.9200 ± 0.79 [b]	**<0.001** *	31	1.7300 ± 0.53 [a]	25	2.0000 ± 0.62 [a]	20	2.7300 ± 0.73 [b]	**<0.001** *
FADS1	rs174545	C/G	30	2.0000 ± 0.64 [a]	40	2.4900 ± 0.54 [b]	17	2.9000 ± 0.81 [b]	**<0.001** *	31	1.7300 ± 0.53 [a]	27	2.0500 ± 0.63 [a]	20	2.7300 ± 0.73 [b]	**<0.001** *
FADS1	rs174546	C/T	30	2.0000 ± 0.64 [a]	40	2.4900 ± 0.54 [b]	18	2.9200 ± 0.79 [b]	**<0.001** *	31	1.7300 ± 0.53 [a]	27	2.0500 ± 0.63 [a]	20	2.7300 ± 0.73 [b]	**<0.001** *
FADS1	rs174548	C/G	33	1.9200 ± 0.63 [a]	40	2.5000 ± 0.54 [b]	21	2.8700 ± 0.78 [b]	**<0.001** *	28	1.8000 ± 0.56 [a]	27	2.0500 ± 0.62 [a]	17	2.7500 ± 0.73 [b]	**<0.001** *
FADS1	rs174553	A/G	30	2.0000 ± 0.64 [a]	40	2.4900 ± 0.54 [b]	18	2.9200 ± 0.79 [b]	**<0.001** *	31	1.7300 ± 0.53 [a]	27	2.0500 ± 0.63 [a]	20	2.7300 ± 0.73 [b]	**<0.001** *
FADS2	rs1535	A/G	30	2.0000 ± 0.64 [a]	40	2.4900 ± 0.54 [b]	18	2.9200 ± 0.79 [b]	**<0.001** *	31	1.7300 ± 0.53 [a]	27	2.0600 ± 0.63 [a]	20	2.7300 ± 0.73 [b]	**<0.001** *
FADS2	rs174570	C/T	44	1.9600 ± 0.60 [a]	53	2.4100 ± 0.58 [b]	28	2.9500 ± 0.75 [c]	**<0.001** *	17	1.6200 ± 0.52 [a]	13	1.8900 ± 0.57 [ab]	10	2.4300 ± 0.64 [b]	**0.006**
FADS2	rs2072114	A/G	47	1.8700 ± 0.61 [a]	54	2.4400 ± 0.53 [b]	30	2.8500 ± 0.76 [b]	**<0.001** *	14	1.8400 ± 0.56 [a]	13	1.8100 ± 0.69 [a]	8	2.6800 ± 0.75 [b]	**0.007**
C22:6n3 (DHA)																
FADS1	rs174537	G/T	30	0.5100 ± 0.24 [a]	41	0.9900 ± 0.22 [b]	18	1.2300 ± 0.42 [b]	**<0.001** *	31	0.4500 ± 0.25 [a]	25	0.7900 ± 0.27 [b]	20	1.1800 ± 0.46 [c]	**<0.001** *
FADS1	rs174545	C/G	30	0.5100 ± 0.24 [a]	40	0.9900 ± 0.22 [b]	17	1.2000 ± 0.43 [b]	**<0.001** *	31	0.4500 ± 0.25 [a]	27	0.8200 ± 0.28 [b]	20	1.1800 ± 0.46 [c]	**<0.001** *
FADS1	rs174546	C/T	30	0.5100 ± 0.24 [a]	40	0.9900 ± 0.22 [b]	18	1.2300 ± 0.42 [b]	**<0.001** *	31	0.4500 ± 0.25 [a]	27	0.8200 ± 0.28 [b]	20	1.1800 ± 0.46 [c]	**<0.001** *
FADS1	rs174548	C/G	33	0.4900 ± 0.24 [a]	40	0.9900 ± 0.22 [b]	21	1.2000 ± 0.43 [b]	**<0.001** *	28	0.4600 ± 0.26 [a]	27	0.8200 ± 0.29 [b]	17	1.2000 ± 0.45 [c]	**<0.001** *
FADS1	rs174553	A/G	30	0.5100 ± 0.24 [a]	40	0.9900 ± 0.22 [b]	18	1.2300 ± 0.42 [b]	**<0.001** *	31	0.4500 ± 0.25 [a]	27	0.8200 ± 0.28 [b]	20	1.1800 ± 0.46 [c]	**<0.001** *
FADS2	rs1535	A/G	30	0.5100 ± 0.24 [a]	40	0.9900 ± 0.22 [b]	18	1.2300 ± 0.42 [b]	**<0.001** *	31	0.4500 ± 0.25 [a]	27	0.8200 ± 0.28 [b]	20	1.1800 ± 0.46 [c]	**<0.001** *
FADS2	rs174570	C/T	44	0.5000 ± 0.25 [a]	53	0.9500 ± 0.22 [b]	28	1.3000 ± 0.42 [c]	**<0.001** *	17	0.4200 ± 0.21 [a]	13	0.7700 ± 0.33 [b]	10	0.9200 ± 0.35 [b]	**<0.001** *
FADS2	rs2072114	A/G	47	0.4700 ± 0.24 [a]	54	0.9600 ± 0.25 [b]	30	1.2300 ± 0.45 [b]	**<0.001** *	14	0.5100 ± 0.28 [a]	13	0.7600 ± 0.26 [b]	8	1.0900 ± 0.38 [b]	**<0.001** *

Values are means ± standard deviations. The general linear model and Bonferroni post-hoc test were applied. The analysis was corrected for potential confounders such as pre-gestational IMC, smoking, education and age of mother and infant gender. p-values < 0.05 are highlighted in bold and significant differences that persisted after Bonferroni corrections are additionally denoted by asterisks (* $p < 0.005$). Different superscript letter indicate which groups are different from the others. M: Major allele; m: minor allele; SNP, single nucleotide polymorphism; AA: Arachidonic Acid; DHA: docosahexaenoic Acid.

4. Discussion

The present study analyzed the influence of an infant formula, supplemented with AA + DHA, on LCPUFA levels in infants with different FADS genotype. A number of studies have investigated the association between variants in the FADS gene cluster and FA levels in human tissue [13,14,22–24]; however, little information is available on the neonatal population. Other studies have analyzed the effect of LCPUFA supplementation in early life [9,39–41], but no association with FADS SNPs has been investigated whatsoever. Our study contributes to generating new evidence in this matter.

FADS minor alleles have shown to decrease the desaturase activity [13,16,17,42–46], compromising LCPUFA production. Some authors have demonstrated that FADS SNPs lower proportions of GLA, AA, and EPA, and accumulate the LCPUFA precursors LA and ALA [11,46,47]. Others have demonstrated that FADS minor allele carriers exhibit lower AA:DGLA and EPA:ALA indexes [48,49]. As mentioned before, some studies include indexes of AA to LA, as well as EPA and DHA to ALA in order to use them as markers of the activity of fatty acids desaturation mediated by the enzymes D5D and D6D, respectively; in our study, we use GLA:AA and DGLA:LA to indicate D6D activity, whereas D5D activity is reflected by the ratio of AA to DGLA, and we consider it relevant to record if an infant formula supplemented with LCPUFA can influence the enzymatic activity of infants compared with non-supplemented, to allow a possible comparison for future studies. Moreover, it has been established that the AA is the most severely affected FA [13]. In our study, infants from the BF group carrying FADS minor alleles were not associated with FAs, which suggests that desaturase activity is not affected by FADS genotype when infants are exclusively breastfed.

However, infants carrying FADS minor alleles in the EF and SF groups were associated with decreased D5D and D6D activities, which is in line with the previous studies [46,50–52]. The most affected group was the EF, where infants carrying minor alleles of rs173547 (FADS1) had decreased levels of LA, AA and DHA, and minor allele carriers of rs2072114 (FADS2) were negatively associated with AA and the D5D and D6D desaturases activity (AA:LA index) ($p < 0.005$). Accordingly, the nominal associations ($p < 0.05$) were also inclined to decrease the desaturase activities when infants presented FADS minor alleles. In the EF group this was observed with n6 PUFAs (LA, DGLA, AA, AdA, DPAn6, AA:DGLA), EPA and DHA. Moreover, in the SF group the SNP rs174570 (FADS2) stood out by associating with decreased levels of AA, GLA:LA, DGLA:LA, AA:LA and EPA:ALA. These results suggest that the infants without AA and DHA supplementation were the least affected in terms of FA levels by FADS genetic variants. To make a proper interpretation of the results, it is of interest to take into account the different effect size among the study groups. For instance, the strongest association was found within the EF group, where minor allele carriers of rs2072114 showed the highest negative association with AA (βc -0.522, $p < 0.001$).

In our study, AA and DHA levels, in spite of the genotype, showed a gradient of SF < EF < BF. More specifically, among major homozygotes of FADS SNPs (except rs174570), AA and DHA concentrations were closer between the EF and the BF groups, and higher compared to SF infants, which shows the expected effect of the infant formula supplementation. Nevertheless, when carrying minor alleles, the EF group did not reach similar levels to the BF infants. In summary, Table 4 should be interpreted with caution due to effect size differences among study groups (e.g., the difference between the FA means of EF and BF groups is narrower when infants carry major homozygotes, and these differences increase among minor allele carriers).

This study exposes minor allele carriers as a potential vulnerable group since the same supplementation might not be enough for them, especially in the case of AA that showed the same levels than the SF group, whereas the DHA was at least higher than them.

Increasing the supplemented dose of preformed LCPUFAs may compensate for the effect of FADS minor alleles. According to Miklavcic et al., increasing the formula supplementation to AA 34 mg/100 kcal and DHA 17 mg/100 kcal prevents the reduction in AA by minor alleles [53]. However, in our study, the EF group received a supplementation of 23.2 mg/100 kcal of AA and 15.5 mg/100 kcal of DHA, which could be a reason for their suggested high SNP influence. As for the SF infants, their

AA and DHA levels were almost unaffected by minor alleles. Since previous evidence suggested that high supplementation levels of AA and DHA could lessen the influence of FADS SNPs on LCPUFA levels, we somewhat expected a gradient effect of SNPs of SF > EF > BF. However, this expectation was not determined since the SF group was not supplemented at all. The gradient resulted in EF > SF > BF. It is interesting how the LCPUFA levels of the SF group were less influenced by the FADS SNPs than the EF group. We could speculate some kind of protection effect (e.g., a more effective synthesis in the absence of preformed AA and DHA intake [54]) against FADS SNPs when infants have low LCPUFA levels. It is important to remember that, even though the EF group was more influenced by FADS SNPs than the SF group, infants from the EF group still presented higher AA and DHA levels. Corresponding to the theory of the higher the LCPUFA supply the less SNP influence, AA and DHA levels of BF infants were not perceptibly affected by genotype, possibly because they had the highest LCPUFA concentrations related to the high content in breast milk. One should consider that mean fat content of human milk may vary considerably between individuals as well as between study populations from affluent or developing countries [55]. Maternal factors, such as diet and weight gain during pregnancy, and sampling procedures have distinct impact on fat levels [56]. Additionally, DHA levels in breast milk are quite sensitive to maternal diet [4] and maternal FADS genotypes are associated with breast-milk AA concentration and this might therefore influence the supply of breast milk FAs [42].

Several authors have demonstrated that FADS SNPs affect FA levels and are associated with health conditions [13,39,57–62]. The major contribution of our study is providing evidence in infants below 6 months of age, identifying a potential vulnerable group of infants who could benefit from more personalized nutrition, and contributing to defining the ideal AA and DHA supplementation of infant formulas. This line of research merits further attention because early life nutrient exposure can program future health. We acknowledge some limitations, such as the lack of information on maternal dietary intake and supplementation, and the relatively small sample size of our population. We should also take into consideration the estimation of effect size to interpret the influence of SNPs on LCPUFA levels according to the study group. Now that we have evidence for each individual SNP, it is of interest to perform a FADS haplotype analysis to compare the results. The strengths of our study include the double-blinded cohort study design and the participation of three infant groups with different feeding practices. It is important to mention that the infant formulas were created previous to the implementation of the Commission Delegated Regulation (EU) 2016/127 [8] when DHA supplementation was not mandatory.

5. Conclusions

In conclusion, formula fed infants with FADS minor alleles, especially those with AA and DHA supplementation, were associated with decreased desaturase activity and lower AA and DHA levels. Breastfed infants were not affected, possibly due to the high LCPUFA content in breast milk. The AA and DHA supplementation of the infant formula provided the infants carrying major allele homozygotes with closer levels to those obtained with breastfeeding. This exposes minor alleles as a potential factor of vulnerability since the same supplementation might not be enough for them. Considering infant FADS genotype to meet the individual needs could contribute to narrow the gap of AA and DHA concentrations between breastfed and formula fed infants. A new LCPUFA supplementation dose should be explored to determine if an increased supplementation of AA and DHA might prevent the reduction of these FAs observed in the presence of FADS minor alleles. However, when breastfeeding is not possible, supplemented formulas should be considered as the second choice since they provide better AA and DHA concentrations compared to infants without supplementation.

Author Contributions: Cristina Campoy designed and coordinated the project; A.N., F.H. and E.D. performed the follow-up of the children, collected data and prepared the samples for later analysis; I.S.L. and A.d.l.G.P. performed the experimental procedures; M.C.L.-S., A.I.C., M.R.-P., I.S.L., A.M.C.T. and A.d.l.G.P. analyzed the data and designed the manuscript; A.M.C.T., I.S.L. and A.d.l.G.P. conducted the statistical analysis, interpretation of results and drafting of the manuscript. All authors read and approved the final manuscript.

Acknowledgments: The authors want to acknowledge the parents and children who participated in the study and also Ordesa laboratories, S.L. Barcelona, Spain. We are also grateful to personnel, scientists, staff and all people involved in the COGNIS team who have made this research possible.

References

1. Abedi, E.; Sahari, M.A. Long-chain polyunsaturated fatty acid sources and evaluation of their nutritional and functional properties. *Food Sci. Nutr.* **2014**, *2*, 443–463. [CrossRef]
2. Richard, C.; Lewis, E.D.; Field, C.J. Evidence for the essentiality of arachidonic and docosahexaenoic acid in the postnatal maternal and infant diet for the development of the infant's immune system early in life. *Appl. Physiol. Nutr. Metab.* **2016**, *41*, 461–475. [CrossRef] [PubMed]
3. Koletzko, B. Human milk lipids. *Ann. Nutr. Metab.* **2017**, *69*, 28–40. [CrossRef] [PubMed]
4. Grote, V.; Verduci, E.; Scaglioni, S.; Vecchi, F.; Contarini, G.; Giovannini, M.; Koletzko, B.; Agostoni, C. Breast milk composition and infant nutrient intakes during the first 12 months of life. *Eur. J. Clin. Nutr.* **2015**, *70*, 1–7. [CrossRef]
5. World Health Organization How to Prepare Powdered Infant Formula in Care Settings Formula Is Not Sterile. Available online: http://www.who.int/foodsafety/publications/micro/PIF_Care_en.pdf (accessed on 20 August 2008).
6. Brenna, J.T.; Varamini, B.; Jensen, R.G.; Diersen-schade, D.A.; Boettcher, J.A.; Arterburn, L.M. Docosahexaenoic and arachidonic acid concentrations in humanbreast milk worldwide. *Am. J. Clin. Nutr.* **2007**, *85*, 1457–1464. [CrossRef]
7. Scientific opinion on the essential composition of infant and follow-on formulae. *EFSA J.* **2014**, *1212*. [CrossRef]
8. European Union Law Reglamento Delegado (UE) 2016/127 de la Comisión, de 25 de Septiembre de 2015, que Complementa el Reglamento (UE) n° 609/2013 del Parlamento Europeo y del Consejo en lo que Respecta a Los Requisitos Específicos de Composición e Información Aplicables a lo. Available online: https://eur-lex.europa.eu/legal-content/es/TXT/?uri=CELEX:32016R0127 (accesed on 11 March 2019).
9. Liao, K.; Mccandliss, B.D.; Carlson, S.E.; Colombo, J.; Shaddy, D.J.; Kerling, E.H.; Lepping, R.J.; Sittiprapaporn, W.; Cheatham, C.L.; Gustafson, K.M. Event-related potential differences in children supplemented with long-chain polyunsaturated fatty acids during infancy. *Dev. Sci.* **2016**, 1–16. [CrossRef]
10. Birch, E.E.; Garfield, S.; Hoffman, D.R.; Uauy, R.; Birch, D.G. A randomized controlled trial of early dietary supply of long-chain polyunsaturated fatty acids and mental development in term infants. *Dev. Med. Child Neurol.* **2000**, *42*, 174–181. [CrossRef]
11. CI, J.; Kiliaan, A.J. Long-chain polyunsaturated fatty acids (LCPUFA) from genesis to senescence: The influence of LCPUFA on neural development, aging, and neurodegeneration. *Prog. Lipid Res.* **2014**, *53*, 1–17. [CrossRef]
12. Demmelmair, H.; Baumheuer, M.; Koletzko, B.; Dokoupil, K.; Kratl, G. Metabolism of U13C-labeled linoleic acid in lactating women. *J. Lipid Res.* **1998**, *39*, 1389–1396. [PubMed]
13. Schaeffer, L.; Gohlke, H.; Müller, M.; Heid, I.M.; Palmer, L.J.; Kompauer, I.; Demmelmair, H.; Illig, T.; Koletzko, B.; Heinrich, J. Common genetic variants of the FADS1 FADS2 gene cluster and their reconstructed haplotypes are associated with the fatty acid composition in phospholipids. *Hum. Mol. Genet.* **2006**, *15*, 1745–1756. [CrossRef] [PubMed]
14. Glaser, C.; Heinrich, J.; Koletzko, B. Role of FADS1 and FADS2 polymorphisms in polyunsaturated fatty acid metabolism. *Metabolism.* **2010**, *59*, 993–999. [CrossRef] [PubMed]
15. Glaser, C.; Lattka, E.; Rzehak, P.; Steer, C.; Koletzko, B. Genetic variation in polyunsaturated fatty acid metabolism and its potential relevance for human development and health. *Matern. Child Nutr.* **2011**, *7*, 27–40. [CrossRef]

16. Lattka, E.; Illig, T.; Koletzko, B.; Heinrich, J. Genetic variants of the FADS1 FADS2 gene cluster as related to essential fatty acid metabolism. *Curr. Opin. Lipidol.* **2010**, *21*, 64–69. [CrossRef] [PubMed]

17. Rzehak, P.; Thijs, C.; Standl, M.; Mommers, M.; Glaser, C.; Jansen, E.; Klopp, N.; Koppelman, G.H.; Singmann, P.; Postma, D.S.; et al. Variants of the FADS1 FADS2 gene cluster, blood levels of polyunsaturated fatty acids and eczema in children within the first 2 years of life. *PLoS ONE* **2010**, *5*, e13261. [CrossRef]

18. Zhang, J.Y.; Qin, X.; Liang, A.; Kim, E.; Lawrence, P.; Park, W.J.; Kothapalli, K.S.D.; Thomas Brenna, J. Fads3 modulates docosahexaenoic acid in liver and brain. *Prostaglandins Leukot Essent Fat. Acids* **2017**, *123*, 25–32. [CrossRef] [PubMed]

19. Fahmida, U.; Htet, M.K.; Adhiyanto, C.; Kolopaking, R.; Yudisti, M.A.; Maududi, A.; Suryandari, D.A.; Dillon, D.; Afman, L.; Müller, M. Genetic variants of FADS gene cluster, plasma LC-PUFA levels and the association with cognitive function of under-two-year-old Sasaknese Indonesian children. *Asia Pac. J. Clin. Nutr.* **2015**, *24*, 323–328. [CrossRef]

20. Morales, E.; Bustamante, M.; Gonzalez, J.R.; Guxens, M.; Torrent, M.; Mendez, M.; Garcia-Esteban, R.; Julvez, J.; Forns, J.; Vrijheid, M.; et al. Genetic variants of the FADS gene cluster and ELOVL gene family, colostrums LC-PUFA levels, breastfeeding, and child cognition. *PLoS ONE* **2011**, *6*, e17181. [CrossRef] [PubMed]

21. Lattka, E.; Illig, T.; Heinrich, J.; Koletzko, B. Do FADS genotypes enhance our knowledge about fatty acid related phenotypes? *Clin. Nutr.* **2010**, *29*, 277–287. [CrossRef] [PubMed]

22. Baylin, A.; Ruiz-narvaez, E.; Kraft, P.; Campos, H. α-Linolenic acid, Δ6-desaturase gene polymorphism, and the risk of nonfatal myocardial infarction. *Am. J. Clin. Nutr.* **2007**, *85*, 554–560. [CrossRef] [PubMed]

23. Moltó-Puigmartí, C.; Plat, J.; Mensink, R.P.; Müller, A.; Jansen, E.; Zeegers, M.P.; Thijs, C. FADS1 FADS2 gene variants modify the association between fish intake and the docosahexaenoic acid proportions in human milk. *Am. J. Clin. Nutr.* **2010**, *91*, 1368–1376. [CrossRef] [PubMed]

24. Gieger, C.; Geistlinger, L.; Altmaier, E.; De Angelis, M.H.; Kronenberg, F.; Meitinger, T.; Mewes, H.W.; Wichmann, H.E.; Weinberger, K.M.; Adamski, J.; et al. Genetics meets metabolomics: A genome-wide association study of metabolite profiles in human serum. *PLoS Genet.* **2008**, *4*, e1000282. [CrossRef] [PubMed]

25. Aulchenko, Y.S.; Ripatti, S.; Lindqvist, I.; Boomsma, D.; Iris, M. Europe PMC funders group loci influencing lipid levels and coronary heart disease risk in 16 european population cohorts. *Nat Genet.* **2009**, *41*, 47–55. [CrossRef] [PubMed]

26. Jensen, H.A.R.; Harsløf, L.B.S.; Nielsen, M.S.; Christensen, L.B.; Ritz, C.; Michaelsen, K.F.; Vogel, U.; Lauritzen, L. FADS single-nucleotide polymorphisms are associated with behavioral outcomes in children, and the effect varies between sexes and is dependent on PPAR genotype. *Am. J. Clin. Nutr.* **2014**, *100*, 826–832. [CrossRef] [PubMed]

27. Molto-Puigmarti, C.; Jansen, E.; Heinrich, J.; Standl, M.; Mensink, R.P.; Plat, J.; Penders, J.; Mommers, M.; Koppelman, G.H.; Postma, D.S.; et al. Genetic variation in FADS genes and plasma cholesterol levels in 2-year-old infants: KOALA birth cohort study. *PLoS ONE* **2013**, *8*, e61671. [CrossRef]

28. Standl, M.; Sausenthaler, S.; Lattka, E.; Koletzko, S.; Bauer, C.P.; Wichmann, H.E.; von Berg, A.; Berdel, D.; Krämer, U.; Schaaf, B.; et al. FADS gene variants modulate the effect of dietary fatty acid intake on allergic diseases in children. *Clin. Exp. Allergy* **2011**, *41*, 1757–1766. [CrossRef] [PubMed]

29. Lepping, R.J.; Honea, R.A.; Martin, L.E.; Liao, K.; Choi, I.-Y.; Lee, P.; Papa, V.B.; Brooks, W.M.; Shaddy, D.J.; Carlson, S.E.; et al. Long-chain polyunsaturated fatty acid supplementation in the first year of life affects brain function, structure, and metabolism at age nine years. *Dev. Psychobiol.* **2018**, 1–12. [CrossRef]

30. de la Garza Puentes, A.; Montes Goyanes, R.; Chisaguano Tonato, A.M.; Castellote, A.I.; Moreno-Torres, R.; Campoy Folgoso, C.; López-Sabater, M.C. Evaluation of less invasive methods to assess fatty acids from phospholipid fraction: Cheek cell and capillary blood sampling. *Int. J. Food Sci. Nutr.* **2015**, *66*, 936–942. [CrossRef] [PubMed]

31. Bondia, E.M.; Castellote, A.I.; Lopez, M.; Rivero, M. Determination of plasma fatty acid composition gas chromatography in neonates by gas chromatography. *J. Chromatogr. B* **1994**, *4347*, 369–374. [CrossRef]

32. Hong, S.H.; Kwak, J.H. Association of polymorphisms in FADS gene with age-related changes in serum phospholipid polyunsaturated fatty acids and oxidative stress markers in middle-aged nonobese men. *Clin. Interv. Aging* **2013**, *13*, 585–596.

33. Cormier, H.; Rudkowska, I.; Thifault, E.; Lemieux, S.; Couture, P.; Vohl, M.C. Polymorphisms in Fatty Acid Desaturase (FADS) gene cluster: Effects on glycemic controls following an omega-3 Polyunsaturated Fatty Acids (PUFA) supplementation. *Genes (Basel)* **2013**, *4*, 485–498. [CrossRef] [PubMed]

34. Harsløf, L.B.S.; Larsen, L.H.; Ritz, C.; Hellgren, L.I.; Michaelsen, K.F.; Vogel, U.; Lauritzen, L. FADS genotype and diet are important determinants of DHA status: A cross-sectional study in Danish infants. *Am. J. Clin. Nutr.* **2013**, *97*, 1403–1410. [CrossRef] [PubMed]

35. Groen-blokhuis, M.M.; Franic, S.; Van Beijsterveldt, C.E.M.; De Geus, E.; Bartels, M.; Davies, G.E.; Ehli, E.A.; Xiao, X.; Scheet, P.A.; Althoff, R.; et al. Neuropsychiatric Genetics A Prospective Study of the Effects of Breastfeeding and FADS2 Polymorphisms on Cognition and Hyperactivity/Attention Problems. *Am. J. Med. Genet.* **2013**, *162*, 457–465. [CrossRef] [PubMed]

36. Al-hilal, M.; Alsaleh, A.; Maniou, Z.; Lewis, F.J.; Hall, W.L.; Sanders, T.A.B.; Dell, S.D.O. Genetic variation at the FADS1-FADS2 gene locus infl uences delta-5 desaturase activity and LC-PUFA proportions after fi sh oil supplement. *J. Lipid Res.* **2013**, *54*, 542–551. [CrossRef] [PubMed]

37. Gillingham, L.G.; Harding, S.V.; Rideout, T.C.; Yurkova, N.; Cunnane, S.C.; Eck, P.K.; Jones, P.J.H. Dietary oils and FADS1–FADS2 genetic variants modulate [^{13}C]α-linolenic acid metabolism and plasma fatty acid composition. *Am. J. Clin. Nutr.* **2013**, *97*, 195–207. [CrossRef] [PubMed]

38. One, Y.S.; Ido, T.K.; Inuki, T.A.; Onoda, M.S.; Chi, I.I. Genetic variants of the fatty acid desaturase gene cluster are associated with plasma LDL cholesterol levels in japanese males. *J. Nutr. Sci. Vitaminol.* **2013**, *59*, 325–335.

39. Colombo, J.; Carlson, S.E.; Cheatham, C.L.; Fitzgerald-gustafson, K.M.; Kepler, A.; Doty, T. Long Chain Polyunsaturated Fatty Acid Supplementation in Infancy Reduces Heart Rate and Positively Affects Distribution of Attention. *Pediatr. Res.* **2012**, *70*, 406–410. [CrossRef]

40. Carlson, S.E.; Colombo, J. Docosahexaenoic Acid and Arachidonic Acid Nutrition in Early Development. *Adv. Pediatr.* **2016**, *63*, 453–471. [CrossRef]

41. Uhl, O.; Fleddermann, M.; Hellmuth, C.; Demmelmair, H.; Koletzko, B. Phospholipid species in newborn and 4 month old infants after consumption of different formulas or breast milk. *PLoS ONE* **2016**, *11*, e0162040. [CrossRef]

42. Jakobik, V.; Weck, M.; Weyermann, M.; Grallert, H.; Lattka, E.; Rzehak, P. Genetic variants in the FADS gene cluster are associated with arachidonic acid concentrations of human breast milk at 1.5 and 6 mo postpartum and influence the course of milk dodecanoic, tetracosenoic, and trans-9-octadecenoic acid concentrations. *Am. J. Clin. Nutr.* **2011**, *93*, 382–391. [CrossRef]

43. Wu, Y.; Zeng, L.; Chen, X.; Xu, Y.; Ye, L.; Qin, L.; Chen, L.; Xie, L. Association of the FADS gene cluster with coronary artery disease and plasma lipid concentrations in the northern Chinese Han population. *Prostaglandins Leukot. Essent. Fat. Acids* **2017**, *117*, 11–16. [CrossRef] [PubMed]

44. Hester, A.G.; Murphy, R.C.; Uhlson, C.J.; Ivester, P.; Lee, T.C.; Sergeant, S.; Miller, L.R.; Howard, T.D.; Mathias, R.A.; Chilton, F.H. Relationship between a common variant in the fatty acid desaturase (FADS) cluster and eicosanoid generation in humans. *J. Biol. Chem.* **2014**, *289*, 22482–22489. [CrossRef] [PubMed]

45. Martinelli, N.; Girelli, D.; Malerba, G.; Guarini, P.; Illig, T.; Trabetti, E.; Sandri, M.; Friso, S.; Pizzolo, F.; Schaeffer, L.; et al. FADS genotypes and desaturase activity estimated by the ratio of arachidonic acid to linoleic acid are associated with inflammation and coronary artery disease. *Am. J. Clin. Nutr.* **2008**, *88*, 941–949. [CrossRef]

46. Zietemann, V.; Kröger, J.; Enzenbach, C.; Jansen, E.; Fritsche, A.; Weikert, C.; Boeing, H.; Schulze, M.B. Genetic variation of the FADS1 FADS2 gene cluster and n-6 PUFA composition in erythrocyte membranes in the European Prospective Investigation into Cancer and Nutrition-Potsdam study. *Br. J. Nutr.* **2010**, *104*, 1748–1759. [CrossRef]

47. Meldrum, S.J.; Li, Y.; Zhang, G.; Heaton, A.E.M.; D'Vaz, N.; Manz, J.; Reischl, E.; Koletzko, B.V.; Prescott, S.L.; Simmer, K. Can polymorphisms in the fatty acid desaturase (FADS) gene cluster alter the effects of fish oil supplementation on plasma and erythrocyte fatty acid profiles? An exploratory study. *Eur. J. Nutr.* **2017**, 1–12. [CrossRef] [PubMed]

48. Koletzko, B.; Lattka, E.; Zeilinger, S.; Illig, T.; Steer, C. Genetic variants of the fatty acid desaturase gene cluster predict amounts of red blood cell docosahexaenoic and other polyunsaturated fatty acids in pregnant women: Findings from the Avon Longitudinal Study of Parents and Children. *Am. J. Nutr.* **2011**, *93*, 211–219. [CrossRef] [PubMed]

49. Barman, M.; Nilsson, S.; Naluai, Å.T.; Sandin, A.; Wold, A.E.; Sandberg, A.S. Single nucleotide polymorphisms in the FADS gene cluster but not the ELOVL2 gene are associated with serum polyunsaturated fatty acid composition and development of allergy (in a Swedish birth cohort). *Nutrients* **2015**, *7*, 10100–10115. [CrossRef] [PubMed]

50. Ding, Z.; Liu, G.-L.; Li, X.; Chen, X.-Y.; Wu, Y.-X.; Cui, C.-C.; Zhang, X.; Yang, G.; Xie, L. Association of polyunsaturated fatty acids in breast milk with fatty acid desaturase gene polymorphisms among Chinese lactating mothers. *Prostaglandins Leukot. Essent. Fat. Acids* **2016**, *109*, 66–71. [CrossRef]

51. Hellstrand, S.; Ericson, U.; Gullberg, B.; Hedblad, B.; Orho-melander, M.; Sonestedt, E. Genetic Variation in FADS1 Has Little Effect on the Association between Dietary PUFA Intake and Cardiovascular Disease. *J. Nutr.* **2014**, *144*, 1356–1363. [CrossRef]

52. Roke, K.; Mutch, D.M. The role of FADS1/2 polymorphisms on cardiometabolic markers and fatty acid profiles in young adults consuming fish oil supplements. *Nutrients* **2014**, *6*, 2290–2304. [CrossRef]

53. Miklavcic, J.J.; Larsen, B.M.K.; Mazurak, V.C.; Scalabrin, D.M.F.; MacDonald, I.M.; Shoemaker, G.K.; Casey, L.; Van Aerde, J.E.; Clandinin, M.T. Reduction of Arachidonate Is Associated With Increase in B-Cell Activation Marker in Infants: A Randomized Trial. *J. Pediatr. Gastroenterol. Nutr.* **2017**, *64*, 446–453. [CrossRef] [PubMed]

54. Schwartz, J.; Drossard, C.; Dube, K.; Kannenberg, F.; Kunz, C.; Kalhoff, H.; Kersting, M. Dietary intake and plasma concentrations of PUFA and LC-PUFA in breastfed and formula fed infants under real-life conditions. *Eur. J. Nutr.* **2010**, *49*, 189–195. [CrossRef] [PubMed]

55. Michaelsen, K.F.; Skafte, L.; Badsberg, J.H.; Jørgensen, M. Variation in macronutrients in human bank milk: Influencing factors and implications for human milk banking. *J. Pediatr. Gastroenterol. Nutr.* **1990**, *11*, 229–239. [CrossRef]

56. Stam, J.; Sauer, P.J.; Boehm, G. Can we define an infant's need from the composition of human milk? *Am. J. Clin. Nutr.* **2013**, *98*, 521S–528S. [CrossRef]

57. Moon, Y.-A.; Hammer, R.E.; Horton, J.D. Deletion of ELOVL5 leads to fatty liver through activation of SREBP-1c in mice. *J. Lipid Res.* **2009**, *50*, 412–423. [CrossRef]

58. Hallmann, J.; Kolossa, S.; Gedrich, K.; Celis-Morales, C.; Forster, H.; O'Donovan, C.B.; Woolhead, C.; Macready, A.L.; Fallaize, R.; Marsaux, C.F.M.; et al. Predicting fatty acid profiles in blood based on food intake and the FADS1 rs174546 SNP. *Mol. Nutr. Food Res.* **2015**, *59*, 2565–2573. [CrossRef] [PubMed]

59. Field, C.J.; Van Aerde, J.E.; Robinson, L.E.; Clandinin, M.T. Effect of providing a formula supplemented with long-chain polyunsaturated fatty acids on immunity in full-term neonates. *Br. J. Nutr.* **2008**, *99*, 91–99. [CrossRef] [PubMed]

60. Ward, G.R.; Huang, Y.S.; Bobik, E.; Xing, H.C.; Mutsaers, L.; Auestad, N.; Montalto, M.; Wainwright, P. Long-chain polyunsaturated fatty acid levels in formulae influence deposition of docosahexaenoic acid and arachidonic acid in brain and red blood cells of artificially reared neonatal rats. *J. Nutr.* **1998**, *128*, 2473–2487. [CrossRef] [PubMed]

61. Janssen, C.I.F.; Zerbi, V.; Mutsaers, M.P.C.; de Jong, B.S.W.; Wiesmann, M.; Arnoldussen, I.A.C.; Geenen, B.; Heerschap, A.; Muskiet, F.A.J.; Jouni, Z.E.; et al. Impact of dietary n-3 polyunsaturated fatty acids on cognition, motor skills and hippocampal neurogenesis in developing C57BL/6J mice. *J. Nutr. Biochem.* **2015**, *26*, 24–35. [CrossRef] [PubMed]

62. Lauritzen, L.; Sørensen, L.B.; Harsløf, L.B.; Ritz, C.; Stark, K.D.; Astrup, A.; Dyssegaard, C.B.; Egelund, N.; Michaelsen, K.F.; Damsgaard, C.T. Mendelian randomization shows sex-specific associations between long-chain PUFA-related genotypes and cognitive performance in Danish schoolchildren. *Am. J. Clin. Nutr.* **2017**, *106*, 88–95. [CrossRef]

12

Point of Care Quantitative Assessment of Muscle Health in Older Individuals: An Investigation of Quantitative Muscle Ultrasound and Electrical Impedance Myography Techniques

Lisa D Hobson-Webb [1,*], **Paul J Zwelling** [1], **Ashley N Pifer** [1], **Carrie M Killelea** [2,3], **Mallory S Faherty** [2,3], **Timothy C Sell** [2,3] and **Amy M Pastva** [2,4]

[1] Duke University Department of Neurology/Neuromuscular Division, Durham, NC 27710, USA; paul.zwelling@duke.edu (P.J.Z.); ashley.pifer@duke.edu (A.N.P.)

[2] Duke University Department of Orthopaedic Surgery, Durham, NC 27710, USA; carolyn.killelea@duke.edu (C.M.K.); mallory.faherty@duke.edu (M.S.F.); tcs30@duke.edu (T.C.S.); amy.pastva@duke.edu (A.M.P.)

[3] Michael W. Krzyzewski Human Performance Laboratory, Durham, NC 27710, USA

[4] Duke University Claude D. Pepper Older American Independence Center Durham, NC 27710, USA

* Correspondence: lisa.hobsonwebb@duke.edu

Abstract: *Background:* Muscle health is recognized for its critical role in the functionality and well-being of older adults. Readily accessible, reliable, and inexpensive methods of measuring muscle health are needed to advance research and clinical care. *Methods:* In this prospective, blinded study, 27 patients underwent quantitative muscle ultrasound (QMUS), standard electrical impedance myography (sEIM), and handheld electrical impedance myography (hEIM) of the anterior thigh musculature by two independent examiners. Subjects also had dual-energy X-ray absorptiometry (DEXA) scans and standardized tests of physical function and strength. Data were analyzed for intra- and inter-rater reliability, along with correlations with DEXA and physical measures. *Results:* Measures of intra- and inter-rater reliability were excellent (>0.90) for all QMUS, sEIM, and hEIM parameters except intra-rater reliability of rectus femoris echointensity (0.87–0.89). There were moderate, inverse correlations between QMUS, sEIM, and hEIM parameters and measures of knee extensor strength. Moderate to strong correlations (0.57–0.81) were noted between investigational measures and DEXA-measured fat mass. *Conclusions:* QMUS, sEIM and hEIM were highly reliable in a controlled, same-day testing protocol. Multiple correlations with measures of strength and body composition were noted for each method. Point-of-care technologies may provide an alternative means of measuring health.

Keywords: elderly; aging; muscle; ultrasound; electrical impedance myography; point of care; TUG; frailty

1. Introduction

Muscle health is recognized for its critical role in the well-being and functionality of older adults [1]. Aging is associated with loss of muscle mass, known as sarcopenia, and loss of muscle quality, manifesting as replacement of healthy muscle tissue by adipose and water. Both have been associated with limitations in physical activity and function, including the performance of routine activities of daily required for independent living [2,3]. To date, muscle health assessment has primarily focused on muscle quantity; however, this assessment alone may overestimate the amount of functional muscle. Computed tomography (CT), magnetic resonance imaging (MRI), and dual energy X-ray absorptiometry (DEXA) scans are gold standard measures used to assess the quantity and quality of muscle [4]. CT has most frequently been used to assess fatty infiltration of muscle, which manifests as a reduced attenuation coefficient [5]. However, given that these scans are expensive, not readily accessible in the outpatient or community setting, or well-suited for home use, there is a need for novel means of measuring muscle health for both clinical and research purposes.

Ultrasound provides a rapid, non-invasive, portable and inexpensive means of evaluating muscle. Although new approaches, including shear wave elastography, are being investigated, measures of muscle size and signal are traditionally used. Muscle size is often expressed as thickness or cross-sectional area of the muscle, while signal is described in terms of echointensity (EI). As expected, reduced muscle size at select sites has been linked to an overall reduction in muscle mass. Studied primarily in disease states, elevated EI represents increased intramuscular fibrous composition and generally correlates with worsening muscle health [6]. Other factors that can affect EI include ultrasound system settings, aging, sex and level of conditioning, making its interpretation somewhat challenging [7,8].

A number of recent studies have explored the role of quantitative muscle ultrasound (QMUS) in the critically ill, but less is known about the role of muscle health in community-dwelling elderly individuals [9,10]. An early study of 92 elderly Japanese patients demonstrated moderate inverse correlations between EI and quadriceps strength among middle-aged and elderly individuals, independent of age or muscle thickness [11]. More recently, Mirón Mombiela et al. examined EI as biomarker of frailty in a study of patients aged 20 to 90 years [12]. The group found, similar to the aforementioned study, moderate, inverse correlations between EI and quadriceps strength. Higher EI values were also associated with greater frailty.

Electrical impedance myography (EIM) is another technology receiving recent attention for measurement of muscle health. Differing EIM devices are available, but the basic principle is that these systems measure the muscle impedance to flow of a painless, electrical current. Impedance is not very high in healthy muscle but is known to increase in conditions that impact normal muscle architecture [13]. Prior studies in amyotrophic lateral sclerosis (ALS) and Duchenne muscular dystrophy (DMD) demonstrate the promise of this technique [14–16]. Unlike imaging studies, EIM can be performed with little training. It is portable and hand-held devices are available. The equipment is inexpensive; some consumer-marketed devices are available for less than US $100. These advantages are appealing, but data on reliability, longitudinal change, correlation with established measures of strength, and the impact of patient positioning, hydration and many other factors are lacking.

Given the need for improved muscle health data and the advantages of QMUS and EIM, the current study was designed to investigate the feasibility of using both technologies in the community-dwelling elderly. The aims of the current study were to determine the inter-rater reliability and reproducibility of QMUS and EIM. In addition, we examined the correlations between QMUS, EIM and currently accepted measures of physical strength, physical function, and muscle mass. The findings demonstrate that both QMUS and EIM are reliable tools that correlate with functional and DEXA measures.

2. Materials and Methods

2.1. Research Cohort

The Duke Institutional Review Board approved the current study (Duke IRB Protocol 00076633). Twenty-seven subjects were recruited through use of the Pepper Center (Duke IRB Protocol 00016209)/Duke Aging Center Subject Registry (Duke IRB Pro00005016) from January to December 2017. Subjects were recruited through letters sent to individuals that had previously consented to being listed in the Duke Aging Center Subject Registry. Flyers were also posted at geriatric clinics and in physical therapy clinics around campus. Interested subjects replied to the study coordinator to learn more about the study before the informed consent process took place.

Inclusion criteria were age >65 years and the ability to provide informed consent. Those unable to provide informed consent were excluded. Patients with known active malignancy, myositis, motor neuron disease, inability to ambulate independently or taking daily steroids were also excluded as these factors can affect muscle bulk rapidly.

Upon providing informed consent to participate in the study, subjects underwent testing (estimated time involvement 3–4 h) over 1–2 site visits. All study activities were completed within a 7-day period. QMUS and EIM were performed on the same day for all patients studied.

2.2. Investigational Techniques

2.2.1. Quantitative Muscle Ultrasonography (QMUS)

QMUS of the right rectus femoris and vastus intermedius complex was performed at one-third the distance between the patella and anterior superior iliac spine. The subject was positioned at rest in the supine position with the knee in passive extension. Two independent examiners (LHW, PJZ) each collected three separate images at this site. LHW is a neurologist with 14 years of experience in neuromuscular ultrasound, while PJZ is an electrodiagnostic technician trained to perform muscle ultrasound for the purpose of the current study. PJZ had 2 weeks of training prior to study initiation, provided by LHW. The examiners were blinded to the results of each other's imaging and other study results.

A Esaote MyLabSIX Ultrasound system was used, equipped with a 6–18 MHz linear array probe. Probe frequency was held at 6 MHz with constant gain, compression, and time gain compensation settings. Depth was adjusted as needed to accommodate the size of the patient imaged. Ultrasound data were digitally stored in the ultrasound system and processed off-line after each subject's visit was complete.

Both examiners performed off-line independent, analysis of images. Subcutaneous fat thickness was calculated by measuring the distance from the skin surface to the superficial fascia of the muscles using on-screen calipers. Thickness of the rectus femoris and vastus intermedius was then measured in a similar manner using the femoral border and muscle fascia as landmarks. EI was measured by exporting the still images to Adobe Photoshop (Adobe Systems Incorporated, San Jose, CA, USA) for gray scale analysis scoring. The gray scale ranges from 0 to 255 (0 = black, 255 = white). A region of interest (ROI) was drawn as large as possible for each muscle, making effort to exclude fascial borders, bone and any artifact present in the image. As each examiner generated three measurements for each parameter recorded, the mean was calculated for thickness, while the mean, standard deviation, and median were calculated for gray scale scoring.

2.2.2. Electrical Impedance Myography (EIM)—Standard Equipment (sEIM)

sEIM was performed over the right rectus femoris/vastus intermedius complex, as outlined in the QMUS section. sEIM was conducted with a device (SFB7 Impedimed, Inc., Pinkenba, Australia) previously used in the assessment of neuromuscular disease. The device provides a painless, surface alternating current over muscle with four adhesive electrodes placed across the muscle for recording. Measurements were taken over the muscles' axial plane, which is the accepted standard. Three measures each of resistance (R) and reactance (Xc) and phase (θ) were recorded for each muscle at 50 kHz and 200 kHz then averaged for the mean value of each. The subjects had sEIM performed by two independent examiners (LHW, PJZ), creating two complete sets of measures. Neither examiner had experience with this device prior to the current study and were self-trained using the company provided instructional materials. The examiners were blinded to the results of each other's testing and other study results.

2.2.3. Electrical Impedance Myography (hEIM)-Handheld Device

A handheld, portable, commercially available fitness tracker device was used (Chisel, Skulpt, Inc., San Franscisco, CA, USA). This smart-phone sized device uses the same methods as previously described for sEIM but has incorporated fixed electrodes and provides users with both a body fat measurement for each muscle assessed, as well as a Muscle Quality (MQ) score derived from raw EIM data. The frequencies used with the handheld system are proprietary and cannot be selected or altered by the user. MQ is derived from resistance and reactance measures, but the values are not available on the commercial display. The MQ scale ranges from 0 to 100, with 100 being the best score possible. The scoring system is as follows: 0–20 Needs Work, 20–40 Good, 60–80 Fit, and 80–100 Athletic.

The hEIM electrodes on the device were moistened with water and then placed over the right rectus femoris/vastus intermedius complex for approximately 5 s, while measurements were made. The subjects had three hEIM measurements performed by two independent clinicians (LHW, PJZ). Neither examiner had experience with this device prior to the current study and were self-trained using the company provided instructional materials. The examiners were blinded to the results of each other's testing and other study results.

2.2.4. Standard Clinical Measures

Age, sex, height, and weight were recorded for each subject on the day of their first study visit.

2.2.5. Lower Extremity Strength and Physical Function Testing

Quantitative testing of lower extremity strength was performed by personnel at the Duke Sports Science Institute's Michael W. Krzyzewski Human Performance Lab, under the direction of authors (AMP, TCS, MSF, CMK). Personnel were blinded to other study results.

An isokinetic dynamometer (Biodex System 3 Multi-Joint Testing and Rehabilitation System, White Plains, NY, USA) was used to measure leg strength and data were assessed using the system's proprietary software. The test protocol was maintained for all subjects as follows: concentric (CON) at 180°/s and isometric (ISO) at 0°/s at a ~60° knee angle. Subjects were placed in a comfortable, seated position on the Biodex System 3 chair and secured using thigh, pelvic and torso straps in order to minimize accessory body movements and isolate performance at the knee. The lateral femoral epicondyle was used as the bony landmark for aligning the axis of rotation of the knee joint with the axis of rotation of the dynamometer axis. Subjects were provided a warm-up session of three repetitions at 50% of maximum effort and three repetitions at 100% of maximum effort for both the ISO and CON tests. A one-minute rest period was provided prior to the actual testing and between the two different test modes (ISO and CON). Subjects were instructed to give maximum effort throughout the entire test. For the CON test, five maximal quadriceps contractions at 180°/s were performed. For the ISO test, the leg was flexed to 60°. Subjects completed five repetitions (5-s hold for each rep) with 10 s of rest between repetitions. The Timed Up and Go test (TUG) was included as a standardized and validated physical function task measure in older adults. The test measures the time taken to arise from a chair, walk three meters, turn around, walk back to the chair, and sit down.

2.2.6. Imaging Studies

Whole-body dual energy X-ray absorptiometry (DEXA) was performed on all subjects and considered to be the gold standard for muscle mass and fat calculations of the proximal right lower extremity (thigh). Staff radiologists blinded to other study results interpreted the DEXA scans.

2.3. Data Analysis

Study data were collected and managed using REDCap electronic data capture tools hosted at Duke University. REDCap (Research Electronic Data Capture) is a secure, web-based application designed to support data capture for research studies, providing (1) an intuitive interface for validated data entry; (2) audit trails for tracking data manipulation and export procedures; (3) automated export procedures for seamless data downloads to common statistical packages; and (4) procedures for importing data from external sources.

QMUS and EIM measures were analyzed for inter-rater reliability as measured by the InterClass correlation. Intra-rater reliability was also assessed. For QMUS, muscle thickness, subcutaneous fat thickness and muscle EI were examined for correlation with patient demographics, DEXA measures of muscle mass, and the results of isokinetic and isometric testing. For sEIM, the impedance measures were analyzed for correlation with the same set of clinical measures. For the hEIM, the correlation between clinical measures and both the MQ score and muscle fat percentage were assessed.

Statistical significance was set at $p \leq 0.05$, while a trend is defined as $p = 0.051\text{--}0.10$.

3. Results

Twenty-seven volunteers were recruited and enrolled for the study. No participants were excluded upon contact with the study coordinator. The cohort was 70% male with mean age of 72.6 years. More detailed demographics and details on the absolute QMUS values are shown in Table 1. For each subject, all testing was completed within a 7-day window. QMUS and EIM were always performed on the same day and examiner 1 and 2's measurements were separated by a period of at least 15 min.

Table 1. Subject demographics and group quantitative muscle ultrasound (QMUS) results.

Male/Female	19 (70%)/8 (30%)
Age (years)	72.6 ± 5 (range 65–82 years)
Height (cm)	172.2 ± 11 (range 152–200 cm)
Weight (kg)	83.3 kg ± 19 (range 52–131 kg)
BMI (kg/m^2)	28.1
Ultrasound Measurements	
Fat thickness (mm)	8.8 ± 7 (range 0.6–23.5)
RF thickness (mm)	13.7 ± 6 (range 1.2–23.5)
VI thickness (mm)	13.2 ± 6 (range 0.9–22.7)
Echointensity RF	94.16 ± 20 (range 68.8–167.5)
VI	62.6 ± 32 (range 10.3–121.2)

3.1. Intra- and Inter-Rater Reliability

Intra-and inter-rater reliability data for all investigational techniques are summarized in Table 2.

Table 2. Intra- and inter-rater reliability.

Test	Intra-Rater		Inter-Rater
	Examiner 1	**Examiner 2**	
QMUS			
SQ thickness	0.98 *	0.99 *	0.99 *
RF thickness	0.98 *	0.98 *	0.98 *
VI thickness	0.98 *	0.99 *	0.97 *
RF echointensity	0.89 *	0.87 *	0.94 *
VI echointensity	0.93 *	0.93 *	0.96 **
sEIM			
50 kHz R	1.0 *	1.0 *	1.0 *
50 kHz Xc	1.0 *	1.0 *	0.99 *
50 kHz θ	1.0 *	0.99 *	0.99 *
200 kHz R	1.0 *	1.0 *	1.0 *
200 kHz Xc	1.0 *	0.99 *	0.99 *
200 kHz θ	0.97 *	0.99 *	0.98 *
hEIM			
Fat %	0.99 *	0.99 *	0.98 *
Muscle Quality	0.99 *	0.99 *	0.98 *

hEIM: handheld electrical impedance myography; Hz: hertz; QMUS: quantitative muscle ultrasound; R: resistance; RF: rectus femoris; sEIM: standard electrical impedance myography; SQ: subcutaneous tissue; VI: vastus intermedius; Xc: reactance; θ = phase; *: $p < 0.0001$; **: $p = 0.005$.

3.1.1. QMUS

Intra-rater reliability for subcutaneous fat thickness was excellent ($r = 0.98$, $p < 0.0001$ for examiner 1 and $r = 0.99$, $p < 0.0001$ for examiner 2). Rectus femoris thickness reliability was high for both examiners ($r = 0.98$, $p < 0.0001$). Vastus intermedius thickness had good agreement ($r = 0.98$, $p < 0.0001$ for examiner 1 and $r = 0.99$, $p < 0.0001$ for examiner 2). Intra-rater reliability for rectus femoris echointensity was high for both examiners ($r = 0.89$, $p < 0.0001$ for examiner 1 and $r = 0.87$, $p < 0.0001$ for examiner 2). For vastus intermedius echointensity, intra-rater agreement was similar ($r = 0.93$, $p < 0.0001$ for examiner 1 and $r = 0.93$, $p < 0.0001$ for examiner 2).

Inter-rater reliability for subcutaneous fat thickness was excellent ($r = 0.99$, $p < 0.0001$). Rectus femoris and vastus intermedius thickness demonstrated similar results ($r = 0.98$, $p < 0.0001$ and $r = 0.97$, $p < 0.0001$, respectively). Unexpectedly, mean muscle echointensity measures for vastus intermedius had excellent agreement ($r = 0.96$, $p = 0.005$), as did rectus femoris ($r = 0.94$, $p < 0.0001$).

No significant differences between examiners were found for any QMUS parameter.

3.1.2. sEIM

Intra-rater reliability measures were extremely high for 50 kHz, which was not unexpected as all measures occurred within a one-second-measurement period that required no movement of electrodes. Examiner 1 performed well for R, Xc and θ. ($r = 1.0$, $p < 0.0001$). For examiner 2, R and Xc had extraordinary reliability ($r = 1.0$, $p < 0.0001$), with θ performing only slightly worse ($r = 0.99$, $p < 0.0001$). Examiner 1 intra-rater reliability at 200 kHz was the same for R and Xc ($r = 1.0$, $p < 0.0001$). There was slightly lower agreement for θ ($r = 0.97$, $p < 0.0001$) that appeared to be secondary to a single outlying value related to patient movement. For examiner 2, reliability was also high for R ($r = 1.0$, $p < 0.0001$), Xc ($r = 0.99$, $p < 0.0001$) and θ ($r = 0.99$, $p < 0.0001$).

Inter-rater measurements were separated by several minutes, but performed well. The 50-kHz sEIM had excellent inter-rater reliability for R ($r = 1.0$, $p < 0.0001$), Xc ($r = 0.99$, $p < 0.0001$) and θ ($r = 0.99$, $p < 0.0001$). For 200 Hz, measures were similar for R ($r = 1.0$, $p < 0.0001$), Xc ($r = 0.99$, $p < 0.0001$) and θ ($r = 0.98$, $p < 0.0001$). Please note that a single data point from subject 1, examiner 1 200 kHz Xc was excluded due to a data entry error and concerns over accuracy.

No significant differences were found between examiners for any sEIM parameter at either 50 or 200 kHz.

3.1.3. hEIM

hEIM performed well on intra-rater reliability measures. Examiner 1 performed well on muscle quality ($r = 0.99$, $p < 0.0001$) and muscle fat % ($r = 0.99$, $p < 0.0001$). Examiner 2 did just as well for muscle quality ($r = 0.99$, $p < 0.0001$) and muscle fat % ($r = 0.99$, $p < 0.0001$). Inter-rater reliability for muscle quality was excellent ($r = 0.98$, $p < 0.0001$), as was muscle fat % ($r = 0.98$, $p < 0.0001$). It is not surprising that the reliability was essentially identical for the two measures, given that they are inter-related and reported simultaneously. No significant differences were found between examiners for hEIM-measured muscle quality or muscle fat %.

3.2. Correlations

Detailed information on all correlations between investigational measures can be found in Tables 3 and 4.

Table 3. Correlations between test results and functional measures.

Test	Isometric Normalized Peak Torque	Isokinetic Normalized Peak Torque	Timed Up and Go (TUG)
QMUS			
SQ thickness	-0.56, $p = 0.002$	-0.50, $p = 0.08$	—
RF thickness	—	—	-0.37, $p = 0.06$
VI thickness	—	—	—
RF echointensity	-0.48, $p = 0.01$	—	—
VI echointensity	—	—	—
sEIM			
50 kHz R	-0.46, $p = 0.016$	—	—
50 kHz Xc	—	—	—
50 kHz θ	-0.45, $p = 0.02$	—	0.35, $p = 0.07$
200 kHz R	-0.57, $p = 0.01$	-0.53, $p = 0.01$	0.45, $p = 0.04$
200 kHz Xc	—	—	—
200 kHz θ	-0.54, $p = 0.01$	-0.51, $p = 0.02$	0.49, $p = 0.02$
50/200 kHz θ Ratio	—	—	—
200/50 kHz Phase Ratio	0.50, $p = 0.01$	0.44, $p = 0.027$	—
hEIM			
Fat %	-0.49, $p = 0.009$	—	—
Muscle Quality	—	—	—
DEXA			
Thigh muscle mass	—	—	—
Thigh fat mass	-0.52, $p = 0.005$	-0.39, $p = 0.04$	—

hEIM: handheld electrical impedance myography; Hz: hertz; QMUS: quantitative muscle ultrasound; R: resistance; RF: rectus femoris; sEIM: standard electrical impedance myography; SQ: subcutaneous tissue; VI: vastus intermedius; Xc: reactance; θ: phase; —: no significant correlations observed.

Table 4. Correlations between investigational tests and DEXA results.

Test	DEXA-Measured Right Thigh Fat Mass	DEXA-Measured Right Thigh Muscle Mass
QMUS		
SQ thickness	**0.81, $p < 0.0001$**	—
RF thickness	—	**0.53, $p = 0.0045$**
VI thickness	—	**0.54, $p = 0.004$**
RF echointensity	*0.35, $p = 0.07$*	*−0.33, $p = 0.09$*
VI echointensity	—	**−0.52, $p = 0.006$**
sEIM		
50 kHz R	**0.65, $p = 0.0003$**	—
50 kHz Xc	—	—
50 kHz θ	**0.57, $p = 0.002$**	*−0.37, $p = 0.06$*
200 kHz R	**0.70, $p < 0.0001$**	*−0.26, $p = 0.06$*
200 kHz Xc	—	**−0.46, $p = 0.016$**
200 kHz θ	**0.72, $p < 0.001$**	*−0.34, $p = 0.09$*
50/200 kHz θ Ratio	—	—
200/50 kHz θ Ratio	**−0.41, $p = 0.041$**	—
hEIM		
Fat %	**0.74, $p < 0.0001$**	**−0.38, $p = 0.0492$**
Muscle Quality	**−0.72, $p < 0.0001$**	—

hEIM: handheld electrical impedance myography; Hz: hertz; QMUS: quantitative muscle ultrasound; R: resistance; RF: rectus femoris; sEIM: standard electrical impedance myography; SQ: subcutaneous tissue; VI: vastus intermedius; Xc: capacitance; θ; phase; —: no significant correlations observed.

3.2.1. QMUS

Rectus femoris and vastus intermedius thickness did not correlate with isokinetic normalized peak torque. However, there was a negative correlation with subcutaneous fat thickness ($r = -0.50$, $p = 0.008$). The same pattern was evident for isometric normalized peak torque, with an inverse correlation present for subcutaneous fat thickness ($r = -0.56$, $p = 0.002$). TUG time trended toward a correlation with rectus femoris thickness ($r = -0.37$, $p = 0.06$), but there were no correlations with vastus intermedius or subcutaneous fat thickness.

Rectus femoris thickness correlated with DEXA measured right thigh muscle mass ($r = 0.53$, $p = 0.0045$), as did vastus intermedius thickness ($r = 0.54$, $p = 0.004$). There was no correlation observed with subcutaneous fat thickness. For DEXA measured right thigh fat mass, there was a strong correlation with subcutaneous fat thickness ($r = 0.81$, $p < 0.0001$). There were no correlations between DEXA measured right thigh fat mass and muscle thickness.

Muscle echointensity measures were also analyzed. Rectus femoris echointensity did not correlate with isokinetic normalized peak torque or TUG time, but did inversely correlate with isometric normalized peak torque ($r = -0.48$, $p = 0.01$). Vastus intermedius echointensity did not correlate with isokinetic normalized peak torque, isometric peak torque or TUG time. There was a trend between rectus femoris echointensity and DEXA-measured fat mass of the right leg ($r = 0.35$, $p = 0.07$) that was not seen for vastus intermedius. Similarly, a trend toward an inverse correlation between rectus femoris echointensity and DEXA-measured muscle mass of the right thigh was present ($r = -0.33$, $p = 0.09$). In addition, there was an inverse correlation between vastus intermedius echointensity and DEXA-measured muscle mass of the right thigh ($r = -0.52$, $p = 0.006$)

3.2.2. sEIM

At 50 kHz, moderate negative correlations were noted between isometric normalized peak torque of knee extension and R ($r = -0.46$, $p = 0.016$) and phase ($r = -0.45$, $p = 0.02$), but not for Xc. No correlations were observed between the 50 kHz measures and isokinetic normalized peak torque of knee extension. No significant correlations were found between the 50 kHz measures and TUG time, although a trend was seen for θ ($r = 0.35$, $p = 0.07$).

For DEXA measured right leg muscle mass and 50 kHz measures, there was a trend toward a negative correlation with θ ($r = -0.37$, $p = 0.06$), but not for R or Xc. For right leg fat mass, there were correlations with R ($r = 0.65$, $p = 0.0003$) and θ ($r = 0.57$, $p = 0.002$), but not Xc.

At 200 kHz, negative correlations were again noted between isometric normalized peak torque of knee extension and R ($r=-0.57$, $p = 0.01$), as well as θ ($r = -0.54$, $p = 0.01$), but not Xc. There were also negative correlations with isokinetic normalized peak torque of knee extension and R ($r = -0.53$, $p = 0.01$), as well as θ ($r = -0.51$, $p = 0.02$). There was no correlation between Xc and isokinetic normalized peak torque of the anterior quadriceps. For TUG time, there was a positive correlation with R ($r = 0.45$, $p = 0.04$) and θ ($r = 0.49$, $p = 0.02$), but not Xc.

For DEXA measured right leg muscle mass and 200 kHz measures, there was a moderate negative correlation with Xc ($r = -0.46$, $p = 0.016$). There was a trend toward a negative correlation with R ($r = -0.26$, $p = 0.06$) and θ ($r = -0.34$, $p = 0.09$). For right leg fat mass, there were correlations with R ($r = 0.70$, $p < 0.0001$) and θ ($r = 0.72$, $p < 0.001$), but not Xc.

Use of the 50/200 kHz phase ratio negated all correlations, while a 200/50 kHz θ ratio gave nearly identical results to the 50 and 200 kHz measures for correlation with functional testing (Table 3) but performed worse for correlation with DEXA-estimated thigh fat and muscle mass.

Based upon these observations, the 200 kHz setting correlated best with measures of physical function and body composition.

3.2.3. hEIM

There was no correlation between isokinetic normalized peak torque of the quadriceps and either MQ or muscle fat %. For isometric normalized peak torque, there was an inverse correlation with muscle fat % ($r = -0.49$, $p = 0.009$). TUG time did not correlate with either parameter.

MQ did not correlate with DEXA-measured muscle mass of the right thigh but had a strong inverse correlation with fat mass ($r = -0.72$, $p < 0.0001$). Muscle fat % had a strong correlation with DEXA-measured fat mass of the thigh ($r = 0.74$, $p < 0.0001$) and a weaker inverse correlation with muscle mass ($r = -0.38$, $p = 0.0492$).

3.2.4. DEXA Correlation with Strength and Functional Measures

DEXA-measured muscle mass did not correlate with isometric normalized peak torque, isokinetic normalized peak torque or TUG time. DEXA-measured thigh fat mass had moderate, negative correlations with both isometric ($r = -0.52$, $p = 0.005$) and isokinetic ($r = -0.39$, $p = 0.04$) normalized peak torque, but not TUG time.

Of little surprise, isometric and isokinetic normalized peak torque correlated with TUG time ($r = -0.61$, $p = 0.001$; $r = -0.37$, $p = 0.01$).

4. Discussion

In this pilot study, we aimed to determine if QMUS, sEIM or hEIM would be feasible tools for assessing muscle health and function in older adults. Validating each of these techniques first required an assessment of intra- and inter-rater reliability, followed by analysis of correlations with accepted measures of muscle mass, strength, and physical function. The results show that each method was reliable within and between examiners after minimal training and correlated with both DEXA and functional measures. Our study was unique in that it examined intra- and inter-rater agreement and included a mixed population of community dwelling older adults. The population consisted of both men and women; those with chronic medical conditions were not excluded. In the following sections, the results of each investigational technique are analyzed separately and compared with prior literature.

4.1. QMUS

The QMUS portion of our study was unique in that it examined intra- and inter-rater agreement in a mixed population of community dwelling older adults. Subcutaneous fat thickness was also measured, which has not been a focus of prior publications. Additionally, our study compared QMUS results to standard physical rehabilitation-administered strength testing, functional task measures and DEXA scans.

The intra-rater and inter-rater reliability in the current study were excellent for all tissue thickness measures (0.97–0.99). These are very similar to a recent study examining reliability for rectus femoris measurements [17]. Multiple other publications have reported similar results for anterior thigh imaging [18–21]. The intra- and inter-rater agreement for EI in the current study (0.87–0.96) aligned with previous publications. For example, Ishida et al. found an inter-rater reliability of 0.96 for EI of the rectus femoris, while we found a value of 0.94 [17]. Other recent studies have found similar values. These findings provide reassurance that QMUS measures are accurate and repeatable between examinations, as long as the imaging is performed according to a standardized protocol.

In comparing the current QMUS with prior publications, our findings align well with the previously mentioned Fukumoto study of 92 elderly women in regards to patient age, muscle thickness, and EI [11]. This is encouraging when considering the possibility of generalizing results, as the two studies were performed in different patient populations and with different ultrasound systems. The correlations noted between QMUS parameters and strength measurements are also similar.

Lopez et al. examined the relationship between quadriceps echointensity and functional measures in 50 healthy, elderly men [22]. The quadriceps were considered as a group for the purpose of analyzing EI and the mean value was 69.78 ± 11.4, different than seen in the current study (94.16 ± 20 for rectus femoris and 62.6 ± 32 for vastus intermedius). This may reflect the inclusion of only healthy patients, a younger population, lower BMI, the averaging of all quadriceps musculature in calculating the EI and differences in ultrasound systems. Despite the differences in absolute values, the authors found similar, moderate inverse correlations between EI and strength [20].

Similar to other studies [12,22,23], we found that EI correlated better with strength measures than did muscle thickness. In their discussion, Lopez et al. note that the presence of adipose tissue might be more relevant to age-related reductions in strength than the loss of muscle mass alone. Further supporting this hypothesis is our finding that subcutaneous fat thickness had moderate, inverse correlations with muscle strength ($r = -0.50$ to -0.56). This QMUS finding is felt to be accurate, given the strong correlation ($r = 0.81$) with the gold standard DEXA measurement of right thigh fat mass. As QMUS measured subcutaneous fat thickness is much more easily obtained than DEXA measures, QMUS may provide an excellent clinical and research tool for monitoring body fat composition.

4.2. sEIM

sEIM performed extremely well in parameters of intra- and inter-rater reliability (range 0.97–1.0). This was not unexpected given the short interval between trials, the easily accessible muscle chosen for analysis and the standardized protocol. Over the years, different sEIM devices have been assessed, some with fixed electrodes and some using the disposable electrode method described here. A fixed electrode array would be expected to reduce error and improve results.

Both 50 and 200 kHz frequencies were tested in the current study. Most early work focused on use of the 50 kHz frequency in sarcopenia [13]. Aaron et al. 2006 found aging to be associated with reductions in muscle impedance, specifically, the 50-kHz phase, in a cross-sectional study of 100 people [24]. This was most pronounced in men and those over age 60, but only 4 people older than

75 years were included in the study. A follow-up study demonstrated lower 50 kHz reactance, not phase, with aging. Again, men seemed to suffer more decline than women [25].

In our study, moderate, inverse correlations were found between isometric normalized peak torque and both resistance and phase at 50 and 200 kHz (Table 3). The relationship was somewhat stronger for 200 kHz measures, which also displayed similar correlations with normalized isokinetic peak torque. Only the 200 kHz measures had a moderate correlation with TUG time, although a weaker trend was observed for 50 kHz phase.

Good correlations were found between both 50 and 200 kHz resistance and phase with DEXA measured fat mass (Table 4). Again, 200 kHz measures performed better. There were trends toward correlation with muscle mass, but only 200 kHz fat mass reached statistical significance.

4.3. hEIM

To the best of our knowledge, there is only one other published study on the direct-to-consumer hEIM device used here [26]. The purpose of testing the device was to determine if it could be deployed in homes and possibly used by patients and research subjects for longitudinal monitoring of muscle health. No modifications were made to the system and there were no attempts to extract and analyze raw data. Intra-and inter-rater reliability was excellent (0.98–0.99) for muscle quality and % fat as measured by the device. This indicates that with minimal training, the measures are reliable for use in an outpatient clinical setting, warranting larger trials.

hEIM % fat had a moderate inverse correlation with isometric normalized peak torque, but muscle quality's correlation with this measure did not reach clinical significance. There was a strong correlation between hEIM measured % fat and DEXA measured right thigh fat mass (0.74) and a weaker correlation with the TUG time (−0.38). Again, this suggests that increased body and muscle fat have a more profound negative impact on function than muscle mass alone.

The findings here are similar to that found by McLester et al., who studied a population of healthy young adults (mean age 24–25 years). Their study found high agreement between examiners and also found hEIM to be a viable alternative for measuring body fat % [24].

4.4. Study Limitations

The current study is not without limitations and poses new questions. Methodologically, the frequencies used by the hEIM were not available, so a direct comparison between the sEIM and hEIM devices could not be performed. This pilot study had a small sample size ($n = 27$), but a larger cohort would be more likely to strengthen the correlations and trends seen here rather than weaken them. Using multiple muscles, as opposed to a single muscle may alter observed correlations as well. In addition, the study was not powered to detect differences between men and women, which may have been missed in this group. Furthermore, the extremely high reliability seen between examiners is likely related to the strict training provided and the fact that all investigative measures were performed on the same day.

Additional studies are needed to determine the reliability of electrical impedance myography measures over multiple visits, although data by Geisbush et al. suggest high reliability when electrical impedance measurements are separated by 3–7 days [27]. Muscle ultrasound has also demonstrated high reliability when performed on separate days [28]. The effects of hydration, changes in skin impedance and activity prior to testing may affect reliability and should be addressed in future projects. As a final note, the hEIM device was not deployed into subjects' homes to see if they were able to use the device with ease. Future studies will require a lapse of days to weeks prior to determining the real-world reliability of QMUS, sEIM, and hEIM.

5. Conclusions

QMUS, sEIM and hEIM all demonstrated excellent intra- and inter-rater reliability in a controlled, same-day testing protocol. Furthermore, multiple correlations with measures of muscle strength and body composition were noted for each method. Of particular interest is the finding that in older adults, the quality of muscle (i.e., lower % muscle fat) had stronger correlations with strength and function than muscle mass alone. This was true for QMUS, sEIM, and hEIM parameters. DEXA measures of lower extremity fat and muscle mass did not outperform ultrasound or EIM in this regard, suggesting that point-of-care, non-radiating inexpensive technologies may one day replace it as the gold standard.

The current findings require replication and further analysis in larger studies but suggest that interventions to reduce body fat may improve the health of elderly individuals.

Author Contributions: Conceptualization, L.DH.-W. and A.M.P.; Methodology, L.DH.-W. and A.M.P.; Validation, L.DH.-W., P.J.Z., A.N.P., T.C.S., A.M.P.; Formal analysis, L.DH.-W.; Investigation, L.DH.-W., P.J.Z., T.C.S., M.S.F., C.M.K., A.M.P.; Resources, L.DH.-W. and T.C.S.; Data curation, L.DH.-W., A.N.P.; Writing—original draft preparation, L.DH.-W.; Writing—review and editing, L.DH.-W., A.M.P., T.C.S., M.S.F., C.M.K.; Visualization, L.DH.-W.; Supervision, L.DH.-W. and A.M.P.; Project administration, L.DH.-W., P.J.Z., A.N.P, T.C.S., C.M.K., A.M.P.; Funding acquisition, L.DH.-W.

Acknowledgments: The authors would like to acknowledge Kevin Caves and Miriam C. Morey of Duke University for their assistance in designing the current study and ensuring its success.

References

1.   Lauretani, F.; Russo, C.R.; Badinelli, S.; Bartali, B.; Cavazzini, C.; Di Iorio, A.; Corsi, A.M.; Rantanen, T.; Guralnik, J.M.; Ferrucci, L. Age-associated changes in skeletal muscles and their effect on mobility: An operational diagnosis of sarcopenia. *J. Appl. Physiol.* **2003**, *95*, 1851–1860. [CrossRef] [PubMed]

2.   Hirani, V.; Blyth, F.; Naganathan, V.; Le Couteur, D.G.; Seibel, M.G.; Waite, M.J.; Handelsman, D.J.; Cumming, R.G. Sarcopenia is associated with incident disability, institutionalization, and mortality in community-dwelling older men: The Concord Health and Ageing in Men Project. *J. Am. Med. Dir. Assoc.* **2015**, *16*, 607–613. [CrossRef] [PubMed]

3.   Visser, M.; Goodpaster, B.H.; Kritchevsky, S.B.; Newman, A.B.; Nevitt, M.; Rubin, S.M.; Simonsick, E.M.; Harris, T.B. Muscle mass, muscle strength, and muscle fat infiltration as predictors of incident mobility limitations in well-functioning older persons. *J. Gerontol. A Biol. Sci. Med. Sci.* **2005**, *60*, 324–333. [PubMed]

4.   Han, A.; Bokshan, S.L.; Marcaccio, S.E.; DePasse, J.M.; Daniels, A.H. Diagnostic criteria and clinical outcomes in sarcopenia research: A literature review. *J. Clin. Med.* **2018**, *7*, 70. [CrossRef] [PubMed]

5.   Goodpaster, B.H.; Thaete, F.L.; Kelley, D.E. Composition of skeletal muscle evaluated with computed tomography. *Ann. N. Y. Acad. Sci.* **2000**, *904*, 18–24. [CrossRef] [PubMed]

6.   Pillen, S.; Tak, R.O.; Zwarts, M.J.; Lammens, M.M.; Verrijp, K.N.; Arts, I.M.; van der Laak, J.A.; Hoogerbruge, P.M.; van Engelen, B.G.; Verrips, A. Skeletal muscle ultrasound: Correlation between fibrous tissue and echo intensity. *Ultrasound Med. Biol.* **2009**, *35*, 443–446. [CrossRef] [PubMed]

7.   Pillen, S.; van Dijk, J.P.; Weijers, G.; Raijmann, W.; de Korte, C.L.; Zwarts, M.J. Quantitative gray-scale analysis in skeletal muscle ultrasound: A comparison study of two ultrasound devices. *Muscle Nerve* **2009**, *39*, 781–786. [CrossRef]

8.   Arts, I.M.; Pillen, S.; Schelhaas, H.J.; Overeem, S.; Zwarts, M.J. Normal values for quantitative muscle ultrasonography in adults. *Muscle Nerve* **2010**, *41*, 32–41. [CrossRef]

9.   Parry, S.M.; El-Ansary, D.; Cartwright, M.S.; Sarwal, A.; Berney, S.; Koopman, R.; Annoni, R.; Puthucheary, Z.; Gordon, I.R.; Morris, P.E.; et al. Ultrasonography in the intensive care setting can be used to detect changes in the quality and quantity of muscle and is related muscle strength and function. *J. Crit. Care* **2015**, *30*, e9–e14. [CrossRef]

10.   Puthucheary, Z.A.; Phadke, R.; Rawal, J.; McPhail, M.J.; Sidhu, P.S.; Rowlerson, A.; Moxham, J.; Harridge, S.; Hart, N.; Montgomery, H.E. Qualitative ultrasound in acute critical illness muscle wasting. *Crit. Care Med.* **2015**, *43*, 1603–1611. [CrossRef]

11.   Fukumoto, Y.; Ikezoe, T.; Yamada, Y.; Tsukagoshi, R.; Nakamura, M.; Mori, N.; Kimura, M.; Ichihashi, N. Skeletal muscle quality assessed from echo intensity is associated with muscle strength of middle-aged and elderly persons. *Eur. J. Appl. Physiol.* **2012**, *112*, 1519–1525. [CrossRef] [PubMed]

12.   Mirón Mombiela, R.; Facal de Castro, F.; Moreno, P.; Borras, C. Ultrasonic echo intensity as a new noninvasive in vivo biomarker of frailty. *J. Am. Geriatr. Soc.* **2017**, *65*, 2685–2690. [CrossRef] [PubMed]

13. Sanchez, B.; Rutkove, S.B. Electrical impedance myography and its applications in neuromuscular disorders. *Neurotherapeutics* **2017**, *14*, 107–118. [CrossRef]

14. Shefner, J.M.; Rutkove, S.B.; Caress, J.B.; Benatar, M.; David, W.S.; Cartwright, M.C.; Macklin, E.A.; Bohoroquez, J.L. Reducing sample size requirements for future ALS clinical trials with a dedicated electrical impedance myography system. *Amyotroph. Lateral Scler. Frontotemporal Degener.* **2018**, *28*, 1–7. [CrossRef] [PubMed]

15. Rutkove, S.B.; Kapur, K.; Zaidman, C.M.; Wu, J.S.; Paternak, A.; Madabusi, L.; Yim, S.; Pacheck, A.; Szelag, H.; Harrington, T.; et al. Electrical impedance myography for assessment of Duchenne muscular dystrophy. *Ann. Neurol.* **2017**, *81*, 622–632. [CrossRef] [PubMed]

16. Zaidman, C.M.; Wang, L.L.; Connolly, A.M.; Florence, J.; Wong, B.L.; Parsons, J.A.; Apkon, S.; Goyal, N.; Williams, E.; Escolar, D.; et al. Electrical impedance myography in Duchenne muscular dystrophy and healthy controls: A multicenter study of reliability and validity. *Muscle Nerve* **2015**, *52*, 592–597. [CrossRef] [PubMed]

17. Ishida, H.; Suehiro, T.; Suzuki, K.; Watanabe, S. Muscle thickness and echo intensity measurements of the rectus femoris muscle of healthy subjects: Intra and interrater reliability of transducer tilt during ultrasound. *J. Bodyw. Mov. Ther.* **2018**, *22*, 657–660. [CrossRef]

18. Toledo, D.O.; Silva, D.C.L.E.; Santos, D.M.D.; Freitas, B.J.; Dib, R.; Cordioli, R.L.; Figueiredo, E.J.A.; Piovacari, S.M.F.; Silva, J.M., Jr. Bedside ultrasound is a practical measurement tool for assessing muscle mass. *Revista Brasileira de Terapia Intensiva* **2017**, *29*, 476–480. [CrossRef]

19. Hadda, V.; Khilnani, G.C.; Kumar, R.; Dhungana, A.; Mittal, S.; Khan, M.A.; Madan, K.; Mohan, A.; Guleria, R. Intra- and inter-observer reliability of quadriceps muscle thickness measured with bedside ultrasonography by critical care physicians. *Indian J. Crit. Care Med.* **2017**, *21*, 448–452. [CrossRef]

20. Thoirs, K.; English, C. Ultrasound measures of muscle thickness: Intra-examiner reliability and influence of body position. *Clin. Physiol. Funct. Imaging* **2009**, *29*, 440–446. [CrossRef]

21. Tillquist, M.; Kutsogiannis, D.J.; Wischmeyer, P.E.; Kummerlen, C.; Leung, R.; Stollery, D.; Karvellas, C.K.; Preiser, J.C.; Bird, N.; Kozar, R.; et al. Bedside ultrasound is a practical and reliable measurement tool for assessing quadriceps muscle layer thickness. *JPEN J. Parenter. Enteral Nutr.* **2014**, *38*, 886–890. [CrossRef] [PubMed]

22. Lopez, P.; Wilhelm, E.N.; Rech, A.; Minozzo, F.; Radaelli, R.; Pinto, R.S. Echo intensity independently predicts functionality in sedentary older men. *Muscle Nerve* **2017**, *55*, 9–15. [CrossRef] [PubMed]

23. Rech, A.; Radaelli, R.; Goltz, F.R.; da Rosa, L.H.; Schneider, C.D.; Pinto, R.S. Echo intensity is negatively associated with functional capacity in older women. *Age* **2014**, *36*, 9708. [CrossRef]

24. Aaron, R.; Esper, G.J.; Shiffman, C.A.; Bradonjic, K.; Lee, K.S.; Rutkove, S.B. Effects of age on muscle as measured by electrical impedance myography. *Physiol. Meas.* **2006**, *27*, 953–959. [CrossRef]

25. Kortman, H.G.; Wilder, S.C.; Geisbush, T.R.; Narayanaswami, P.; Rutkove, S.B. Age- and gender-associated differences in electrical impedance values of skeletal muscle. *Physiol. Meas.* **2013**, *34*, 1611–1622. [CrossRef]

26. McLester, C.N.; Dewitt, A.D.; Rooks, R.; McLester, J.R. An investigation of the accuracy and reliability of body composition assessed with a handheld electrical impedance myography device. *Eur. J. Sport Sci.* **2018**, *18*, 763–771. [CrossRef]

27. Geisbush, T.R.; Visyak, N.; Madabusi, L.; Rutkove, S.B.; Darras, B.T. Inter-session reliability of electrical impedance myography in children in a clinical trial setting. *Clin. Neurophysiol.* **2015**, *126*, 1790–1796. [CrossRef] [PubMed]

28. O'Brien, T.G.; Cazares Gonzalez, M.L.; Ghosh, P.S.; Mandrekar, J.; Boon, A.J. Reliability of a novel ultrasound system for gray-scale analysis of muscle. *Muscle Nerve* **2017**, *56*, 408–412. [CrossRef]

13

Fruit and Vegetable Consumption and Potential Moderators Associated with All-Cause Mortality in a Representative Sample of Spanish Older Adults

Beatriz Olaya [1,2,*], Cecilia A. Essau [3], Maria Victoria Moneta [1,2], Elvira Lara [2,4,5], Marta Miret [2,4,5], Natalia Martín-María [2,4,5], Darío Moreno-Agostino [2,4,5], José Luis Ayuso-Mateos [2,4,5], Adel S. Abduljabbar [6] and Josep Maria Haro [1,2,6]

[1] Research, Innovation and Teaching Unit, Parc Sanitari Sant Joan de Déu, Carrer Doctor Pujadas 42, 08830 Sant Boi de Llobregat, Spain
[2] Instituto de Salud Carlos III, Centro de Investigación Biomédica en Red de Salud Mental (CIBERSAM), Calle Monforte de Lemos 3–5, 28029 Madrid, Spain
[3] Department of Psychology, University of Roehampton, Whitelands College, London SW15 4JD, UK
[4] Department of Psychiatry, Instituto de Investigación Sanitaria, Hospital Universitario de La Princesa (IIS-Princesa), Calle de Diego de León 62, 28006 Madrid, Spain
[5] Department of Psychiatry, Universidad Autónoma de Madrid, Madrid, Calle Arzobispo Morcillo 4, 28029 Madrid, Spain
[6] Psychology Deparment, King Saud University, Riyadh 11451, Saudi Arabia
* Correspondence: beatriz.olaya@pssjd.org

Abstract: This study sought to determine the association between levels of fruit and vegetable consumption and time to death, and to explore potential moderators. We analyzed a nationally-representative sample of 1699 older adults aged 65+ who were followed up for a period of 6 years. Participants were classified into low (≤3 servings day), medium (4), or high (≥5) consumption using tertiles. Unadjusted and adjusted cox proportional hazard regression models (by age, gender, cohabiting, education, multimorbidity, smoking, physical activity, alcohol consumption, and obesity) were calculated. The majority of participants (65.7%) did not meet the recommendation of five servings per day. High fruit and vegetable intake increased by 27% the probability of surviving among older adults with two chronic conditions, compared to those who consumed ≤3 servings per day (HR = 0.38, 95%CI = 0.21–0.69). However, this beneficial effect was not found for people with none, one chronic condition or three or more, indicating that this protective effect might not be sufficient for more severe cases of multimorbidity. Given a common co-occurrence of two non-communicable diseases in the elderly and the low frequency of fruit and vegetable consumption in this population, interventions to promote consuming five or more servings per day could have a significant positive impact on reducing mortality.

Keywords: survival; fruit and vegetable consumption; interaction; older adults; multimorbidity

1. Introduction

Fruit and vegetable consumption has consistently been associated with beneficial effects on health [1,2]. Several meta-analyses have indicated a reduced risk of non-communicable diseases such as cancer [3], stroke [4], diabetes [5], hypertension [6], and heart diseases [3]. According to the WHO, 16 million disability-adjusted life-years (DALYs) and 1.7 million deaths worldwide are attributable to low fruit and vegetable consumption [7]. High fruit and vegetable intake has been associated with a reduced risk of all-cause mortality [8,9] due to cardiovascular diseases (CVD) [10], but also to other non-cardiovascular diseases [11], such as cancer [12], although findings are inconsistent [13]. Many public health guidelines recommend a daily intake of a minimum of five servings per day of fruit and vegetable, although these recommendations vary across regions. For example, the Eurodiet core report [14], the World Cancer Research Fund [15], and the WHO/FAO [16] recommend at least 400 g/day, 600 g/day in Denmark [17], and 640/800 g/day in the USA [3].

Older adults have unique nutritional needs that might require special adaptations of the nutritional clinical guidelines and public health policies addressed to this population [18]. Chronic diseases, multimorbidity, and geriatric conditions such as polypharmacy, mobility-difficulties, and oral problems, are common in older adults and might be associated with malnutrition [19]. The majority of studies of the health benefits of fruit and vegetable consumption have traditionally focused on children, adolescents, or young adults, but few have included older adults [18]. These few studies seem to suggest that fruit and vegetable intake can prevent the onset of depression [20], cognitive decline [21], disability [22], and frailty [23], and can decrease the risk of disease-specific and all-cause mortality in this population [18]. Moreover, the potential benefit of fruit and vegetable intake in reducing the risk of mortality in older adults might depend on various circumstances. For example, a study conducted in several population-based cohorts from Eastern Europe [24] reported that fruit and vegetable consumption was strongly and inversely associated with risk of total and CVD mortality among smokers, compared with non-smokers.

The present study sought to determine the association between different levels of fruit and vegetable consumption and risk of all-cause mortality in a representative sample of Spanish community-dwelling older adults and to determine potential moderators of this association, including multimorbidity and other lifestyle factors such as smoking, alcohol consumption, and physical activity.

2. Methods

Study Sample

This study used data from the "Edad con Salud", a longitudinal household survey of the non-institutionalized adult population in Spain. The first wave took place between 2011 and 2012 and was part of the Collaborative Research on Ageing in Europe (COURAGE) study [25]. The participants were re-evaluated twice, between 2014 and 2015, and in 2018. A stratified multistage clustered design was used, in which strata included Autonomous Communities except Ceuta and Melilla. People aged 50+ were oversampled. The Spanish Statistical Office provided a list of households, and individuals were randomly selected from within the household by the interviewer. A total of 4753 persons participated at baseline with a final response rate of 69.9%.

Interviews were conducted face to face by trained lay interviewers using Computer-Assisted Personal Interviewing (CAPI) at respondents' homes. Participants answered a questionnaire adapted from the Study on global AGEing and adult health [26] (SAGE) which was translated from English into Spanish using World Health Organization translation guidelines for assessment instruments [27]. Quality control procedures were implemented during the fieldwork [28]. At the beginning of the interview, the interviewer judged whether the selected person had cognitive limitations that would prevent correct understanding of the survey questions. In such cases, a proxy respondent answered a short version of the interview. Proxy interviews were excluded from the present analysis ($n = 170$). We focused on people aged 65 or older with complete data in all the covariates at baseline, resulting in a final n of 1699. Ethical approval was obtained from the Clinical Investigation Ethics Committee, Parc Sanitari Sant Joan de Déu, Barcelona (PIC-12-11; PIC-71-12) and from the Clinical Investigation Ethics Committee, Hospital Universitario la Princesa, Madrid (PI-364; 2399). Informed consent was obtained from each participant.

3. Measures

3.1. Fruit and Vegetable Consumption

Participants were asked the following questions: *"How many servings of fruit do you eat on a typical day?"* and *"How many servings of vegetables do you eat on a typical day?"*. Respondents were shown a card indicating with pictures and in written explanation what was considered a serving of fruit and vegetables, according to the WHO recommendations [7]. One standard serving (portion) included 80 g, translated into different units of cups depending on the type of fruit and vegetable and standard cup measures available in the country. For example, a piece of banana or apple was considered as one serving. Tubers (such as potatoes) were not included. The total number of fruit and vegetables was added up (ranging from 0 to 18), and a categorical variable was created to indicate the level of consumption using tertiles: low (≤3 servings day), medium (4 servings day), and high (≥5 servings day).

3.2. Other Covariates

Socio-demographic information at baseline included age, gender, educational level (no education/primary school, secondary school, and high school/university studies), and current marital status (never married, widowed, separated or divorced, recorded as "not cohabiting", and married or cohabiting with someone, recorded as "cohabiting"). A binary variable (*ever smoked*) was created including those who had never smoked and those who were current smokers or ex-smokers (including smoking tobacco or using smokeless tobacco). Level of physical activity was evaluated with the Global Physical Activity Questionnaire [29], and participants were classified into high, medium, and low levels [30]. Respondents were asked if they had ever consumed alcohol, the number of days, and standard drinks on average. They were classified as lifetime abstainers (never consumed alcohol), occasional drinkers (did not consume alcohol in the last 30 days or in the last 7 days), non-heavy drinkers (did consume alcohol in the last 30 days and in the last 7 days), infrequent heavy drinkers (did consume alcohol 1–2 days per week, with five or more standard drinks in the last 7 days for men and four or more for women), and frequent heavy drinkers (did consume alcohol 3 or more days per week with five or more standard drinks in the last 7 days for men and four or more for women). Due to the low frequency of heavy drinkers in our sample, non-heavy drinkers, infrequent, and frequent heavy-drinkers were merged into the single category of "frequent drinker".

A combined method, consisting of self-reported physician's diagnosis and/or symptom-based algorithms [31], was used to assess the following medical conditions: arthritis, asthma, chronic obstructive pulmonary disease (COPD), angina pectoris, stroke, hypertension, and diabetes. For diabetes, only a self-reported diagnosis was considered. The presence of hypertension was based on self-reported diagnosis or presence of systolic blood pressure ≥ 140 mmHg or diastolic blood pressure ≥ 90 mmHg measured at the time of the interview [32,33]. The number of chronic conditions (CC) was calculated (none or one, 2, and 3 or more CC). Interviewers measured participants' height and weight using a stadiometer and a routinely calibrated electronic weighing scale, respectively. Body Mass Index (BMI) was calculated as weight (in kilograms) divided by the square of height (in meters). A BMI of 30 or higher was used as cut-off point for obesity [34].

3.3. Mortality

The National Death Index, a civil registry for all Spanish residents, was used to ascertain the vital status and date of death for all participants from 25 July 2011 to March 2018. Vital status was also updated during household visits in the follow-up assessment by asking respondents' relatives. A final update was conducted on the 31 October 2018 by once again consulting the National Death Index. Twelve participants that appeared as deceased had no information about their date of death. Thus, we estimated their date of death as occurring at the mid-point between the date of interview at baseline and 31 October 2018.

3.4. Statistical Analysis

Unweighted frequencies, weighted proportions, and means were used for descriptive analyses. Distinct levels of fruit and vegetable consumption were compared using the Rao-Scott chi-squared test statistic (which adjusts for complex sample design) [35] for categorical variables and one-way ANOVA test for continuous variables.

Mortality was the outcome for the analyses. Kaplan–Meier survival curves and log-rank test statistics were used to estimate the time to death (from the first interview) stratified by levels of fruit and vegetable consumption. Participants who were alive at the end of the observational period (31 October 2018) were censored.

We conducted unadjusted and adjusted Cox proportional hazards regression models to explore the association between fruit and vegetable consumption and risk of all-cause mortality. The adjusted model included levels of fruit and vegetable consumption (with "low" level as the reference category) plus other potential confounders at baseline (gender, age, educational level, cohabiting, smoking status, level of physical activity, obesity, and number of chronic conditions). Interactions between levels of fruit and vegetable consumption and covariates were explored in the adjusted models. Hazard ratios (HRs) with their 95% confidence intervals (CI) were calculated.

The assumption of proportionality was explored by calculating plots of cumulative hazard functions across the independent variables. Violation in the assumption was not found. All analyses were performed using Stata version 13 for Windows (SE version 13, StataCorp: College Station, TX, USA) taking into account complex sampling design. Weights were used to adjust for differential probabilities of selection within households, and post-stratification corrections to the weights were made to match the samples to the socio-demographic distributions of the Spanish population. Statistical significance was set at $p < 0.05$.

3.5. Results

The mean age of the total sample was 74.8 years (95% CI = 74.49–75.12) ranging from 65 to 104, with 54.8% females, 54.7% cohabiting with someone, and 46.3% reporting low levels of education (Table 1). Some 37.2% reported being smokers or ex-smokers, 33.4% presented obesity, and 33.2% had low levels of physical activity. A total of 56.2% reported having two or more chronic conditions. Fruit and vegetable servings per day ranged from 0 to 18, with a mean of four servings (95% CI = 3.82–4.19). Participants with lower consumption (equal to or less than three servings per day) were more likely to be men, smokers, not frequently engaging in physical activity, frequent drinkers, and have a low educational level.

The minimum number of days of survival was 19 and the maximum 2688, with a mean of 2323.94 days (SD = 553.7). We observed 322 confirmed deceased cases (132 women and 190 men). The Kaplan–Meier estimated curves (Figure 1) showed that the level of fruit and vegetable consumption had a significant negative effect on survival. In the adjusted Cox proportional hazards regression model, only the interaction term *fruit and vegetable consumption* * *number of chronic conditions* was found to be significant ($p = 0.035$). Table 2 presents the unadjusted and adjusted HRs and 95%CI. In the unadjusted model, both medium (HR = 1.68, 95%CI = 1.3–2.18) and high fruit (HR = 1.12, 95%CI = 1.1–1.14) consumption were significantly associated with higher risk of death. Other significant predictors of higher risk of mortality were being male, low levels of physical activity (compared with high), lower levels of education, being a smoker (current or past), and having three or more chronic conditions. The adjusted model including the interaction term between fruit and vegetable consumption and number of chronic conditions is presented in Table 2. In order to interpret the effect of fruit and vegetable consumption on time to death in the presence of interaction, HRs were calculated according to the number of chronic conditions (Table 3). The proportion of deceased people was significantly higher ($p < 0.001$) among those who had three or more CCs ($n = 112$, 25.8%) compared to those with none or one CC ($n = 127$, 16.3%) or two CCs ($n = 83$, 15.5%). Subjects who consumed five or more servings of fruit and vegetable per day and had two chronic conditions were at 27% less risk of mortality (HR = 0.38, 95%CI = 0.21–0.69, *p* = 0.002) compared with participants consuming three or fewer servings, while other covariates held constant. However, fruit and vegetable consumption had no impact on time to death among subjects who reported none or one CC, or three or more.

Table 1. Baseline characteristics of the sample and comparison between levels of fruit and vegetable consumption.

	Fruit & Vegetable Consumption				
	Total Sample (*n* = 1699)	Low (*n* = 669, 39.6%)	Medium (*n* = 448, 26.1%)	High (*n* = 582, 34.3%)	*p* Value
Death, *n* (%)	322 (18.6)	150 (21.9)	78 (18.7)	94 (14.7)	0.019
Age, *mean* (95%CI)	74.80 (74.49–75.12)	74.98 (74.46–75.5)	75.06 (74.43–75.68)	74.4 (73.57–75.24)	0.476
Females, *n* (%)	956 (54.8)	341 (49.7)	266 (58.8)	349 (57.6)	0.013
Cohabiting, *n* (%)	935 (54.7)	376 (54.4)	254 (56.9)	305 (53.4)	0.653
Educational level, *n* (%)					0.023
No education/Primary school	804 (46.3)	343 (51.7)	216 (47.5)	245 (39)	-
Secondary school	492 (30.1)	181 (27)	125 (30.6)	186 (33.4)	-
High school/University	403 (23.6)	145 (21.3)	107 (22)	151 (27.6)	0.791
Ever smoked, *n* (%)	620 (37.2)	278 (41.8)	150 (32.5)	192 (35.5)	0.008
Obesity, *n* (%)	606 (33.4)	237 (33.8)	156 (34.5)	213 (32.1)	0.803
Alcohol consumption, *n* (%)					<0.001
Lifetime abstainer	618 (36.5)	218 (31.9)	167 (38.7)	233 (40.1)	-
Occasional drinker	524 (31)	197 (28.6)	138 (30.4)	189 (34.2)	-
Frequent drinker	557 (32.5)	254 (39.5)	143 (30.9)	160 (25.7)	-
Number CC, *n* (%)					0.369
None or one	780 (43.8)	305 (43.9)	197 (42.2)	278 (44.9)	-
Two	482 (29.7)	188 (28.5)	130 (28.6)	164 (31.8)	-
Three or more	437 (26.5)	176 (27.6)	121 (29.2)	140 (23.3)	-
Level PA, *n* (%)					0.011
High	427 (25.2)	151 (21.6)	108 (21)	168 (32.7)	-
Medium	700 (41.6)	268 (40.6)	185 (45.1)	247 (40.1)	-
Low	572 (33.2)	250 (37.8)	155 (33.9)	167 (27.2)	-

Note: CC = Chronic conditions; PA = Physical activity; 95% CI = 95% Confidence interval; Unweighted frequencies, weighted proportions and means.

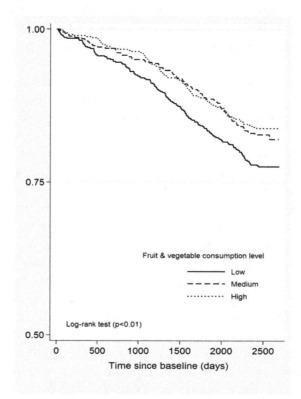

Figure 1. Kaplan–Meier estimated curves for cumulative survival by levels of fruit and vegetable consumption.

Table 2. Hazard ratios, Confidence intervals and p values for the unadjusted and adjusted Cox proportional hazards models ($n = 1699$).

	Unadjusted		Adjusted [a]	
	HR (95% CI)	p Value	HR (95% CI)	p Value
Fruit & veg consumption				
Low (ref.)	-	-	-	-
Medium	0.83 (0.61–1.13)	0.802	1.0 (0.62–1.60)	0.989
High	**1.68 (1.3–2.18)**	**<0.001**	1.11 (0.70–1.74)	0.659
Age	**1.12 (1.1–1.14)**	**<0.001**	**1.13 (1.1–15)**	**<0.001**
Gender				
Female (ref.)	-	-	-	-
Male	**1.96 (1.49–2.57)**	**<0.001**	**3.31 (2.21–4.99)**	**<0.001**
Marital status				
Not cohabiting (ref.)	-	-	-	-
Cohabiting	0.84 (0.66–1.1)	0.169	0.9 (0.66–1.24)	0.523
Educational level				
No education/Primary school	-	-	-	-
Secondary school	**0.57 (0.39–0.83)**	**0.004**	0.77 (0.54–1.11)	0.168
High school/University	**0.67 (0.49–0.92)**	**0.013**	1.0 (0.74–1.35)	0.997
Level PA				
High (ref.)	-	-	-	-
Medium	1.45 (0.99–2.13)	0.056	1.28 (0.84–1.93)	0.246
Low	**2.3 (1.59–3.32)**	**<0.001**	**1.61 (1.07–2.43)**	**0.021**
Smoking status		-	-	-
Never smoked	-	-	-	-
Ever smoked	**1.38 (1.07–1.78)**	**0.013**	1.01 (0.73–1.39)	0.973
Alcohol consumption				
Lifetime abstainer (ref.)	-	-	-	-
Occasional drinker	1.13 (0.84–1.5)	0.414	0.97 (0.69–1.36)	0.87
Frequent drinker	0.93 (0.69–1.24)	0.625	**0.64 (0.46–0.91)**	**0.012**
Obesity				
Non-obese (ref.)	-	-	-	-
Obese	1.14 (0.82–1.57)	0.43	1.11 (0.8–1.55)	0.515
Number CC				
None/one (ref.)	-	-	-	-
Two	0.95 (0.67–1.37)	0.802	1.56 (0.91–2.65)	0.102
Three or more	**1.68 (1.3–2.18)**	**<0.001**	1.47 (0.99–2.18)	0.056
Fruit & veg × number CC				
Medium/two CC	-	-	0.63 (0.31–1.28)	0.199
Medium/three+ CC	-	-	0.97 (0.47–2.0)	0.930
High/two CC	-	-	**0.34 (0.18–0.65)**	**0.001**
High/three+ CC	-	-	0.74 (0.39–1.42)	0.360

Note: HR = Hazard ratio; 95% CI = 95% Confidence interval; CC = Chronic conditions; PA = Physical activity. In bold, significant effect. [a] The adjusted model included all the variables and the interaction term simultaneously.

Table 3. Adjusted hazard ratios of the effect of fruit and vegetable consumption by number of chronic conditions on all-cause mortality. Cox regression model ($n = 1,699$).

Level of Fruit & Vegetable Consumption	None or One CC				Two CC				Three or More CC			
	HR	95%CI		p Value	HR	95%CI		p Value	HR	95%CI		p Value
Low (ref.)	-	-	-	-	-	-	-	-	-	-	-	-
Medium	1.0	0.62	1.6	0.989	0.63	0.33	0.19	0.151	0.96	0.54	0.73	0.905
High	1.11	0.7	1.74	0.659	**0.38**	**0.21**	**0.69**	**0.002**	0.82	0.5	1.35	0.428

Note: HR = Hazard ratio; 95%CI = 95% Confidence interval; CC = Chronic conditions. In bold, significant HR. Model included the *fruit & vegetable consumption*number CC* interaction term and the following variables: age, gender, educational level, cohabiting, ever smoked, obesity, alcohol consumption, and level of physical activity (see Table 2).

Comparison between "medium" and "high" levels of fruit and vegetable consumption; (1) in the none or one CC group: $p = 0.66$; (2) in the two CC: $p = 0.13$; (3) and in the three or more CC: $p = 0.596$

Survival curves as a function of levels of fruit and vegetable consumption and number of chronic conditions are displayed in Figure 2 for a specific pattern of covariates (i.e., females, not cohabiting, never smoked, no education/primary school studies, non-obese, lifetime abstainers, high level of physical activity, and age 74.8 years old). For people with two chronic conditions, the probability of surviving until the end of the study was significantly greater if they consumed five or more servings per day of fruit and vegetables, compared with those who ate three or fewer.

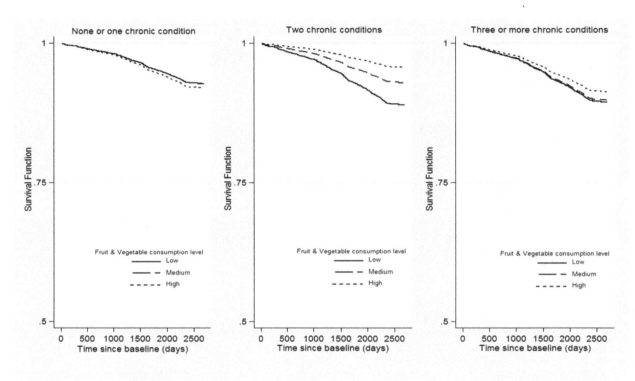

Figure 2. Survival function according to the level of fruit and vegetable consumption and number of chronic conditions ($n = 1699$). The first subfigure (left) shows the survival curves according to the three levels of fruit and vegetable intake for people with none or one chronic condition, the second (middle) for those with two chronic conditions and the third (right) shows survival curves associated with fruit and vegetable consumption for respondents with three or more chronic conditions. Note: Survival functions calculated from the adjusted Cox proportional hazards model presented in Table 2. All covariates were set equal to zero.

4. Discussion

This study sought to determine the effect of fruit and vegetable consumption on all-cause mortality in a representative sample of Spanish community-dwelling older adults who were followed up for a period of approximately 6 years. Our results show that consuming five or more servings per day increases the probability of surviving in the general older population with two chronic conditions by 27%, compared to those who consume three or fewer servings per day. However, this beneficial effect of fruit and vegetable consumption is not found among participants with none or one chronic condition, or three or more.

Most participants (65.7%) in the study did not adhere to the WHO recommendation of consuming a minimum of five servings of fruit and vegetables per day, with the median of servings per day being four. In a very large Spanish sample of university graduates, the mean consumption of fruits and vegetables was 343 g/day and 525 g/day [36], respectively, with an equivalence of approximately four and six portions of 80 g. However, few epidemiological studies have described the patterns of fruit and vegetable consumption among the older Spanish population. For example, in the Seniors-ENRICA study, a population-based cohort of Spanish older adults aged 60+, a total of 22.5% participants reported having five or more portions of fruit and vegetables a day [23], slightly inferior to the 34.3% found in our study. These discrepancies could be explained by the different tools used to assess fruit and vegetable consumption.

Previous population-based studies have repeatedly reported an inverse association between fruit and vegetable consumption, and all-cause and disease-specific mortality in the older population [37–39], although some studies have reported inconsistent findings about whether this greater risk of all-cause mortality might be mainly due to CVD-related or non-cardiovascular-related deaths, such as cancer [40]. Our findings contribute to this evidence by showing that this effect is exerted through a protective effect in the presence of multimorbidity. Additionally, the consumption of both fruit and vegetables rather than the consumption of only fruit or vegetables seems to be especially beneficial for reducing the risk of CVD [39] and non-cardiovascular diseases [3]. Our findings also support the recommendation of a minimum of five servings per day of fruit and vegetables whereas there were no differences in terms of increased risk of mortality among older adults with low (equal to or less than three servings/d) or medium (four servings/d) consumption. This is in line with previous studies that investigated the risk of all-cause mortality associated with a dose-response of fruit and vegetable consumption in a large population-based cohort aged 45–83 [8]. The authors found that consuming fewer than five servings a day was associated with progressively shorter survival and higher mortality rate, whereas consuming more than five servings did not add any benefits with respect to survival.

A systematic review conducted by Nunes et al [41] showed an overall positive association between multimorbidity (defined as the presence of two or more chronic diseases) and mortality (HR = 1.44, 95%CI = 134–1.55). In the unadjusted model, we found that only three or more chronic conditions were related to a 62% higher probability of having a shorter survival and dying, compared to those with none or one chronic condition. We found that the beneficial effect of consuming five or more fruit and vegetable servings per day is exerted in those having two CCs, but not three or more. Additionally, this protective effect seems to be beyond the confounding effects of other risk factors, such as obesity, physical activity, smoking, gender, or educational level. Participants suffering from three or more chronic conditions might represent complex patients, who might be in need of intensive care. The presence of multiple diseases is related to interactions between morbidities, inadequate use of medication, polypharmacy [42], and frailty [43]. Thus, the protective effect of high intake of fruit and vegetables might not be sufficient to reduce the risk of death in people with three or more CCs. It is also possible that older adults with three or more CCs have been given a prescription of a balanced diet, or have been advised to quit or reduce smoking and alcohol intake [44], which might in turn explain the lack of association between fruit and vegetable intake and time to death in this particular subgroup. Despite this, the beneficial effect of consuming five or more servings per day of fruit and vegetables could be huge. Taking into account that an important proportion of Spanish older adults do not reach the recommended five servings per day of fruit and vegetables along with the high prevalence of multimorbidity in this population, interventions promoting fruit and vegetable consumption among older adults might have a positive impact on reducing the risk of death and increasing their quality of life. Future research is needed to learn whether fruit and vegetable intake is particularly beneficial in reducing the risk of death for a particular pair of diseases.

There are several mechanisms by which fruit and vegetable consumption can reduce the risk of mortality in older adults. Fruit and vegetables contain a variety of nutrients and phytochemicals (i.e., fibre, vitamin C, carotenoids, antioxidants, potassium, and flavonoids) that act through several biological mechanisms to reduce the risk of chronic conditions and premature mortality [3]. Greater intake of fruit and vegetables has also been linked to a greater adherence to the Mediterranean diet in older adults (characterized by abundant consumption of olive oil, minimally processed, locally grown vegetables, fruits, nuts, legumes, and cereals, and proteins coming mainly from fish and shellfish) [45] and to reduced consumption of sweet foods [46] which in turn might also prevent

CVD [47], several types of cancer [48,49], cognitive decline, and dementia [50,51], while increasing longevity [52]. Our study did not include data on adherence to the Mediterranean diet or other potential dietary risk factors for non-communicable diseases and risk of mortality, such as consumption of red and processed meat [53] or ultraprocessed food [54]. More studies are needed to determine whether the beneficial effect of fruit and vegetable intake on the probability of survival among people with multimorbidity is maintained or attenuated by the presence of these diet-related risk factors. Additionally, the way in which fruits and vegetables are consumed (e.g., raw or cooked) might also play an important role in the potential protective factor among older adults with chronic conditions. Another mechanism by which fruit and vegetable consumption might impact the risk of mortality among older adults is the presence of unhealthy lifestyles among those who consume less fruit and vegetables. Previous research has indicated an inverse association between fruit and vegetable intake and smoking [55], alcohol consumption [56], obesity [57], and sedentarism [58]. The beneficial effects of consuming fruit and vegetables, such as lower systemic inflammation [59], reduced oxidative stress [60], and decreased platelet aggregation [61], may partially reduce the effects of smoking and alcohol intake [55,56]. However, we did not find significant interactions between fruit and vegetable consumption and smoking status, alcohol consumption, obesity, or low levels of physical activity. Future research is needed to replicate these results.

Our study had some limitations. First, health variables, such as fruit and vegetable consumption, tobacco and physical activity, were self-reported, thus potentially leading to measurement errors or misclassification. Additionally, recall bias might also be present. Second, it was assumed that the fruit and vegetable intake pattern was unchanged during the follow-up period. Third, it is possible that the beneficial effect of fruit and vegetable consumption is not observed among participants with none or one chronic condition because they are more likely to survive during the follow-up period. Thus, longer periods of follow-up might be needed. Fourth, measuring fruit and vegetable consumption might be problematic. For example, the study did not extensively measure the dietary habits of the sample through a 24-hour dietary recall or a frequency questionnaire; thus, some measurement bias might have been introduced. Questions concerning the number of fruit and vegetable servings were asked once, yet they may be prone to seasonable bias as well. Additionally, these questions were aggregated, and the effect of this variable could be due to specific sorts of fruits and vegetables. Fourth, residual confounding might explain our findings. For example, consuming vitamin supplements or specific diet patterns such as the Mediterranean diet could be related to both fruit and vegetable consumption and mortality. However, findings were adjusted for several potential confounders, such as smoking status, alcohol consumption, physical activity, and obesity.

In sum, the finding that a high level of fruit and vegetable consumption (reaching the threshold of five or more servings per day) significantly reduces the risk of mortality among older adults with two chronic conditions has several implications. As has been shown in the present study, fruit and vegetable intake in the general population of older adults does not approach recommended levels. Interventions to increase fruit and vegetable intake in older adults should take into account their unique nutritional needs and barriers, as well as several characteristics that might influence their fruit and vegetable intake, such as appetite loss, tooth loss and oral problems, changes in perception of hunger, taste acuity and sense of smell (sometimes associated with drugs' side effects), and mobility difficulties in shopping [18]. These factors should be taken into account when designing interventions to promote fruit and vegetable consumption geared to the older population.

Author Contributions: Conceptualization, B.O., C.A.E., J.L.A.-M., and J.M.H.; Methodology, B.O., M.V.M., E.L., M.M., N.M.M., D.M.-A., J.L.A.-M., and J.M.H.; Formal analysis, B.O. and M.V.M.; Investigation, B.O., M.V.M., E.L., M.M., N.M.M., D.M.-A., J.L.A.-M., and J.M.H.; Resources, B.O., M.V.M., E.L., M.M., N.M.M., D.M.-A., J.L.A.-M., and J.M.H.; Data curation, B.O., M.V.M., E.L., N.M.M., D.M.-A.; Writing–Original draft preparation, B.O., C.A.E. and A.A.; Writing–Review & Editing, all authors; Supervision, C.A.E., J.L.A.-M., and J.M.H.; Project administration, B.O., E.L., M.M., N.M.M., D.M.-A., J.L.A.-M., and J.M.H., Funding acquisition, M.M., J.L.A.-M., and J.M.H.

References

1. Fulton, S.L.; McKinley, M.C.; Young, I.S.; Cardwell, C.R.; Woodside, J.V. The effect of increasing fruit and vegetable consumption on overall diet: A systematic review and meta-analysis. *Crit. Rev. Food Sci. Nutr.* **2016**, *56*, 802–816. [CrossRef] [PubMed]

2. Mytton, O.T.; Nnoaham, K.; Eyles, H.; Scarborough, P.; Ni Mhurchu, C. Systematic review and meta-analysis of the effect of increased vegetable and fruit consumption on body weight and energy intake. *BMC Public Health* **2014**, *14*, 886.

3. Aune, D.; Giovannucci, E.; Boffetta, P.; Fadnes, L.T.; Keum, N.N.; Norat, T.; Greenwood, D.C.; Riboli, E.; Vatten, L.J.; Tonstad, S. Fruit and vegetable intake and the risk of cardiovascular disease, total cancer and all-cause mortality—A systematic review and dose-response meta-analysis of prospective studies. *Int. J. Epidemiol.* **2017**, *46*, 1029–1056. [CrossRef] [PubMed]

4. Hu, D.; Huang, J.; Wang, Y.; Zhang, D.; Qu, Y. Fruits and vegetables consumption and risk of stroke. *Stroke* **2014**, *45*, 1613–1619. [CrossRef] [PubMed]

5. Li, M.; Fan, Y.; Zhang, X.; Hou, W.; Tang, Z. Fruit and vegetable intake and risk of type 2 diabetes mellitus: Meta-analysis of prospective cohort studies. *BMJ Open* **2014**, *4*, e005497. [PubMed]

6. Li, B.; Li, F.; Wang, L.; Zhang, D. Fruit and vegetables consumption and risk of hypertension: A meta-analysis. *J. Clin. Hypertens.* **2016**, *18*, 468–476.

7. WHO, Promoting Fruit and Vegetable Consumption Around the World. Available online: https://www.who.int/dietphysicalactivity/fruit/en/index2.html (accessed on 5 June 2019).

8. Bellavia, A.; Larsson, S.C.; Bottai, M.; Wolk, A.; Orsini, N. Fruit and vegetable consumption and all-cause mortality: A dose-response analysis. *Am. J. Clin. Nutr.* **2013**, *98*, 454–459. [PubMed]

9. Buil-Cosiales, P.; Zazpe, I.; Toledo, E.; Corella, D.; Salas-Salvadó, J.; Diez-Espino, J.; Ros, E.; Navajas, J.F.C.; Santos-Lozano, J.M.; Arós, F.; et al. Fiber intake and all-cause mortality in the Prevención con Dieta Mediterránea (PREDIMED) study. *Am. J. Clin. Nutr.* **2014**, *100*, 1498–1507. [CrossRef] [PubMed]

10. Wang, X.; Ouyang, Y.; Liu, J.; Zhu, M.; Zhao, G.; Bao, W.; Hu, F.B. Fruit and vegetable consumption and mortality from all causes, cardiovascular disease, and cancer: Systematic review and dose-response meta-analysis of prospective cohort studies. *BMJ* **2014**, *349*, g4490. [CrossRef]

11. Miller, V.; Mente, A.; Dehghan, M.; Rangarajan, S.; Zhang, X.; Swaminathan, S.; Dagenais, G.; Gupta, R.; Mohan, V.; Lear, S.; et al. Fruit, vegetable, and legume intake, and cardiovascular disease and deaths in 18 countries (PURE): A prospective cohort study. *Lancet* **2017**, *390*, 2037–2049. [CrossRef]

12. Oyebode, O.; Gordon-Dseagu, V.; Walker, A.; Mindell, J.S. Fruit and vegetable consumption and all-cause, cancer and CVD mortality: Analysis of health survey for England data. *J. Epidemiol. Community Health* **2014**, *68*, 856–862. [CrossRef] [PubMed]

13. Liu, Y.; Sobue, T.; Otani, T.; Tsugane, S. Vegetables, fruit consumption and risk of lung cancer among middle-aged Japanese men and women: JPHC study. *Cancer Causes Control* **2004**, *15*, 349–357. [CrossRef] [PubMed]

14. Rajala, M. Nutrition and diet for healthy lifestyles in Europe: Science and policy implications. *Public Health Nutr.* **2001**, *4*, 339–340. [PubMed]

15. World Cancer Research Fund; American Institute for Cancer Research. *Diet Nutrition Physical Activity and Cancer: A Global Perspective*; Continuous Update Project Expert Report 2018; World Cancer Research Fund/American Institute for Cancer Research: Washington, DC, USA, 2018. Available online: http://dietandcancerreport.org (accessed on 27 April 2019).

16. WHO/FAO. *Expert Report on Diet, Nutrition and the Prevention of Chronic Diseases*; Technical Report Series 916; World Health Organisation: Geneva, Switzerland, 2003.

17. Yngve, A.; Wolf, A.; Poortvliet, E.; Elmadfa, I.; Brug, J.; Ehrenblad, B.; Franchini, B.; Haraldsdóttir, J.; Krølner, R.; Maes, L.; et al. Fruit and vegetable intake in a sample of 11-year-old children in 9 European countries: The pro children cross-sectional survey. *Ann. Nutr. Metab.* **2005**, *49*, 236–245. [CrossRef] [PubMed]

18. Nicklett, E.J.; Kadell, A.R. Fruit and vegetable intake among older adults: A scoping review. *Maturitas* **2013**, *75*, 305–312. [PubMed]

19. Amarya, S.; Singh, K.; Sabharwal, M. Changes during aging and their association with malnutrition. *J. Clin. Gerontol. Geriatr.* **2015**, *6*, 78–84.

20. Tsai, A.C.; Chang, T.-L.; Chi, S.-H. Frequent consumption of vegetables predicts lower risk of depression in older Taiwanese—Results of a prospective population-based study. *Public Health Nutr.* **2012**, *15*, 1087–1092. [CrossRef]

21. Loef, M.; Walach, H. Fruit, vegetables and prevention of cognitive decline or dementia: A systematic review of cohort studies. *J. Nutr. Health Aging* **2012**, *16*, 626–630. [CrossRef]

22. Gopinath, B.; Russell, J.; Flood, V.M.; Burlutsky, G.; Mitchell, P. Adherence to dietary guidelines positively affects quality of life and functional status of older adults. *J. Acad. Nutr. Diet.* **2014**, *114*, 220–229. [CrossRef]

23. García-Esquinas, E.; Rahi, B.; Peres, K.; Colpo, M.; Dartigues, J.-F.; Bandinelli, S.; Feart, C.; Rodríguez-Artalejo, F. Consumption of fruit and vegetables and risk of frailty: A dose-response analysis of 3 prospective cohorts of community-dwelling older adults. *Am. J. Clin. Nutr.* **2016**, *104*, 132–142. [CrossRef]

24. Stefler, D.; Pikhart, H.; Kubinova, R.; Pajak, A.; Stepaniak, U.; Malyutina, S.; Simonova, G.; Peasey, A.; Marmot, M.G.; Bobak, M. Fruit and vegetable consumption and mortality in Eastern Europe: Longitudinal results from the health, alcohol and psychosocial factors in Eastern Europe study. *Eur. J. Prev. Cardiol.* **2016**, *23*, 493–501. [CrossRef] [PubMed]

25. Leonardi, M.; Chatterji, S.; Koskinen, S.; Ayuso-Mateos, J.L.; Haro, J.M.; Frisoni, G.; Frattura, L.; Martinuzzi, A.; Tobiasz-Adamczyk, B.; Gmurek, M.; et al. Determinants of health and disability in ageing population: The courage in Europe project (collaborative research on ageing in Europe). *Clin. Psychol. Psychother.* **2014**, *21*, 193–198. [PubMed]

26. Kowal, P.; Chatterji, S.; Naidoo, N.; Biritwum, R.; Fan, W.; Lopez Ridaura, R.; Maximova, T.; Arokiasamy, P.; Phaswana-Mafuya, N.; Williams, S.; et al. Data resource profile: The World Health Organization study on global AGEing and adult health (SAGE). *Int. J. Epidemiol.* **2012**, *41*, 1639–1649. [CrossRef] [PubMed]

27. WHO. Process of Translation and Adaptation of Instruments. Available online: http://www.who.int/ substance_abuse/research_tools/translation/en/ (accessed on 31 March 2019).

28. Üstün, T.; Chatterji, S.; Mechbal, A.; Murray, C.; Groups, W.C. Quality assurance in surveys: Standards, guidelines and procedures. In *Household Sample Surveys in Developing and Transtion Countries*; United Nations: New York, NY, USA, 2005.

29. Bull, F.C.; Maslin, T.S.; Armstrong, T. Global physical activity questionnaire (GPAQ): Nine country reliability and validity study. *J. Phys. Act. Health* **2009**, *6*, 790–804. [CrossRef]

30. Olaya, B.; Moneta, M.V.; Doménech-Abella, J.; Miret, M.; Bayes, I.; Ayuso-Mateos, J.L.; Haro, J.M. Mobility difficulties, physical activity, and all-cause mortality risk in a nationally representative sample of older adults. *J. Gerontol. Ser. A Biol. Sci. Med. Sci.* **2018**, *73*, 1272–1279. [CrossRef]

31. Garin, N.; Koyanagi, A.; Chatterji, S.; Tyrovolas, S.; Olaya, B.; Leonardi, M.; Lara, E.; Koskinen, S.; Tobiasz-Adamczyk, B.; Ayuso-Mateos, J.L.; et al. Global multimorbidity patterns: A cross-sectional, population-based, multi-country study. *J. Gerontol. A Biol. Sci. Med. Sci.* **2016**, *71*, 205–214. [PubMed]

32. Basu, S.; Millett, C. Social epidemiology of hypertension in middle-income countries: Determinants of prevalence, diagnosis, treatment, and control in the WHO SAGE study. *Hypertension* **2013**, *62*, 18–26. [CrossRef]

33. Mancia, G.; Fagard, R.; Narkiewicz, K.; Redón, J.; Zanchetti, A.; Böhm, M.; Christiaens, T.; Cifkova, R.; De Backer, G.; Dominiczak, A.; et al. 2013 ESH/ESC Guidelines for the management of arterial hypertension. *J. Hypertens.* **2013**, *31*, 1281–1357. [CrossRef]

34. World Health Organization WHO. Global Database on Body Mass Index. Available online: http://www.euro. who.int/en/health-topics/disease-prevention/nutrition/a-healthy-lifestyle/body-mass-index-bmi (accessed on 2 May 2019).

35. Rao, J.N.K.; Scott, A.J. On chi-squared tests for multiway contingency tables with cell proportions estimated from survey data. *Ann. Stat.* **1984**, *12*, 46–60. [CrossRef]

36. Buil-Cosiales, P.; Martinez-Gonzalez, M.A.; Ruiz-Canela, M.; Díez-Espino, J.; García-Arellano, A.; Toledo, E. Consumption of fruit or fiber-fruit decreases the risk of cardiovascular disease in a Mediterranean young cohort. *Nutrients* **2017**, *9*, 295. [CrossRef]

37. Hodgson, J.M.; Prince, R.L.; Woodman, R.J.; Bondonno, C.P.; Ivey, K.L.; Bondonno, N.; Rimm, E.B.; Ward, N.C.; Croft, K.D.; Lewis, J.R. Apple intake is inversely associated with all-cause and disease-specific mortality in elderly women. *Br. J. Nutr.* **2016**, *115*, 860–867. [CrossRef]

38. Iimuro, S.; Yoshimura, Y.; Umegaki, H.; Sakurai, T.; Araki, A.; Ohashi, Y.; Iijima, K.; Ito, H. Japanese elderly diabetes intervention trial study group dietary pattern and mortality in Japanese elderly patients with type 2 diabetes mellitus: Does a vegetable- and fish-rich diet improve mortality? An explanatory study. *Geriatr. Gerontol. Int.* **2012**, *12*, 59–67. [CrossRef]

39. Buil-Cosiales, P.; Toledo, E.; Salas-Salvadó, J.; Zazpe, I.; Farràs, M.; Basterra-Gortari, F.J.; Diez-Espino, J.; Estruch, R.; Corella, D.; Ros, E.; et al. Association between dietary fibre intake and fruit, vegetable or whole-grain consumption and the risk of CVD: Results from the PREvención con DIeta MEDiterránea (PREDIMED) trial. *Br. J. Nutr.* **2016**, *116*, 534–546. [CrossRef]

40. Hung, H.-C.; Joshipura, K.J.; Jiang, R.; Hu, F.B.; Hunter, D.; Smith-Warner, S.A.; Colditz, G.A.; Rosner, B.; Spiegelman, D.; Willett, W.C. Fruit and vegetable intake and risk of major chronic disease. *J. Natl. Cancer Inst.* **2004**, *96*, 1577–1584. [CrossRef]

41. Nunes, B.P.; Flores, T.R.; Mielke, G.I.; Thumé, E.; Facchini, L.A. Multimorbidity and mortality in older adults: A systematic review and meta-analysis. *Arch. Gerontol. Geriatr.* **2016**, *67*, 130–138. [CrossRef]

42. Calderón-Larrañaga, A.; Poblador-Plou, B.; González-Rubio, F.; Gimeno-Feliu, L.A.; Abad-Díez, J.M.; Prados-Torres, A. Multimorbidity, polypharmacy, referrals, and adverse drug events: Are we doing things well? *Br. J. Gen. Pract.* **2012**, *62*, e821–e826. [CrossRef]

43. De Mello, C.A.; Engstrom, E.M.; Alves, L.C. Health-related and socio-demographic factors associated with frailty in the elderly: A systematic literature review. *Cad. Saude Publica* **2014**, *30*, 1143–1168. [CrossRef]

44. Hurst, J.R.; Dickhaus, J.; Maulik, P.K.; Miranda, J.J.; Pastakia, S.D.; Soriano, J.B.; Siddharthan, T.; Vedanthan, R.; GACD Multi-Morbidity Working Group. Global alliance for chronic disease researchers' statement on multimorbidity. *Lancet Glob. Health* **2018**, *6*, e1270–e1271. [CrossRef]

45. Trichopoulou, A.; Lagiou, P. Healthy traditional Mediterranean diet: An expression of culture, history, and lifestyle. *Nutr. Rev.* **2009**, *55*, 383–389. [CrossRef]

46. Bermejo, L.M.; Aparicio, A.; Andrés, P.; López-Sobaler, A.M.; Ortega, R.M. The influence of fruit and vegetable intake on the nutritional status and plasma homocysteine levels of institutionalised elderly people. *Public Health Nutr.* **2007**, *10*, 266–272. [CrossRef]

47. Martínez-González, M.A.; Gea, A.; Ruiz-Canela, M. The Mediterranean diet and cardiovascular health: A critical review. *Circ. Res.* **2019**, *124*, 779–798. [CrossRef]

48. Barak, Y.; Fridman, D. Impact of Mediterranean diet on cancer: Focused literature review. *Cancer Genom. Proteom.* **2017**, *14*, 403–408.

49. Schwingshackl, L.; Hoffmann, G. Adherence to Mediterranean diet and risk of cancer: An updated systematic review and meta-analysis of observational studies. *Cancer Med.* **2015**, *4*, 1933–1947. [CrossRef]

50. Samieri, C.; Grodstein, F.; Rosner, B.A.; Kang, J.H.; Cook, N.R.; Manson, J.E.; Buring, J.E.; Willett, W.C.; Okereke, O.I. Mediterranean diet and cognitive function in older age. *Epidemiology* **2013**, *24*, 490–499. [CrossRef]

51. Anastasiou, C.A.; Yannakoulia, M.; Kosmidis, M.H.; Dardiotis, E.; Hadjigeorgiou, G.M.; Sakka, P.; Arampatzi, X.; Bougea, A.; Labropoulos, I.; Scarmeas, N. Mediterranean diet and cognitive health: Initial results from the Hellenic longitudinal investigation of ageing and diet. *PLoS ONE* **2017**, *12*, e0182048. [CrossRef]

52. Trichopoulou, A.; Critselis, E. Mediterranean diet and longevity. *Eur. J. Cancer Prev.* **2004**, *13*, 453–456. [CrossRef]

53. Schwingshackl, L.; Schwedhelm, C.; Hoffmann, G.; Lampousi, A.M.; Knüppel, S.; Iqbal, K.; Bechthold, A.; Schlesinger, S.; Boeing, H. Food groups and risk of all-cause mortality: A systematic review and meta-analysis of prospective studies. *Am. J. Clin. Nutr.* **2017**, *105*, 1462–1473. [CrossRef]

54. Schnabel, L.; Kesse-Guyot, E.; Allès, B.; Touvier, M.; Srour, B.; Hercberg, S.; Buscail, C.; Julia, C. Association between ultraprocessed food consumption and risk of mortality among middle-aged adults in France. *JAMA Intern. Med.* **2019**, *179*, 490–498. [CrossRef]

55. Dauchet, L.; Montaye, M.; Ruidavets, J.-B.; Arveiler, D.; Kee, F.; Bingham, A.; Ferrières, J.; Haas, B.; Evans, A.; Ducimetière, P.; et al. Association between the frequency of fruit and vegetable consumption and cardiovascular disease in male smokers and non-smokers. *Eur. J. Clin. Nutr.* **2010**, *64*, 578–586. [CrossRef]

56. Kesse, E.; Clavel-Chapelon, F.; Slimani, N.; van Liere, M. Do eating habits differ according to alcohol consumption? Results of a study of the French cohort of the European prospective investigation into cancer and nutrition (E3N-EPIC). *Am. J. Clin. Nutr.* **2001**, *74*, 322–327. [CrossRef]

57. Sharma, S.P.; Chung, H.J.; Kim, H.J.; Hong, S.T. Paradoxical effects of fruit on obesity. *Nutrients* **2016**, *8*, 633. [CrossRef]

58. Jezewska-Zychowicz, M.; Gębski, J.; Guzek, D.; Świątkowska, M.; Stangierska, D.; Plichta, M.; Wasilewska, M. The associations between dietary patterns and sedentary behaviors in Polish adults (LifeStyle study). *Nutrients* **2018**, *10*, 1004. [CrossRef]

59. Esmaillzadeh, A.; Kimiagar, M.; Mehrabi, Y.; Azadbakht, L.; Hu, F.B.; Willett, W.C. Fruit and vegetable intakes, C-reactive protein, and the metabolic syndrome. *Am. J. Clin. Nutr.* **2006**, *84*, 1489–1497. [CrossRef]

60. Kris-Etherton, P.M.; Hecker, K.D.; Bonanome, A.; Coval, S.M.; Binkoski, A.E.; Hilpert, K.F.; Griel, A.E.; Etherton, T.D. Bioactive compounds in foods: Their role in the prevention of cardiovascular disease and cancer. *Am. J. Med.* **2002**, *113* (Suppl. 9B), 71S–88S. [CrossRef]

61. Vita, J.A. Polyphenols and cardiovascular disease: Effects on endothelial and platelet function. *Am. J. Clin. Nutr.* **2005**, *81*, 292S–297S. [CrossRef]

14

Comprehensive Geriatric Assessment for Frail Older People in Swedish Acute Care Settings (CGA-Swed)

Katarina Wilhelmson [1,2,3,*], Isabelle Andersson Hammar [1,3], Anna Ehrenberg [4], Johan Niklasson [5], Jeanette Eckerblad [6], Niklas Ekerstad [7,8], Theresa Westgård [1,3], Eva Holmgren [1,3], N. David Åberg [2,9] and Synneve Dahlin Ivanoff [1,3]

[1]   Department of Health and Rehabilitation, Institute of Neuroscience and Physiology, Sahlgrenska Academy, University of Gothenburg, 405 30 Gothenburg, Sweden; isabelle.a-h@neuro.gu.se (I.A.H.); theresa.westgard@neuro.gu.se (T.W.); eva.holmgren@neuro.gu.se (E.H.); synneve.dahlin-ivanoff@neuro.gu.se (S.D.I.)

[2]   Region Västra Götaland, Sahlgrenska University Hospital, Department of Acute Medicine and Geriatrics, 413 45 Gothenburg, Sweden; david.aberg@medic.gu.se

[3]   Centre for Aging and Health—AgeCap, University of Gothenburg, 405 30 Gothenburg, Sweden

[4]   School of Education, Health and Social Studies, Dalarna University, 791 31 Falun, Sweden; aeh@du.se

[5]   Department of Community Medicine and Rehabilitation Geriatric Medicine, Sunderby Research Unit, Umeå University, 901 87 Umeå, Sweden; johan.niklasson@umu.se

[6]   Department of Neurobiology, Care Sciences and Society, Karolinska Institutet, 171 77 Solna, Sweden; jeanette.eckerblad@ki.se

[7]   Region Department of Medical and Health Sciences, Division of Health Care Analysis, Linköping University, 581 83 Linköping, Sweden; niklas.ekerstad@vgregion.se

[8]   Department of Research and Development, NU Hospital Group, 461 73 Trollhättan, Sweden

[9]   Department of Internal Medicine, Institute of Medicine, Sahlgrenska Academy, University of Gothenburg, 405 30 Gothenburg, Sweden

*   Correspondence: katarina.wilhelmson@gu.se

Abstract: The aim of the study is to evaluate the effects of the Comprehensive Geriatric Assessment (CGA) for frail older people in Swedish acute hospital settings – the CGA-Swed study. In this study protocol, we present the study design, the intervention and the outcome measures as well as the baseline characteristics of the study participants. The study is a randomised controlled trial with an intervention group receiving the CGA and a control group receiving medical assessment without the CGA. Follow-ups were conducted after 1, 6 and 12 months, with dependence in activities of daily living (ADL) as the primary outcome measure. The study group consisted of frail older people (75 years and older) in need of acute medical hospital care. The study design, randomisation and process evaluation carried out were intended to ensure the quality of the study. Baseline data show that the randomisation was successful and that the sample included frail older people with high dependence in ADL and with a high comorbidity. The CGA contributed to early recognition of frail older people's needs and ensured a care plan and follow-up. This study is expected to show positive effects on frail older people's dependence in ADL, life satisfaction and satisfaction with health and social care.

Keywords: frail older people; comprehensive geriatric assessment; activities of daily living; geriatric; hospital care

1. Introduction

Even though health care in Sweden is one of the best worldwide [1], many frail older people do not receive appropriate health care. Today's specialised acute care is poorly adapted to the comprehensive care needs of frail older people and, therefore, exposes them to avoidable risks, such as loss of functional capacities, resulting in unnecessary health and social care needs as well as increased mortality [2]. In addition to appropriate specialised care when needed, assessments that are both comprehensive and person-centred are required to provide satisfactory and appropriate care to older people with complex needs [3]. Frailty is a state of decreased reserve resistance to stressors as a result of cumulative decline across multiple physiological systems, causing vulnerability to different outcomes such as falls, hospitalisation, institutionalisation and mortality [3–5]. Frail older people are at risk of further deterioration if their needs are not acknowledged [3]. The prevalence of frailty increases with age and is associated with an elevated risk of adverse health outcomes. Within Europe, the overall prevalence of frailty for people 65 years and older is approximately 10% with the northern countries having lower prevalence than the southern. Sweden has among the lowest, approximately 5% [6,7].

Previous research has found that the Comprehensive Geriatric Assessment (CGA) in acute hospital care is beneficial for frail older patients [8–11] and might be cost effective [12–14]. The CGA adopts a multi-dimensional team approach for assessing medical, functional, psychosocial and environmental needs [15]. The goal is to identify needs and provide support to help older people to be as independent as possible in their daily living. Key components of CGA interventions include coordinated multi-disciplinary assessment; geriatric medicine competence; identification of medical, physical, social and psychological problems; and the formation of a plan for care including appropriate rehabilitation [10]. Other components associated with improved outcomes of CGA are the ability to directly implement treatment recommendations made by the multi-disciplinary team and long-term follow-up [10]. Another key feature is the identification of frail patients. The acute care of older patients currently often takes place in acute care settings with short lengths of stay [16], and the CGA requires time and staff. For efficient use of healthcare resources, it is therefore important to identify those who can benefit the most from such an assessment by screening for frailty [17]. According to consensus from an international expert group, all persons aged ≥70 years should be screened for frailty [3]. Screening for frailty at the emergency department has proven effective [18,19] for identifying those in need of a more comprehensive assessment.

The benefits of CGA are highlighted in systematic reviews by both the Swedish Agency for Health Technology Assessment and Assessment of Social Services (SBU) and the Cochrane Collaboration [8–11]. Positive effects of CGA for frail older patients have been shown in the form of improved functional status, increased ability to remain in own housing and fewer readmissions. These results are important both for the frail older person and for society at large, because the CGA increases the individual's possibility to live independently in their own home and leads to a decreased need for in-hospital and institutional care. However, both reviews state that substantial knowledge gaps concerning the effects of the CGA remain due to the lack of recent studies as well as those evaluating the CGA using validated measures [8,10,11]. Studies on the CGA have been conducted in various countries with different healthcare systems and demographic profiles. The CGA is a complex intervention that is highly dependent upon the context in which it is used [16], and there are very few recent studies carried out within the Swedish healthcare system thus limiting generalisation to the Swedish context.

Swedish healthcare has undergone dramatic changes over the last decades, resulting in decreased numbers of hospital beds and shorter hospital stays [20], especially evident in geriatric hospital care [21]. This has led to Sweden having the lowest per capita hospital bed rate in Europe [20]. Despite the benefits of the CGA, it is a rather unknown concept within Swedish hospital care [11]. Over the past few years, there has been an increased interest, and many geriatric wards have implemented this way of working. However, geriatric hospital care is unevenly distributed within Sweden with a higher density within the bigger cities and university hospitals [11]. The CGA, within a Swedish community setting, has recently proven successful in maintaining/improving independence in activities of daily living (ADL) [22] as has the CGA in outpatient care [23]. One recent controlled study of an acute CGA unit reported the positive effects on health-related quality of life and mortality without higher costs [24]. Besides these studies, recent studies within Swedish acute care are scarce. Other limitations of these reviews are that many of the studies are dated, have limited sample sizes and have other methodological flaws [8–11]. More knowledge is needed on the implementation, effectiveness and cost effectiveness of the CGA in modern acute care settings. There is also a need to further investigate the relationship between frailty and the CGA as pointed out in a recent umbrella review of the CGA by Parker et al. [25]. This review also states that patient-related outcomes of the CGA—such as health-related quality of life, well-being and participation—are scarcely reported.

Thus, there is still a need for studies on the CGA and interventions using the CGA to improve acute care for frail older people in Swedish health care settings. To meet this need, we designed the study "Comprehensive Geriatric Assessment for Frail Older People in Swedish Acute Care Settings (CGA-Swed): A Randomised Controlled Study" with the purpose of improving hospital care for frail older people by implementing the CGA in Swedish acute care and testing the effects of the CGA in a randomised controlled study (RCT). The intervention was planned and elaborated in collaboration between professionals and researchers. The study includes both quantitative and qualitative analyses of the effects of CGA and a process evaluation of the implementation process throughout the intervention period. It started with a pilot and feasibility study that showed that the intervention—the CGA—and the research procedures were feasible [26]. There were also results indicating that the CGA increased patient safety [26]. Qualitative interviews with frail older people receiving care with the CGA at the intervention ward showed that they felt respected as persons when they were enabled to understand, engage in communication and participate in decisions [27]. The process evaluation alongside the RCT will add to the knowledge on the implementation of the CGA.

Aim and Research Questions

The aim of the study was to evaluate the effects of the CGA for frail older people in Swedish acute hospital settings. The study addresses the following research questions:

Can the Comprehensive Geriatric Assessment for frail older people in Swedish acute hospital settings:

1.   Maintain independence in activities of daily living, functional status, health-related quality of life and life satisfaction?
2.   Increase satisfaction with health care?
3.   Reduce hospital and primary health care consumption?

How feasible and acceptable are the study processes and procedures of the CGA from the perspective of care givers and older persons in Swedish settings?

Ethical approval was obtained for the study, ref. no: 4,899-15, Regional Ethical Review Board in Gothenburg. Trial Registration: ClinicalTrials.gov, NCT02773914.

This paper presents the study design, the intervention, baseline characteristics and the outcome measures of the study in accordance with the recommendations for reporting pragmatic randomised controlled trials by CONSORT [28].

2. Material and Methods

2.1. Project Context

The intervention "Comprehensive Geriatric Assessment for frail older people in Swedish acute care settings" took place at Sahlgrenska University Hospital/Sahlgrenska in Gothenburg, Sweden. Gothenburg is the second largest city in Sweden, situated on the west coast. It had 556,000 inhabitants in the year 2016. Sahlgrenska University Hospital is the regional hospital for Gothenburg and the surrounding municipalities, serving a total of almost one million inhabitants in 2016. The percentage of the population of people aged 75 and over for this region was 7.4% in 2016, compared to 8.6% for all of Sweden [29].

2.2. Study Design

The study was a two-armed randomised controlled trial that started with a pilot study in 2016. The CGA is a complex intervention that influences clinicians' cognitive processes, requires multi-disciplinary collaboration and organisation of healthcare and is highly dependent upon the context in which it is used [16]. An RCT conducted in isolation may not be sufficient to provide guidance for decision makers in healthcare on whether or not to implement research findings. In addition, it is of interest to explore why, for whom and under what circumstances the intervention works. Thus, there was a process evaluation alongside the complex intervention as recommended by the Medical Research Council [30]. The pilot study and the process evaluation provide insight into the function and consequences of the intervention—why it works or fails—and help assess the feasibility of the intervention and research procedures. They also provide data on the number of factors that need to be assessed to successfully monitor and evaluate outcomes. This was an important part of the design that will shed light on real-life conditions that may be challenging in implementing the CGA. The pilot study with the first 30 participants showed that both the intervention and the research procedures worked well [26].

2.3. Study Population

The study group included 155 older people who sought acute medical care at the emergency department during the period between March 2016 and December 2018. Inclusion criteria were that participants were to be ≥75 years of age, in need of acute in-hospital care and screened as frail according to the FRESH-screening instrument. This screening instrument was chosen, since it was already implemented in clinical use, has high sensitivity and specificity (81% and 80%) for screening for frailty in acute settings and has an excellent clinical value [19]. It consists of four questions regarding dependence in shopping, tiredness, fatigue and risk of falling. Two or more "yes" responses indicate frailty. Exclusion criteria were not being screened as frail according to the FRESH-screening instrument, being admitted through a "fast track" for direct admission to a designated ward (for predefined diagnosis such as stroke, acute myocardial infarction and hip fracture) and having an acute severe condition requiring a higher level of care (e.g., intensive care) than the intervention ward. Cognitive impairment was not an exclusion criterion, and if the participant could not give informed consent due to the fact of cognitive impairment ($n = 11$), informed consent was obtained from next of kin.

2.4. Intervention Group

The intervention was the ward working according to the Comprehensive Geriatric Assessment. Key components of the CGA are multi-disciplinary teamwork, use of a person-centred approach [31], comprehensive assessments, treatment and rehabilitation, discharge planning and follow-up (see Figure 1). The multi-disciplinary team consisted of a physician, registered nurse (RN), assistant nurse (AN), physiotherapist (PT) and occupational therapist (OT) as well as other team members, such as a social worker (SW) and dietician, if needed. A pharmacist would have been valuable to include in the team, but this is not common in Swedish hospital wards. The senior physicians at the intervention wards were all specialist in geriatrics. The team had primary and continuing responsibility for assessment, planning of hospital care and discharge. Assessments of medical status, self-assessed health, functional status, psychological status, social situation and environment (see Table 1) were administered to ensure a comprehensive evaluation of the health and life situation of the frail older patient. The team used a person-centred approach [31] to individualise the assessment. A team conference was held every weekday to promote the sharing of information, experiences and competences in order to individualise the care for each patient.

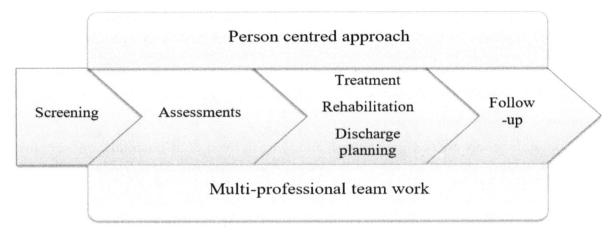

Figure 1. Key components of the Comprehensive Geriatric Assessment (CGA).

The content of the CGA was adapted to local routines and experiences and was elaborated in collaboration between the researchers and those working in the clinical setting where the intervention took place. This was to ensure that the CGA would be both clinically acceptable and evidence based. All personal at the intervention ward received education (i.e., information and workshops) on the CGA prior to the start of the study. During the whole study period, the researchers had meetings with representatives from the different professionals in order to follow how the teams experienced working according to the CGA.

The CGA starts at the intervention ward and continues throughout the hospital stay. It is individualised and unique for each patient, based on the key components in Figure 1 and the assessments in Table 1, providing a comprehensive assessment tailored for each person.

Table 1. Assessments included in the CGA.

Domain	Assessment	Main Professional Responsible
Medical status	Illness burden/medical review	Physician
	Symptoms	Physician/RN
	Somatic status	Physician
	Pharmaceutical review	Physician
	Nutritional status	RN/Dietician
Self-assessed health	Self-assessed health	Physician/RN
Functional status	Activities of daily living	OT
	Physical function	PT
	Sight and hearing	RN/AN
Psychological status	Cognition	OT
	Depression	Physician
Social situation	Social network/informal support	RN/SW
	Formal support	RN/SW
	Financial support	RN/SW
Environment	Living conditions	RN/SW/AN
	Transports	RN/SW/AN
	Accessibility and assistive devices	OT/SW

RN = registered nurse; OT = occupational therapist; PT = physiotherapist; AN = assistant nurse; SW = social worker.

2.5. Control Group

The control group received the usual acute hospital care, i.e., care given at an ordinary medical hospital ward without a specialised multi-disciplinary team approach and without the CGA. The assessments and care provided at the control wards were based on the acute problem/symptom that the patients had and did not include the comprehensive and person-centred approach to the health and life situation of the patient inherent in a CGA. The occupational therapist and the physiotherapist worked more as consultants, and the amount of resources from occupational therapists and physiotherapists were lower at the control wards compared with the intervention wards. At the control ward, they did not perform functional tests, assessments of social network and total disease burden on all frail older patients. The senior physician at the control wards were specialists in internal medicine and were not geriatricians.

2.6. Procedures of the Intervention Study

Older patients who were screened as frail and were in need of in-hospital care were invited to participate in the study during the stay in the Emergency Department (ED). Those who agreed to participate were then randomised into control or intervention groups. Randomisation was done by computer-generated numbers and assigned by one of the researchers using QuickCalcs at GraphPad [32]. The allocation was concealed in numbered opaque envelopes. When a patient consented to participate, the hospital bed coordinator opened the envelope and admitted the patient to the designated ward. The intervention group was admitted to the ward according to the CGA and the control group to a general acute medical ward.

Baseline measures were collected by a research assistant who gathered data from the frail older patient and/or from the medical records during the hospital stay. Six participants were discharged before the baseline interview was completed. For these participants, parts or the whole of the baseline data collection was carried out in the participants' homes as soon as possible after discharge. One participant was discharged to a surgical ward at a different hospital before the baseline interview, suffered a stroke after surgery and, thus, was admitted to the stroke ward at the intervention hospital. For this participant, the baseline interview was conducted retrospectively at the same time as the one-month follow-up which was performed during the stay at the stroke ward.

Follow-up interviews were performed in the older person's home at 1, 6 and 12 months after hospital discharge. The follow-ups were performed using a structured questionnaire including questions about demographic data and assessments of outcome measures. The interviews lasted for approximately 1.5 h. Proxy interviews were done if the participant had a cognitive impairment making them unable to participate in parts or the whole of the baseline/follow-up data collection. No proxy interview was necessary at baseline. However, for a few participants, a next of kin was present during parts of the interview, providing additional information for participants who had difficulties remembering. Next of kin were also present at many follow-up interviews, supplementing the information provided during the interviews. A few of the follow-ups required proxy interviews. Whenever possible, the same person performed all follow-ups for the same participant, minimising the number of people that a frail older participant needed to meet.

The participants could not be blinded to the ward they were being admitted to, but they were not aware at which ward the intervention took place. However, they might have realised if they were administered the CGA. The wards could not be blinded to allocation, because the ward was the allocation. Not all patients at the intervention and control wards were included in the study, and the staff at the wards was not informed which patients were included in the study. In this respect, the staff could be seen as blinded. However, they might have observed the research assistant performing the baseline data collection and thereby understood that the patient was included in the study. Thus, the staff could not be completely blinded to allocation. The researchers performing the baseline interviews could not be blinded. The plan was that the collection of baseline measures and the performance of follow-up interviews were to be carried out by different researchers in order to keep the researchers blinded at the follow-up. However, the participants may have revealed the allocation (i.e., whether administered the CGA or not) during the follow-up interviews, making the interviewers non-blinded. To address this, we added a variable at all follow-ups indicating whether or not the allocation had been revealed which also reflects whether or not the participant was aware of being administered the CGA or not.

Meetings with representatives of all staff categories were regularly held at the intervention ward throughout the entire intervention period. There was a steering group with representatives from the research group and the different clinical care levels (geriatrics, internal medicine and rehabilitation) that met regularly, starting with the planning of the study and lasting throughout the whole study period.

The researchers (occupational therapists, physiotherapists, registered nurses and physicians) performing the interviews and measurements at baseline and follow-ups were all trained in observing and assessing in accordance with the guidelines for the outcome measurements.

2.7. Outcome Measures

For an overview of outcome measures and time of measure, see Table 2.

Table 2. Outcome measures and follow-ups.

Primary Outcomes	Measurement	Baseline	1 Month	6 Months	1 Year
Dependence	ADL-staircase [33]	X	X	X	X
Secondary Outcomes					
Functional status	Timed Up and Go [34]	X	X	X	X
	The Berg Balance Scale [35]	X			X
	Gait Speed 4 m [36]	X	X	X	X
	Grip Strength North Coast Dynamometer [37]	X	X	X	X
Cognition	Mini Mental State Examination (MMSE) [38]	X	X	X	X
Self-rated health	Questionnaire	X	X	X	X
	Symptoms: Göteborg Quality of Life Instrument [39]	X	X	X	X
Life satisfaction	Fugl–Meyer–Lisat-11 Questionnaire [40]	X	X	X	X
Satisfaction with quality of care	Questionnaire	X			
Health care consumption	Register Data				
Home help services	Questionnaire/Register Data	X	X	X	X
Capability	ICECAP-O [41]	X			X
Mortality	Register Data				

2.7.1. The Primary Outcome

Dependence in daily activities was measured using the ADL-staircase assessment [33] by combining both interviews and observations. It includes dependence in nine activities: cleaning, shopping, transportation, cooking, bathing, dressing, going to the toilet, transferring and feeding. Dependence was defined as a state in which another person is involved in the activity by giving personal or directive assistance. The sum of dependence in the nine activities of daily living is calculated, range 0–9, with a clinically significant change of ≥1 unit between baseline and follow-up. At baseline, personal ADL (PADL: bathing, dressing, going to the toilet, transferring and feeding) was inquired for both actual PADL status during the hospital stay and retrospectively for PADL before onset of the acute illness leading to the hospital admission. This was done because the acute illness often leads to a higher dependence in PADL.

2.7.2. The Secondary Outcomes

Functional status was measured using the Timed Up and Go (TUG) test [34], the Berg Balance Scale [35], Gait Speed four-metre walking test [36] and Grip Strength with North Coast Dynamometer [37]. The TUG test measures the time for a person to rise from a chair, walk 3 m, turn around, walk back, and sit down again. It measures both static and dynamic balance. In this study, we defined a change of ≥4 s as a clinically significant difference between baseline and follow-up, with 3.6 s considered as the minimal detectable change for TUG test measurements [42]. For details on Berg Balance Scale, Gait Speed and Grip Strength, see Section 2.8. Cognition was measured using the Mini Mental State Examination [38], see Section 2.8.

Self-rated was measured by the question: "In general, would you say your health is", with the response alternatives: excellent, very good, good, fair, and poor. Clinically significant difference was defined as ≥1 step in the response alternatives between baseline and follow-up. In addition, self-reported symptoms were measured using the Göteborg Quality of Life Instrument [39].

Life satisfaction was measured using the Fugl–Meyer–Lisat-11 Questionnaire [40] which includes 11 items concerning satisfaction with: life as a whole, work, financial situation, leisure, friends and acquaintances, sexual life, functional capacity, family life, partner relationship, physical health and psychological health. Response alternatives included: very dissatisfied, dissatisfied, rather dissatisfied, rather satisfied, satisfied and very satisfied. In the analysis, the responses to each question were dichotomised into satisfied (very satisfied and satisfied) or not satisfied (rather satisfied, rather dissatisfied, dissatisfied and very dissatisfied) as was done in the validation of the questionnaire [40]. The sum of items for which the respondent reported being satisfied were calculated, range 0–11, with a clinically significant change of ≥1 between baseline and follow-up.

Satisfaction with quality of care was measured by the participant's agreement with six statements with a person-centred approach: "I feel that the care given during the hospital stay meets my needs", "I feel that the care planning meeting before discharge was valuable", "I was able to take part in the discussion of my needs in the care planning meeting", "I feel that the actions planned equal my needs", "I feel that the actions delivered equal my needs" and "I am satisfied with the hospital care". The response alternatives were agree completely, agree partly, neither agree nor disagree, disagree, and disagree completely. An answer of agree completely or agree partly were considered as satisfied. These questions were only measured once (at 1 month follow-up) and were used as the difference between intervention and control groups in the proportion of participants being satisfied for each question at follow-up as has been done previously [43].

Outcomes concerning health–economic aspects are health and social care consumption. Data on health care consumption can be retrieved from the regional care databases, including in-hospital and outpatient care, visits to primary healthcare (physicians, physiotherapists, occupational therapists, nurses, and assistant nurses) and home visits by primary healthcare professionals. The number of readmissions, number of in-hospital days, time until first readmission and number of outpatient visits were calculated and compared between intervention and control group for 1 year after study enrolment. Social care consumption was measured by questions about help received for instrumental and personal ADL from the municipality, privately financed help, relatives, friends and/or other. Response alternatives included none, less than once a week, once a week or more and daily. Extent and frequency of help received was calculated and compared between intervention and control groups for 1 year after study enrolment. In addition, questions covered institutional care, such as nursing home, retirement home and sheltered housing, from which the number of days in institutional care were calculated and compared between intervention and control groups for 1 year after study enrolment.

To add to this, we used the ICECAP-O [41,44], which measures capability in older people, for use in the economic evaluation of health and social care interventions. It focuses on well-being defined in a broader sense and covers five attributes: (1) attachment; (2) security; (3) role; (4) enjoyment; and (5) control. The respondent chose one of five statements for each attribute. (1) Attachment: "I can have all the love and friendship that I want"; "I can have a lot of the love and friendship that I want"; "I can have a little of the love and friendship that I want"; "I cannot have any of the love and friendship that I want". (2) Security: "I can think about the future without any concern"; "I can think about the future with only a little concern"; "I can only think about the future with some concern"; "I can only think about the future with a lot of concern". (3) Role: "I am able to do all the things that make me feel valued"; "I am able to do many of the things that make me feel valued"; "I am able to do a few of the things that make me feel valued"; "I am unable to do any of the things that make me feel valued". (4) Enjoyment: "I can have all the enjoyment and pleasure that I want"; "I can have a lot of the enjoyment and pleasure that I want"; "I can have a little of the enjoyment and pleasure that I want"; "I cannot have any of the enjoyment and pleasure that I want". (5) Control: "I am able to be completely independent"; "I am able to be independent in many things"; "I am able to be independent in a few things"; "I am unable to be at all independent".

Mortality rates will be retrieved from the National Cause of Death Registry.

2.8. Measurement of Frailty Indicators

In this study, we used the following measurements and cut-off levels of frailty indicators:

Weakness: Reduced grip strength considered to be below lowest norm range for ages 80–84, 13 kg for women and 21 kg for men for the right hand and below 10 kg for women and 18 kg for men for the left hand, using a North Coast dynamometer [37].

Fatigue: Question from the Göteborg Quality of Life Instrument [39], answering "Yes" to the question "Have you suffered any general fatigue/tiredness over the last three months?"

Weight loss: Question from the Göteborg Quality of Life Instrument [39], answering "Yes" to the question "Have you suffered any weight loss over the last three months?"

Reduced physical activity: Taking 1–2 or less outdoor walks per week.

Impaired balance: The Berg Balance Scale [35,45,46], reduced balance defined as having a value of 47 or less.

Reduced gait speed: Walking four metres with a gait speed of 0.6 metres/second or slower [36].

Visual impairment: The KM chart (Konstantin Moutakis chart) [47], impaired vision defined as having a visual acuity of 0.5 or less.

Impaired cognition: The MMSE [38], impaired cognition defined as having a score below 25.

2.9. Statistical Analysis and Power Calculation

A power calculation was done based on the primary outcome variable, dependence in activities of daily living (range 0–9) with an assumed difference between the intervention and control groups of one dependence (i.e., dependent in one or more activities of daily living, a clinically relevant difference of importance to the individual as well as the caregiver) and a standard deviation of 2 in both groups. To detect a difference between the intervention and control groups with a two-sided test and with a significance level of $\alpha = 0.05$ and 80% power, at least 64 participants were needed in each group. To take a potential loss to follow-up into account, a total of 150 persons (75 in the control group and 75 in the intervention group) were initially planned to be included. This was later revised to allow for a higher loss to follow-up (22%) with 78 + 78, equalling a total of 156 participants. The assumed loss to follow-up and the power calculation were based on previous research on frail older people in need of acute care [48].

Both descriptive and analytical statistics were used in order to compare groups and to analyse changes over time. Non-parametric statistics were used when ordinal data were analysed. Otherwise, parametric statistics were used. Besides descriptive statistics, the chi^2 and Fisher's two-tailed exact tests to test differences in the proportions among the groups were used. A value of $p \leq 0.05$ (two-tailed) were considered significant. The analysis were made on the basis of the intention-to-treat principle, meaning that participants were analysed on the basis of the group to which they were initially randomised. Given the old age of the participants, a relatively high drop-out rate was inevitable. Simply analysing complete cases is not relevant and might lead to bias, especially since missing data would not be at random. Therefore, the approach of data imputation was the replacement of missing values with a value based on the median change of deterioration between baseline and follow-up of all who participated in the follow-up [20]. The reasons for this imputation method were that (1) the study sample (frail older people) was expected to deteriorate over time as a natural course of the ageing process and (2) deteriorated health often is a reason for not fulfilling the follow-ups. Worst-case change was imputed for those who died before follow-up.

2.10. Process Evaluation

The process evaluation aims to provide insight into what is inside "the black box", i.e., shed light on the function and consequences of the intervention—why it works or fails. The process evaluation includes context, recruitment, reach, dose delivered and received and fidelity [49], targeting recruitment and collection of outcome measures during the hospital stay and after discharge. The process evaluation focuses on the following aspects in line with the recommendations of the Medical Research Council [30]:

- The intervention, the actual exposure and the experience of the participants;
- Evaluation of which components of the intervention contributed to its success or failure;
- Description of the conditions under which the intervention is successful/unsuccessful.

The evaluation includes in-depth qualitative interviews with eight to ten participants in the intervention group, focusing on their experiences of receiving care according to the CGA [27]. The experiences of the staff working with to the CGA are explored through focus group discussions in order to gain an understanding of the intervention and its significance as well as its implementation. This includes the respondent's role in working according to the CGA, perceptions about the CGA and its significance and effectiveness and possibilities and challenges involved in working according to the CGA. The focus group methodology distinctly utilises the interaction among participants in order to collect data, encouraging them to clarify not only what they think but also how and why they think in a certain way. The method is suitable for collecting the views and experiences of a selected group and generating a broad knowledge and understanding [50]. In addition, medical records are reviewed to assure that the assessments in the CGA have been conducted as intended, what aspects of CGA has been performed and by whom (i.e., the actual exposure).

2.11. Economic Analysis

The first step in the health–economic evaluation was to conduct a cost-minimisation analysis that compared the total costs between the CGA and CONTROL during the full follow-up period using the healthcare consumption data (measured as the cost of all resources used) as described above. This showed the cost implications for the payers if implementing the CGA or CONTROL.

The second step in the health–economic evaluation was to conduct a cost-effectiveness analysis. The cost-effectiveness of the intervention (versus the control) was evaluated based on the incremental cost-effectiveness ratio (ICER): ICER = (CostCGA – CostCONTROL)/(EffectivenessCGA – EffectivenessCONTROL). The effectiveness measure was based on the score from the ICECAP-O which measures older people's capability for use in economic evaluation [41,44]. The ICER can be interpreted as the cost per one-unit gain in full capability and can, as such, be compared to other interventions using the same outcome measure in order to evaluate the relative cost-effectiveness. Sensitivity analysis and confidence intervals were calculated based on the non-parametric bootstrap approach.

2.12. Time Plan of the Study

The inclusion began in March 2016 and was completed in December 2018. The intervention began when the participant was admitted to the ward and lasted until discharge from the hospital. The follow-ups after one year are planned to be completed in January 2020. See Table 3 for time plan for the study and follow-ups.

Table 3. Time plan for the study and follow-ups.

	Started	Completed	To Be Completed
Inclusion	March 2016	December 2018	
Baseline	March 2016	December 2018	
I month follow-up	April 2016	January 2019	
6 month follow-up	September 2016	July 2019	
12 month follow-up	March 2016		January 2020

3. Results

3.1. Baseline Characteristics

The inclusion and randomisation were carried out by the hospital bed coordinators at the emergency departments, because they are always involved when a patient is admitted to a ward, and they are responsible for coordinating available hospital beds. They had no extra time for this task and presumably did not always remember to inform and ask eligible patients. In addition, in many cases it was not possible to randomise due to the shortage of hospital beds at the wards (as there had to be a vacant bed at both the intervention ward and the control ward to be able to randomise). We asked the hospital bed coordinators to monitor how many patients were eligible and how many declined to participate. Unfortunately, due to their high work load, they only monitored this for approximately half a year. Based on the monitoring that was conducted, we estimated that approximately 210 eligible patients were asked to participate, and 178 of those consented to participate resulting in an estimated participation rate of approximately 85%. For details regarding the number of participants receiving allocated intervention with baseline data and reasons for declining participation, see Figure 2.

The median age of the participants in the inclusion year was 87 years in the control and 87.5 years in the intervention group. There were no statistically significant differences concerning baseline characteristics, frailty indicators and ADL between the control and intervention groups, see Tables 4–6.

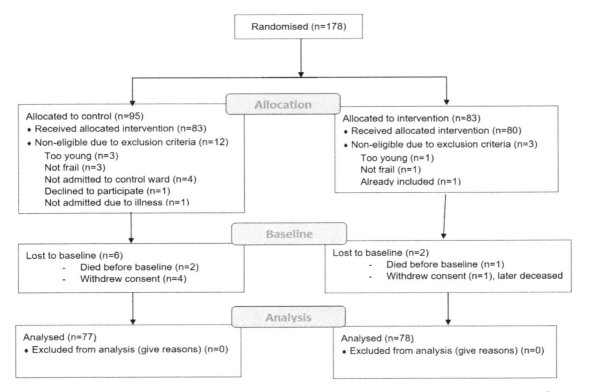

Figure 2. Flowchart of the three phases of the study implementing the "Comprehensive Geriatric Assessment in Swedish Acute Hospital Settings (CGA-Swed): A Randomised Controlled Study", according to CONSORT [28].

Table 4. Baseline characteristics of the study population.

Characteristics	Control Group N = 77	Intervention Group N = 78	p-Value
Age, mean (range)	86.2 (76–98)	87.5 (75–101)	0.17
Female, % (n)	55.8 (43)	60.3 (47)	0.58
Living alone, % (n)	62.3 (48)	65.4 (51)	0.70
Academic education, % (n)	20.1 (16)	10.3 (8)	0.07
Good self-rated health, % (n) *	27.3 (21)	33.3 (26)	0.41
CIRS-G ≥ 3 in any category, % **	93.5 (72)	98.7 (77)	0.26
CIRS-G, median number of ratings 3–4 (range)	3 (0–9)	3 (0–7)	

* Excellent, very good or good. ** Cumulative Illness Rating Scale for Geriatrics. Rating 3 = severe/constant significant disability/uncontrollable chronic problem and rating 4 = extremely severe/immediate treatment required/end-organ failure/severe impairment in function [51].

Table 5. Frailty indicators.

Frailty Indicator	Control Group N = 77	Intervention group N = 78	p-Value
Fatigue, % (n) [1]	90.9 (70)	87.2 (68)	0.46
Weight loss, % (n) [2]	50.0 (38)	51.9 (40)	0.81
Weakness, % (n) [3]	28.6 (22)	36.0 (27)	0.33
Reduced physical activity, % (n) [4]	71.1 (54)	68.0 (51)	0.68
Impaired balance, % (n) [5]	86.8 (66)	94.8 (73)	0.09
Reduced gait speed, % (n) [6]	75.3 (58)	84.2 (64)	0.17
Visual impairment, % (n) [7]	80.0 (60)	78.7 (59)	0.84
Impaired cognition, % (n) [8]	48.1 (37)	52.0 (39)	0.63
Number of frailty indicators [9]			
1, % (n)	1.3 (1)	0	0.88
2, % (n)	6.5 (5)	3.8 (3)	
3, % (n)	11.7 (9)	9.0 (7)	
4, % (n)	11.7 (9)	14.1 (11)	
5, % (n)	19.5 (15)	21.8 (17)	
6, % (n)	20.8 (16)	26.9 (21)	
7, % (n)	20.8 (16)	16.7 (13)	
8, % (n)	7.8 (6)	7.7 (6)	

[1] Answering "Yes" to the question "Have you suffered any general fatigue/tiredness over the last three months?" (Part of the Göteborg Quality of Life Instrument [39]). [2] Answering "Yes" to the question "Have you suffered any weight loss over the last three months?" (Part of the Göteborg Quality of Life Instrument [39]). Missing 1 in the control. [3] Reduced grip strength: below 13 kg for women and 21 kg for men for the right hand and below 10 kg for women and 18 kg for men for the left hand, using a North Coast dynamometer [37]. Missing 3 in the intervention. [4] Taking outdoor walks 1–2 times a week or less. Missing 1 in the control and 3 in the intervention. [5] Having a value of 47 or less on the Berg Balance Scale [35,45,46]. Missing 1 in the control and 1 in the intervention. [6] Walking four metres with a gait speed of 0.6 metres/second or slower [36]. Missing 2 in the control and 2 in the intervention. [7] Having a visual acuity of 0.5 or less using the KM chart [47]. Missing 2 in the control and 3 in the intervention. [8] Scoring below 25 on the Mini Mental State Examination (MMSE) [38]. Missing 3 in the intervention. [9] Missing information on 1–4 frailty indicators for 13 participants.

3.2. Process Evaluation during Inclusion Period

There was a period (approximately half a year) with very high work strain for the CGA staff during the inclusion. The ward had to open up ten additional hospital beds within a couple of days due to the shortage of beds available at the hospital. This led to the need of hiring staff that did not have the knowledge and experience of working according to the CGA. Therefore, it is probable that a majority of the participants in the intervention group during this period did not receive a full CGA. Through the medical record review, we will investigate the extent to which the CGA was documented for each participant in order to be able to estimate the completeness of the CGA actually received by each participant in the intervention group.

In addition, there have been many readmissions during the follow-up period, in many cases to a different ward than during the inclusion. Thus, several participants in the control group may have received care at the CGA ward during the year after inclusion. This also needs to be considered when analysing follow-up data.

Table 6. ADL dependence at baseline.

Number of Dependences		Control Group N = 77	Intervention Group N = 78	p-Value
IADL dependence, % (n)	0	9.1 (7)	6.4 (5)	0.11
	1	19.5 (15)	7.7 (6)	
	2	18.2 (14)	14.1 (11)	
	3	20.8 (16)	21.8 (17)	
	4	32.5 (25)	50.0 (39)	
PADL dependence before onset of illness, % (n)	0	61.0 (47)	52.6 (41)	0.83
	1	15.6 (12)	16.7 (13)	
	2	7.8 (6)	12.8 (10)	
	3	7.8 (6)	7.7 (6)	
	4	5.2 (4)	5.1 (4)	
	5	2.6 (2)	5.1 (4)	
PADL dependence during hospital stay, % (n)	0	31.2 (24)	23.1 (18)	0.38
	1	20.8 (16)	11.5 (9)	
	2	9.1 (7)	12.8 (10)	
	3	9.1 (7)	10.3 (8)	
	4	24.7 (19)	33.3 (26)	
	5	5.2 (4)	9.0 (7)	

4. Discussion

The study "CGA-Swed" was designed to evaluate the effects of the CGA for frail older people in Swedish acute hospital settings. The primary outcome was dependence in ADL, as this has been pointed out as an important aspect for frail older people in previous research [52,53]. Secondary outcomes include other important aspects and patient-related outcomes such as self-rated health, life satisfaction, satisfaction with care, health care consumption and cost-effectiveness. Another strength of the study was the process evaluation alongside the RCT, adding to the knowledge on the implementation of the CGA and, thus, filling a knowledge gap pointed out by the Cochrane reviews of the CGA [9,10].

The randomisation seems to have been successful, as the baseline characteristics were similar between the intervention and control groups with no statistically significant differences among the two groups. Unfortunately, we do not know how many eligible participants could have been asked to participate nor how many in fact were asked to participate. This limitation could be seen as a consequence of performing a complex intervention in "real life", being dependent on clinical staff performing parts of the research process. In our study, we were dependent on the hospital bed coordinators asking eligible participants beyond their ordinary duties as hospital bed coordinators and with no extra time or reward given. Similarly, it was not possible for us to have a researcher designated for the inclusion, since this would have required too much time and resources. Our estimate of a participation rate of 85% may seem high but seems realistic to us after discussion with the hospital bed coordinators. However, some of the participants had not fully understood what they had consented to, as they were asked about participation when seeking care for an acute medical problem. There is a risk that some were so comforted by being admitted to a ward that they consented out of pure relief. However, the researcher doing the baseline interview repeated the information about the study and asked once again about consent to participate, and very few participants declined participation at this occasion.

The baseline characteristics show that our sample was frail and had a high morbidity and high degree of dependence in activities of daily living. This is not surprising, since they all were screened as frail and in need of acute in-hospital care. The prevalence of frailty is known to be high among patients in internal medicine wards and especially in geriatric wards [54]. Thus, we argue that our sample is representative for frail older hospital medical in-patients. However, this also indicates a risk of high mortality within the sample, as both frailty and comorbidity are risk factors for high mortality [3,55]. Already during the hospital stay, three participants died, and preliminary data shows a high mortality rate to the follow-ups, higher than we expected based on earlier research [22,48].

The implementation process evaluation alongside the RCT—aiming to provide insight into the function and consequences of the intervention, why it works or fails—is an important part of the design that will contribute with insights into real-life conditions that may be challenging in implementing the CGA. The logistics of the intervention and the research procedures were tested in the pilot study and were found feasible [26]. The major deviation from the plan was the prolonged inclusion period because of the lack of available hospital beds which has prevailed throughout the study. However, we were eventually able to include the first estimated sample size of 150 participants, lacking only one participant to reach the revised estimated sample size of 156 participants. The process evaluation is a strength of the study, enabling us to generate knowledge on the process of the implementation of the CGA which has been pointed out as a knowledge gap by the Cochrane reviews of the CGA [9,10]. The results of the implementation process evaluation are planned to be presented in a forthcoming paper. There were some obvious threats to the study during the inclusion period and the follow-up period that we already observed and which may hamper our ability to demonstrate positive outcomes. The period with high work strain at the intervention ward is very likely to have led to CGAs of both lower quantity and quality than what was planned for. The patient medical record review will help us identify those not receiving a full CGA and allow us to adjust the analysis accordingly. However, this will probably lead to lower ability to detect a true difference between the groups. In addition, the fact that participants in the control group might have been admitted to the intervention group during the follow-up period needs to be accounted for in the analysis. As this can make the sample in each group smaller, this might also lead to lower power.

Findings on how frail older persons experience receiving care according to the CGA have already been published elsewhere based on this study, showing that they experienced being seen as a person while being admitted to a CGA ward [27].

To a large extent, we used the same questionnaires, measurements, manuals and outcomes as in our previous studies "Elderly Persons in the Risk Zone" [56] and "Continuum of Care for Frail Elderly People" [48]. This gives us the opportunity to compare among the studies with different levels of frailty within the samples, with the sample in "Elderly Persons in the Risk Zone" being prefrail [56] and the sample in "Continuum of Care" being less frail [48] than the sample in the current study. The outcome measures for the studies were carefully selected to make sure that they are valid and reliable for the target group and covering different components and levels of frailty.

We planned to have different researchers doing the baseline interviews and the follow-ups so as to be able to keep the researcher blinded at the follow-ups. However, in many cases it has been and will be the same research assistant doing the follow-up interviews who also conducted the baseline interview. Thus, we have not been able to keep the researcher blinded at the follow-up. The research assistant has, however, conducted most of the baseline interviews ($n = 155$) and in most cases did not remember the group assignment. It can also be seen as a strength that the same person carries out most interviews and assessments, as this ensures that the questions and assessments are done similarly at all occasions, thus enhancing the reliability of the assessments. In addition, having the same person in the follow-ups minimises the number of persons the participant has to meet. This might increase the chance of the participant remaining in the study, as they already are familiar with the person asking to do the follow-up. Since we had a variable at the follow-up regarding whether or not the researcher was aware of the allocation or whether the participant had revealed the allocation during the interview, we will know to what extent the researcher was blinded.

The intervention was planned in collaboration with representatives from the Department of Geriatrics (i.e., intervention ward), the Department of Medicine (i.e., control wards) and the Department of Occupational Therapy and Physiotherapy. Regular meetings were held, starting with the planning of the study and lasting throughout the intervention period to discuss the content of the intervention and the research procedures which enhanced the implementation and strengthened the study. Both the research group and the group of professionals carrying out the intervention are multi-professional which is important since the CGA implies multi-professional team collaboration.

In summary, this study evaluated the CGA in current Swedish acute hospital settings employing a randomised controlled design, adding to the knowledge of the effects of the CGA in today's hospital care which is characterised by shorter hospital stays and fewer available hospital beds than before. The results are expected to optimise the implementation of future complex interventions and lead to the improvement of care, support and rehabilitation of frail older people with complex needs. The process evaluation, aiming to provide insights into the function and consequences of the intervention—why it works or fails—is an important part of the design that will contribute with insights into real life conditions that may be challenging in implementing the CGA. This study is expected to show positive effects on frail older people's dependence in activities of daily living, an outcome that is important for both the person and society. In addition, the CGA has potential to increase the satisfaction with care, life satisfaction and self-rated health as well as prevent deterioration in functional status and to be cost effective.

Author Contributions: K.W. led the intervention of the study and was the primary author of the manuscript. K.W., A.E. and S.D.I. participated in the research design. K.W., A.E., J.N., J.E., N.E. and S.D.I. participated in the planning of the study. K.W., I.A.H., T.W., E.H., N.D.Å. and S.D.I. participated in the implementation of the study. K.W., I.A.H., T.W. and E.H. collected data. All authors contributed to the writing and review of the manuscript and approved the submitted version of the manuscript. All authors have read and agreed to the published version of the manuscript.

Acknowledgments: Special thanks to the hospital bed coordinators at Sahlgrenska University Hospital, Catarina Söderström and Jenny Midsem, for their participation in the inclusion of participants, and to research assistant Katharina Sjöberg for data collection.

References

1. Barber, R.M.; Fullman, N.; Sorensen, R.J.; Bollyky, T.; McKee, M.; Nolte, E.; Abajobir, A.A.; Abate, K.H.; Abbafati, C.; Abbas, K.M. Healthcare Access and Quality Index based on mortality from causes amenable to personal health care in 195 countries and territories, 1990–2015: A novel analysis from the Global Burden of Disease Study 2015. *Lancet* **2017**, *390*, 231–266. [CrossRef]

2. Lafont, C.; Gérard, S.; Voisin, T.; Pahor, M.; Vellas, B. Reducing "iatrogenic disability" in the hospitalized frail elderly. *J. Nutr. Health Aging* **2011**, *15*, 645–660. [CrossRef] [PubMed]

3. Morley, J.E.; Vellas, B.; Van Kan, G.A.; Anker, S.D.; Bauer, J.M.; Bernabei, R.; Cesari, M.; Chumlea, W.; Doehner, W.; Evans, J. Frailty consensus: A call to action. *J. Am. Med. Dir. Assoc.* **2013**, *14*, 392–397. [CrossRef] [PubMed]

4. McMillan, G.; Hubbard, R. Frailty in older inpatients: What physicians need to know. *QJM Int. J. Med.* **2012**, *105*, 1059–1065. [CrossRef] [PubMed]

5. Clegg, A.; Young, J.; Iliffe, S.; Rikkert, M.O.; Rockwood, K. Frailty in elderly people. *Lancet* **2013**, *381*, 752–762. [CrossRef]

6. Castell, M.V.; Van Der Pas, S.; Otero, A.; Siviero, P.; Dennison, E.; Denkinger, M.; Pedersen, N.; Sanchez-Martinez, M.; Queipo, R.; Van Schoor, N. Osteoarthritis and frailty in elderly individuals across six European countries: Results from the European Project on OSteoArthritis (EPOSA). *BMC Musculoskelet. Dis.* **2015**, *16*, 359. [CrossRef] [PubMed]

7. Haider, S.; Grabovac, I.; Dorner, T.E. Fulfillment of physical activity guidelines in the general population and frailty status in the elderly population. *Wiener Klin. Wochenschr.* **2019**, *131*, 288–293. [CrossRef]

8. Ekdahl, A.; Sjöstrand, F.; Ehrenberg, A.; Oredsson, S.; Stavenow, L.; Wisten, A.; Wårdh, I.; Ivanoff, S.D. Frailty and comprehensive geriatric assessment organized as CGA-ward or CGA-consult for older adult patients in the acute care setting: A systematic review and meta-analysis. *Eur. Geriatr. Med.* **2015**, *6*, 523–540. [CrossRef]

9.   Ellis, G.; Gardner, M.; Tsiachristas, A.; Langhorne, P.; Burke, O.; Harwood, R.H.; Conroy, S.P.; Kircher, T.; Somme, D.; Saltvedt, I. Comprehensive geriatric assessment for older adults admitted to hospital. *Cochrane Database Syst. Rev.* **2017**. [CrossRef]

10. Ellis, G.; Whitehead, M.A.; Robinson, D.; O'Neill, D.; Langhorne, P. Comprehensive geriatric assessment for older adults admitted to hospital: Meta-analysis of randomised controlled trials. *BMJ* **2011**, *343*, d6553. [CrossRef]

11. Swedish Agency for Health Technology Assessment and Assessment of Social Services. Comprehensive Geriatric Assessment and Care of Frail Elderly. SBU Report no 221. 2014. Available online: https://www.sbu.se/sv/publikationer/SBU-utvarderar/omhandertagande-av-aldre-som-inkomm er-akut-till-sjukhus--med-fokus-pa-skora-aldre/ (accessed on 9 December 2019). (In Swedish)

12. Barnes, D.E.; Palmer, R.M.; Kresevic, D.M.; Fortinsky, R.H.; Kowal, J.; Chren, M.-M.; Landefeld, C.S. Acute care for elders units produced shorter hospital stays at lower cost while maintaining patients' functional status. *Health Aff.* **2012**, *31*, 1227–1236. [CrossRef] [PubMed]

13. Ekerstad, N.; Karlson, B.W.; Andersson, D.; Husberg, M.; Carlsson, P.; Heintz, E.; Alwin, J. Short-term resource utilization and cost-effectiveness of comprehensive geriatric assessment in acute hospital care for severely frail elderly patients. *J. Am. Med. Dir. Assoc.* **2018**, *19*, 871–878.e872. [CrossRef] [PubMed]

14. Melis, R.J.; Adang, E.; Teerenstra, S.; van Eijken, M.I.; Wimo, A.; Achterberg, T.V.; Lisdonk, E.H.V.d.; Rikkert, M.G.O. Multidimensional geriatric assessment: Back to the future cost-effectiveness of a multi-disciplinary intervention model for community-dwelling frail older people. *J. Gerontol A Biol. Sci. Med. Sci* **2008**, *63*, 275–282. [CrossRef] [PubMed]

15. Rubenstein, L.; Siu, A.; Wieland, D. Comprehensive geriatric assessment: Toward understanding its efficacy. *Aging Clin. Exp. Res.* **1989**, *1*, 87–98. [CrossRef]

16. Gladman, J.R.; Conroy, S.P.; Ranhoff, A.H.; Gordon, A.L. New horizons in the implementation and research of comprehensive geriatric assessment: Knowing, doing and the 'know-do'gap. *Age Ageing* **2016**, *45*, 194–200. [CrossRef]

17. Graf, C.E.; Zekry, D.; Giannelli, S.; Michel, J.-P.; Chevalley, T. Efficiency and applicability of comprehensive geriatric assessment in the emergency department: A systematic review. *Aging Clin. Exp. Res.* **2011**, *23*, 244–254. [CrossRef]

18. Leichsenring, K. Developing integrated health and social care services for older persons in Europe. *Int. J. Integr. Care* **2004**, *4*. [CrossRef]

19. Eklund, K.; Wilhelmson, K.; Landahl, S.; Ivanoff-Dahlin, S. Screening for frailty among older emergency department visitors: Validation of the new FRESH-screening instrument. *BMC Emerg. Med.* **2016**, *16*, 27. [CrossRef]

20. OECD. Health Statistics. Available online: http://www.oecd.org/els/health-systems/health-data.htm (accessed on 30 August 2017).

21. Borgström, A. Sverige har lägst antalet vårdplatser i Europa. [Sweden has the lowest number of hospital beds in Europe]. *Läkartidningen* **2007**, *104*, 396–397.

22. Eklund, K.; Wilhelmson, K.; Gustafsson, H.; Landahl, S.; Dahlin-Ivanoff, S. One-year outcome of frailty indicators and activities of daily living following the randomised controlled trial: "Continuum of care for frail older people". *BMC Geriatr.* **2013**, *13*, 76. [CrossRef]

23. Ekdahl, A.W.; Alwin, J.; Eckerblad, J.; Husberg, M.; Jaarsma, T.; Mazya, A.L.; Milberg, A.; Krevers, B.; Unosson, M.; Wiklund, R. Long-term evaluation of the ambulatory geriatric assessment: A frailty intervention trial (AGe-FIT): Clinical outcomes and total costs after 36 months. *J. Am. Med. Dir. Assoc.* **2016**, *17*, 263–268. [CrossRef] [PubMed]

24. Ekerstad, N.; Karlson, B.W.; Ivanoff, S.D.; Landahl, S.; Andersson, D.; Heintz, E.; Husberg, M.; Alwin, J. Is the acute care of frail elderly patients in a comprehensive geriatric assessment unit superior to conventional acute medical care? *Clin. Interv. Aging* **2017**, *12*, 1. [CrossRef] [PubMed]

25. Parker, S.; McCue, P.; Phelps, K.; McCleod, A.; Arora, S.; Nockels, K.; Kennedy, S.; Roberts, H.; Conroy, S. What is comprehensive geriatric assessment (CGA)? An umbrella review. *Age Ageing* **2017**, *47*, 149–155. [CrossRef] [PubMed]

26. Westgård, T.; Ottenvall Hammar, I.; Holmgren, E.; Ehrenberg, A.; Wisten, A.; Ekdahl, A.W.; Dahlin-Ivanoff, S.; Wilhelmson, K. Comprehensive geriatric assessment pilot of a randomized control study in a Swedish acute hospital: A feasibility study. *Pilot Feasibility Stud.* **2018**, *4*, 41. [CrossRef]

27. Westgård, T.; Wilhelmson, K.; Dahlin-Ivanoff, S.; Ottenvall Hammar, I. Feeling Respected as a Person: A Qualitative Analysis of Frail Older People's Experiences on an Acute Geriatric Ward Practicing a Comprehensive Geriatric Assessment. *Geriatrics* **2019**, *4*, 16. [CrossRef]

28. Zwarenstein, M.; Treweek, S.; Gagnier, J.J.; Altman, D.G.; Tunis, S.; Haynes, B.; Oxman, A.D.; Moher, D. Improving the reporting of pragmatic trials: An extension of the CONSORT statement. *BMJ* **2008**, *337*, a2390. [CrossRef]

29. Statistics Sweden. Available online: http://www.statistikdatabasen.scb.se (accessed on 28 October 2019).

30. Medical Resarch Council. Available online: http://www.mrc.ac.uk/ (accessed on 30 August 2017).

31. Ekman, I.; Swedberg, K.; Taft, C.; Lindseth, A.; Norberg, A.; Brink, E.; Carlsson, J.; Dahlin-Ivanoff, S.; Johansson, I.-L.; Kjellgren, K. Person-centered care—Ready for prime time. *Eur. J. Cardiovasc. Nurs.* **2011**, *10*, 248–251. [CrossRef]

32. GraphPad. Random Number Generator. Available online: https://graphpad.com/quickcalcs/randomN1.cfm (accessed on 9 December 2019).

33. Sonn, U. Longitudinal studies of dependence in daily life activities among elderly persons. *Scand. J. Rehabil. Med. Suppl.* **1996**, *34*, 1–35.

34. Schoppen, T.; Boonstra, A.; Groothoff, J.W.; de Vries, J.; Göeken, L.N.; Eisma, W.H. The Timed "up and go" test: Reliability and validity in persons with unilateral lower limb amputation. *Arch. Phys. Med. Rehabil.* **1999**, *80*, 825–828. [CrossRef]

35. Berg, K.O.; Wood-Dauphinee, S.L.; Williams, J.I.; Maki, B. Measuring balance in the elderly: Validation of an instrument. *Can. J. Public Health* **1992**, *83*, S7–S11. [PubMed]

36. Peterson, M.J.; Giuliani, C.; Morey, M.C.; Pieper, C.F.; Evenson, K.R.; Mercer, V.; Cohen, H.J.; Visser, M.; Brach, J.S.; Kritchevsky, S.B. Physical activity as a preventative factor for frailty: The health, aging, and body composition study. *J. Gerontol. A Biol. Sci. Med. Sci.* **2009**, *64*, 61–68. [CrossRef] [PubMed]

37. Mathiowetz, V.; Kashman, N.; Volland, G.; Weber, K.; Dowe, M.; Rogers, S. Grip and pinch strength: Normative data for adults. *Arch. Phys. Med. Rehabil.* **1985**, *66*, 69–74.

38. Folstein, M.F.; Folstein, S.E.; McHugh, P.R. "Mini-mental state". A practical method for grading the cognitive state of patients for the clinician. *J. Psychiatr. Res.* **1975**, *12*, 189–198. [CrossRef]

39. Tibblin, G.; Tibblin, B.; Peciva, S.; Kullman, S.; Svardsudd, K. "The Goteborg quality of life instrument"–an assessment of well-being and symptoms among men born 1913 and 1923. Methods and validity. *Scand. J. Prim. Health Care. Suppl.* **1990**, *1*, 33–38.

40. Fugl-Meyer, A.R.; Bränholm, I.-B.; Fugl-Meyer, K.S. Happiness and domain-specific life satisfaction in adult northern Swedes. *Clin. Rehabil.* **1991**, *5*, 25–33. [CrossRef]

41. Coast, J.; Peters, T.J.; Natarajan, L.; Sproston, K.; Flynn, T. An assessment of the construct validity of the descriptive system for the ICECAP capability measure for older people. *Qual Life Res.* **2008**, *17*, 967–976. [CrossRef]

42. Resnik, L.; Borgia, M. Reliability of outcome measures for people with lower-limb amputations: Distinguishing true change from statistical error. *Phys. Ther.* **2011**, *91*, 555–565. [CrossRef]

43. Berglund, H.; Wilhelmson, K.; Blomberg, S.; Duner, A.; Kjellgren, K.; Hasson, H. Older people's views of quality of care: A randomised controlled study of continuum of care. *J. Clin. Nurs.* **2013**, *22*, 2934–2944. [CrossRef]

44. Gustafsson, S.; Hörder, H.; Hammar, I.O.; Skoog, I. Face and content validity and acceptability of the Swedish ICECAP-O capability measure: Cognitive interviews with 70-year-old persons. *Health Psychol. Res.* **2018**, *6*, 6496. [CrossRef]

45. Berg, K.; Wood-Dauphine, S.; Williams, J.; Gayton, D. Measuring balance in the elderly: Preliminary development of an instrument. *Physiother. Can.* **1989**, *41*, 304–311. [CrossRef]

46. Chiu, A.Y.; Au-Yeung, S.S.; Lo, S.K. A comparison of four functional tests in discriminating fallers from non-fallers in older people. *Disabil. Rehabil.* **2003**, *25*, 45–50. [CrossRef]

47. Moutakis, K.; Stigmar, G.; Hall-Lindberg, J. Using the KM visual acuity chart for more reliable evaluation of amblyopia compared to the HVOT method. *Acta Ophthalmol. Scand.* **2004**, *82*, 547–551. [CrossRef]

48. Wilhelmson, K.; Duner, A.; Eklund, K.; Gosman-Hedström, G.; Blomberg, S.; Hasson, H.; Gustafsson, H.; Landahl, S.; Dahlin-Ivanoff, S. Design of a randomized controlled study of a multi-professional and multidimensional intervention targeting frail elderly people. *BMC Geriatr.* **2011**, *11*, 24. [CrossRef] [PubMed]

49. Linnan, L.; Steckler, A. *Process. Evaluation for Public Health Interventions and Research*; Jossey-Bass: San Francisco, CA, USA, 2002.

50. Kitzinger, J. The methodology of focus groups: The importance of interaction between research participants. *Sociol. Health Illn.* **1994**, *16*, 103–121. [CrossRef]

51. Miller, M.D.; Paradis, C.F.; Houck, P.R.; Mazumdar, S.; Stack, J.A.; Rifai, A.H.; Mulsant, B.; Reynolds, C.F., 3rd. Rating chronic medical illness burden in geropsychiatric practice and research: Application of the Cumulative Illness Rating Scale. *Psychiatry Res.* **1992**, *41*, 237–248. [CrossRef]

52. Haak, M.; Fange, A.; Iwarsson, S.; Ivanoff, S.D. Home as a signification of independence and autonomy: Experiences among very old Swedish people. *Scand. J. Occup. Ther.* **2007**, *14*, 16–24. [CrossRef]

53. Häggblom-Kronlöf, G.; Hultberg, J.; Eriksson, B.G.; Sonn, U. Experiences of daily occupations at 99 years of age. *Scand. J. Occup. Ther.* **2007**, *14*, 192–200. [CrossRef]

54. Andela, R.M.; Dijkstra, A.; Slaets, J.P.; Sanderman, R. Prevalence of frailty on clinical wards: Description and implications. *Int. J. Nurs. Pract.* **2010**, *16*, 14–19. [CrossRef]

55. Nunes, B.P.; Flores, T.R.; Mielke, G.I.; Thume, E.; Facchini, L.A. Multimorbidity and mortality in older adults: A systematic review and meta-analysis. *Arch. Gerontol. Geriatr.* **2016**, *67*, 130–138. [CrossRef]

56. Dahlin-Ivanoff, S.; Gosman-Hedstrom, G.; Edberg, A.K.; Wilhelmson, K.; Eklund, K.; Duner, A.; Ziden, L.; Welmer, A.K.; Landahl, S. Elderly persons in the risk zone. Design of a multidimensional, health-promoting, randomised three-armed controlled trial for "prefrail" people of 80+ years living at home. *BMC Geriatr.* **2010**, *10*, 27. [CrossRef] [PubMed]

15

The Convergent Validity of the electronic Frailty Index (eFI) with the Clinical Frailty Scale (CFS)

Antoinette Broad [1], Ben Carter [2], Sara Mckelvie [3,4] and Jonathan Hewitt [5,*]

[1] Community Services, Oxford Health NHS Foundation Trust, Oxford OX3 7JX, UK; antoinette.broad@oxfordhealth.nhs.uk

[2] Department of Biostatistics and Health Informatics, Institute of Psychiatry, Psychology & Neuroscience, King's College London, London SE5 8AF, UK; ben.carter@kcl.ac.uk

[3] Emergency Medical Unit, Oxford Health NHS Foundation Trust, Oxford OX3 7JX, UK; sara.mckelvie@oxfordhealth.nhs.uk or S.Mckelvie@soton.ac.uk

[4] Primary Care Research Group, Faculty of Medicine, University of Southampton, Southampton SO17 1BJ, UK

[5] Division of Population Medicine, Cardiff University, Penarth CF64 2XX, UK

[*] Correspondence: hewittj2@cardiff.ac.uk

Abstract: Background: Different scales are being used to measure frailty. This study examined the convergent validity of the electronic Frailty Index (eFI) with the Clinical Frailty Scale (CFS). **Method:** The cross-sectional study recruited patients from three regional community nursing teams in the South East of England. The CFS was rated at recruitment, and the eFI was extracted from electronic health records (EHRs). A McNemar test of paired data was used to compare discordant pairs between the eFI and the CFS, and an exact McNemar Odds Ratio (OR) was calculated. **Findings:** Of 265 eligible patients consented, 150 (57%) were female, with a mean age of 85.6 years (SD = 7.8), and 78% were 80 years and older. Using the CFS, 68% were estimated to be moderate to severely frail, compared to 91% using the eFI. The eFI recorded a greater degree of frailty than the CFS (OR = 5.43, 95%CI 3.05 to 10.40; $p < 0.001$). This increased to 7.8 times more likely in men, and 9.5 times in those aged over 80 years. **Conclusions:** This study found that the eFI overestimates the frailty status of community dwelling older people. Overestimating frailty may impact on the demand of resources required for further management and treatment of those identified as being frail.

Keywords: clinical Frailty Scale; electronic Frailty Index; community

1. Introduction

Frailty has been defined as a state of vulnerability to adverse outcomes, as a consequence of cumulative decline in physiological systems and homeostatic reserve over the course of an individual's lifetime [1]. Frailty is a distinct syndrome independent of disease [2].

With populations worldwide ageing rapidly frailty is high on everyone's agenda, although the concept is well recognised, an international consensus to define frailty has yet to be reached [3]. In the absence of such a gold standard, many tools have been developed [4]. A standard measurement tool would provide a consistent recognition of frailty [5].

Due to age-related changes, frailty is diagnosed more often in older people [5]. Early identification of frailty can decrease the burden of disease, maintain independence longer and improve quality of life [6]. In response to this increasing evidence, NHS England published a new NHS long term plan [7] which calls for more proactive approaches to targeting interventions appropriately whilst contractually obliging General Practitioners (GPs) to identify patients over the age of 65 with moderate to severe frailty [8]. One frailty measure, the electronic Frailty Index (eFI) can be calculated by GPs using existing software and has become the GPs' preferred frailty tool [9]. The Clinical Frailty Scale (CFS) is another validated measure of frailty based on clinical presentation. It is commonly used in clinical practice to diagnose frailty due to its simplicity [10]. It is essential that frailty is reproducible across different instruments used to identify it (convergent validity).

The study aimed to examine the convergent validity of the electronic Frailty Index (eFI) [11] with the 9- point Clinical Frailty Scale (CFS) [12] on community dwelling older people admitted onto a community nursing caseload.

2. Materials and Methods

2.1. Study Design

An observational design across three sites in the UK. The study was conducted in December 2018. As data used were collected as part of routine care, the study was deemed a service evaluation and was registered locally.

2.2. Participants

Community dwelling people (65 years or over) accepted on to three separate community nursing caseloads during one week in December 2018 were eligible to participate. Selected community nursing caseloads were determined by the following factors: geographical area, number of GP practices and location; city, town or village. Participants excluded from the study were those aged below 65 years.

2.3. Measures

The eFI is a cumulative deficit model that calculates frailty by retrieving patient information recorded from the electronic health record (EHR) [11]. It includes 36 deficit variables derived from diseases, symptoms and clinical signs recorded on the EHR. It can be calculated automatically on the EHR without the oversight of a clinician. Supplementary Table S1 shows the 36 deficits. It includes physical limitations including requirement of care, activity, mobility and transfer problems. It divides the total number of deficits present by the total possible creating a score between 0-1. The deficits each have a binary score of 1 if present and 0 when absent. eFI = Sum of deficits/36 (total number of deficits). The score is categorised accordingly into levels of severity, 0–0.12 = fit; >0.12–0.24 = mild frailty; >0.24–0.36 = moderate frailty and above 0.36 = severely frail [11].

The nine category Clinical Frailty Scale (CFS), is a validated measure of frailty based on clinical presentation. The assessor judges the level of frailty based on clinical findings and includes physical disability, cognition and co morbidity. It scores between one (very fit) to nine (terminally ill with a life expectancy of <6 months) [12]. Each point on the scale corresponds with a picture and written description to assist the clinician to grade the frailty score, a score = or >5 is frail [13]. Supplementary Figure S1 demonstrates the CFS.

2.4. Scoring Frailty

2.4.1. eFI

Trained senior community nurses extracted the participants personal demographic data from community nursing teams' EHR then accessed the participants eFI scores from the GP practice EHR.

2.4.2. CFS

An assessment of frailty using the CFS was completed in the participants' home during routine visits by community nurses within one week of their eFI screening. Training on how to complete the CFS was delivered by the study team. Nurses using the CFS were blinded to the recorded eFI score and classification. Participants were categorised as fit/mild or moderate/severely frail based on their reported scores.

The CFS and eFI were both dichotomised into two comparable scores of fit/mildly frail (CFS very fit, to mildly frail; eFI fit, to mildly frail), and moderately/severely frail (CFS moderately frail to terminally frail; eFI moderate to severely frail).

2.5. Statistical Analysis

Descriptive statistics were used to describe the population demographics and the distribution of frailty. Both the eFI and CFS were categorised into fit/mild, and moderate/severe. Categorisation of CFS followed the literature and 1–5 was compared to CFS 6–9, [14,15]; eFI was less common reported, and we mapped across a consistent threshold for this tool.

The McNemar test was used to test the association between the rating of the two frailty instruments: the eFI and the CFS [16]. The odds ratio (OR) and 95% confidence interval of over estimating frailty was calculated using the discordant pairs (e.g., comparing those more frail in the eFI (but not the CFS), was compared with those more frail in the CFS (but not the eFI)).

A subgroup analysis included patients aged over 80 years, as well as by gender. All analyses were carried out using Stata version 15.0.

3. Results

A total of 365 patients were recorded on the caseload, of which 327 met the eligibility criteria, 62 were removed due to incomplete data. Of those included, 150 (57%) were female, with a mean age of 85.6 years (SD = 7.8), and 78% were 80 years and older. Frailty prevalence estimates of moderate/severe were 91% (eFI), and 68% (CFS). (Table 1). There was a higher proportion of female patients in the moderate/severely frail group, but similar proportions of men and women in the fit/mildly frail group. Association between the frailty instruments was assessed by discordant pair analysis (Table 2).

Table 1. Demographic characteristics of the study population.

Category of Frailty	eFI		CFS	
	Fit/Mild	Moderate/Severe	Fit/Mild	Moderate/Severe
Total patients	23 (9%)	242 (91%)	85 (32%)	180 (68%)
Age (mean)	80.7	86	84.8	85.95
Male	10 (43%)	105 (43%)	43 (51%)	72 (40%)
Female	13 (57%)	137 (57%)	42 (49%)	108 (60%)

Table 2. Association between the electronic Frailty Index (eFI) and the Clinical Frailty Scale (CFS).

		CFS		
	Category of frailty	Fit to Mild	Moderate to Severe	Total
eFI	Fit to Mild	9	14	23
	Moderate to severe	76	166	242
	Total	85	180	265

Looking at the discordant pairs there were 76 patients seen by a clinician and found to have fit/mild frailty via the CFS but recorded moderate/severe frailty using the eFI, and inversely 14 patients scored moderate/severe with the CFS but as fit/mildly frail with the eFI. There was very strong evidence of an association of difference in the rate of discordant pairs ($p < 0.001$), and indication that the eFI is recorded with a greater degree of frailty. A patient being scored as more severely frail using the eFI compared to the CFS exhibited an OR = 5.43, (95%CI 3.05 to 10.40; $p < 0.001$).

Subgroup analysis estimated that this over scoring was more extreme in patients who were over 80 years old ($p < 0.001$), and in men ($p < 0.001$) (Table 3).

Table 3. Subgroup of electronic Frailty Index (eFI) and the Clinical Frailty Scale (CFS) scores by age.

≤80 years	CFS		
eFI	Mild/fit	Moderate/severe	Total
Mild/fit	4 (a)	8 (b)	12 (a + b)
Moderate/severe	19 (c)	39 (d)	58 (c + d)
total	23 (a + c)	47 (b + d)	70
>80 years	CFS		
eFI	Mild/fit	Moderate/severe	Total
Mild/fit	5 (a)	6 (b)	11 (a + b)
Moderate/severe	57 (c)	127 (d)	184 (c + d)
total	62 (a + c)	133 (b + d)	195

4. Discussion

This study found no evidence of convergent validity and the findings suggest that the eFI overestimates frailty among community dwelling older people. This overestimation increased for people greater than 80 years and for men. These findings conflict with recent studies that support the convergent validity of the two instruments [11,17] and endorse the eFI as a valid case finding tool to identify moderate/severely frail patients who may benefit from targeted interventions [11,18,19].

One explanation for the heterogeneity between scores might be that the two frailty instruments are underpinned by two very different theoretical frameworks. The CFS has been used widely (most recently during the COVID-19 pandemic) and has clinical judgement and has good face validity, it requires clinicians to undertake assessments of their patients' comorbidities in real time [20]. Time to complete the CFS assessment and staff training are two main factors that limit the use of the CFS in practice [21]. In contrast the eFI is quick and requires minimal resources to complete; an accumulative deficit tool can be generated automatically on the GP system [11]. Utilising GP records for collecting patient data to assess frailty has been hailed as the gold standard [22]. The eFI is reliant upon clinicians applying clinical judgement and recording patient data accurately, and poor recording on the EHR can lead to absences of deficits or deficits can remain, even for temporary conditions [18]. Deficits no longer relevant to the patient's current health state can lead to the eFI score being a biased estimate, potentially resulting in the reporting of the patient's poorest estimate of frailty.

A second explanation for the divergent scores may be due to the population as housebound populations are often frail [23] so the findings from this study may not be comparable to the other studies that targeted total populations, their findings reported much lower levels of frailty [11]. Participants in the other studies that supported the convergent validity of the eFI and CFS were also less frail and younger than this study population [11,17]. This could offer an explanation as to why the scores were so different in that the eFI exhibited the worst status of the patient's frailty and the convergent validity of the eFI and CFS may only be true for a younger, fit/mildly frail population. This study sample size and targeted population may limit the generalisability of the study findings.

5. Conclusions

The eFI has been recommended as a screening tool for frailty in primary care. This study suggests that the CFS offers current utility and the eFI overestimates the degree of frailty among housebound, older people, so use of the eFI may deplete health resources by directing services to people who do not require them. Thus, CFS should be preferred over the eFI. We recommend replicating this study on a larger scale to explore the above findings in more detail and to investigate the eFI as a case finding tool.

By having a greater understanding of frailty, clinicians can identify those at greatest risk of adverse health outcomes. Assessing frailty in older people over 65 years is now mandated in primary care in

England [8]. The eFI is a popular choice due to its accessibility and ease of use but it may overestimate a patient's true frailty status.

Author Contributions: Conceptualisation, A.B., J.H. and S.M.; methodology, A.B., J.H.; software, A.B., B.C.; validation, A.B., J.H., B.C. and S.M.; formal analysis, A.B., B.C., J.H.; investigation, A.B.; resources, A.B.; data curation; A.B., B.C., J.H.; writing—original draft preparation, A.B..; writing—review and editing, J.H., B.C. and S.M.; supervision, J.H.; project administration, A.B. All authors have read and agreed to the published version of the manuscript.

References

1. Clegg, A.; Rogers, L.; Young, J. Diagnostic test accuracy of simple instruments for identifying frailty in community-dwelling older people: A systematic review. *Age Ageing* **2014**, *44*, 148–152. [CrossRef] [PubMed]
2. Chen, C.Y.; Gan, P.; How, C.H. Approach to frailty in the elderly in primary care and the community. *Singap. Med. J.* **2018**, *59*, 240–245. [CrossRef] [PubMed]
3. John, P.D.S.; McClement, S.S.; Swift, A.U.; Tate, R.B. Older Men's Definitions of Frailty—The Manitoba Follow-up Study. *Can. J. Aging* **2018**, *38*, 13–20. [CrossRef] [PubMed]
4. Gilardi, F.; Capanna, A.; Ferraro, M.; Scarcella, P.; Marazzi, M.C.; Palombi, L.; Liotta, G. Frailty screening and assessment tools: A review of characteristics and use in Public Health. *Ann. Ig.* **2018**, *30*, 128–139. [PubMed]
5. Dent, E.; Kowal, P.; Hoogendijk, E.O. Frailty measurement in research and clinical practice: A review. *Eur. J. Intern. Med.* **2016**, *31*, 3–10. [CrossRef] [PubMed]
6. British Geriatric Society (BGS). Comprehensive Geriatric Assessment Toolkit for Primary Care Practitioners (online). 2019. Available online: https://www.bgs.org.uk/resources/resource-series/comprehensive-geriatric-assessment-toolkit-for-primary-care-practitioners (accessed on 10 July 2020).
7. NHS England. NHS Long Term Plan (online). 2019. Available online: https://www.longtermplan.nhs.uk/online-version/ (accessed on 4 July 2020).
8. NHS England. Supporting Routine Frailty Identification and Frailty through the GP Contract 2017/2018 (online). 2019. Available online: https://www.england.nhs.uk/publication/supporting-routine-frailty-identification-and-frailty-through-the-gp-contract-20172018/ (accessed on 7 July 2020).
9. Stow, D.; Matthews, F.E.; Barclay, S.; Iliffe, S.; Clegg, A.; De Biase, S.; Robinson, L.; Hanratty, B. Evaluating frailty scores to predict mortality in older adults using data from population based electronic health records: Case control study. *Age Ageing* **2018**, *47*, 564–569. [CrossRef] [PubMed]
10. Long, S.; Jelley, B.; Martin, R.; Suter-Jones, V.E. Underestimation of frailty using the 7-point Clinical Frailty Scale: An evaluation of geriatric registrar scoring accuracy. *Age Ageing* **2018**, *47*, ii25–ii39. [CrossRef]
11. Clegg, A.P.; Bates, C.; Young, J.; Ryan, R.; Nichols, L.; Teale, E.A.; Mohammed, M.A.; Parry, J.; Marshall, T. Development and validation of an electronic frailty index using routine primary care electronic health record data. *Age Ageing* **2016**, *45*, 353–360. [CrossRef] [PubMed]
12. Rockwood, K.; Song, X.; Macknight, C.; Bergman, H.; Hogan, D.; McDowell, I.; Mitnitski, A. A global clinical measure of fitness and frailty in elderly people. *Can. Med Assoc. J.* **2005**, *173*, 489–495. [CrossRef] [PubMed]
13. Ozsurekci, C.; Balcı, C.; Kızılarslanoğlu, M.C.; Çalışkan, H.; Doğrul, R.T.; Ayçiçek, G. Şengül; Sümer, F.; Karabulut, E.; Yavuz, B.B.; Cankurtaran, M.; et al. An important problem in an aging country: Identifying the frailty via 9 Point Clinical Frailty Scale. *Acta Clin. Belg.* **2019**, *75*, 200–204. [CrossRef] [PubMed]
14. Owen, R.K.; Conroy, S.P.; Taub, N.; Jones, W.; Bryden, D.; Pareek, M.; Faull, C.; Abrams, K.R.; Davis, D.; Banerjee, J. OUP accepted manuscript. *Age Ageing* **2020**. [CrossRef]
15. Aw, D.; Woodrow, L.; Ogliari, G.; Harwood, R. Association of frailty with mortality in older inpatients with Covid-19: A cohort study. *Age Ageing* **2020**. [CrossRef] [PubMed]
16. Upton, G.J.; Cook, I. *A Dictionary of Statistics*; Oxford University Press: Oxford, UK, 2006.
17. Brundle, C.; Heaven, A.; Brown, L.; Teale, E.; Young, J.; West, R.; Clegg, A. Convergent validity of the electronic frailty index. *Age Ageing* **2018**, *48*, 152–156. [CrossRef] [PubMed]
18. Abbasi, M.; Khera, S.; Dabravolskaj, J.; Vandermeer, B.; Theou, O.; Rolfson, D.; Clegg, A. A cross-sectional study examining convergent validity of a frailty index based on electronic medical records in a Canadian primary care program. *BMC Geriatr.* **2019**, *19*, 109.

19. Lansbury, L.N.; Roberts, H.C.; Clift, E.; Herklots, A.; Robinson, N.; Sayer, A.A. Use of the electronic Frailty Index to identify vulnerable patients: A pilot study in primary care. *Br. J. Gen. Pr.* **2017**, *67*, e751–e756. [CrossRef] [PubMed]
20. Hewitt, J.; Carter, B.; Vilches-Moraga, A.; Quinn, T.J.; Braude, P.; Verduri, A.; Pearce, L.; Stechman, M.; Short, R.; Price, A.; et al. The effect of frailty on survival in patients with COVID-19 (COPE): A multicentre, European, observational cohort study. *Lancet Public Health* **2020**, *5*, e444–e451. [CrossRef]
21. Elliott, A.; Phelps, K.; Regen, E.; Conroy, S.P. Identifying frailty in the Emergency Department—Feasibility study. *Age Ageing* **2017**, *46*, 840–845. [CrossRef] [PubMed]
22. Hale, M.D.; Santorelli, G.; Brundle, C.; Clegg, A. A cross-sectional study assessing agreement between self-reported and general practice-recorded health conditions among community dwelling older adults. *Age Ageing* **2019**, *49*, 135–140. [CrossRef] [PubMed]
23. Qiu, W.; Dean, M.; Liu, T.; George, L.; Gann, M.; Cohen, J.; Bruce, M.L. Physical and mental health of homebound older adults: An overlooked population. *J. Am. Geriatr. Soc.* **2010**, *58*, 2423–2428. [CrossRef] [PubMed]

16

Comprehensive Geriatric Assessment and Nutrition-Related Assessment: A Cross-Sectional Survey for Health Professionals

Junko Ueshima [1,*], Keisuke Maeda [2], Hidetaka Wakabayashi [3], Shinta Nishioka [4], Saori Nakahara [5] and Yoji Kokura [6]

[1] Department of Clinical Nutrition and Food Service, NTT Medical Center Tokyo, Tokyo 141-0022, Japan
[2] Palliative Care Center, Aichi Medical University, Aichi 480-1195, Japan; kskmaeda@aichi-med-u.ac.jp
[3] Department of Rehabilitation Medicine, Yokohama City University Medical Center, Yokohama 232-0024, Japan; noventurenoglory@gmail.com
[4] Department of Clinical Nutrition and Food Services, Nagasaki Rehabilitation Hospital, Nagasaki 850-0854, Japan; shintacks@yahoo.co.jp
[5] Department of Nutrition, Suzuka General Hospital, Suzuka 513-8630, Japan; mikuhiroto1210@gmail.com
[6] Department of Clinical Nutrition, Keiju Medical Center, Nanao 926-8605, Japan; yojikokura@hotmail.com
* Correspondence: j.ueshima@gmail.com

Abstract: (1) Background: It is important to assess physical and nutritional status using the Comprehensive Geriatric Assessment (CGA). However, the correlation between the CGA usage and nutritional-related assessments remain unclear. This study aims to clarify the correlation between the CGA usage and other nutritional-related assessments. (2) Methods: We conducted a questionnaire survey on clinical use of CGA, assessment of sarcopenia/sarcopenic dysphagia/cachexia, and defining nutritional goals/the Nutrition Care Process/the International Classification of Functioning, Disability, and Health (ICF)/the Kuchi–Kara Taberu Index. (3) Results: The number of respondents was 652 (response rate, 12.0%), including 77 who used the CGA in the general practice. The univariate analyses revealed that participants using the CGA tended to assess sarcopenia ($P = 0.029$), sarcopenic dysphagia ($P = 0.001$), and define nutritional goals ($P < 0.001$). Multivariate logistic regression analyses for the CGA usage revealed that using ICF ($P < 0.001$), assessing sarcopenia ($P = 0.001$), sarcopenic dysphagia ($P = 0.022$), and cachexia ($P = 0.039$), and defining nutritional goals ($P = 0.001$) were statistically significant after adjusting for confounders. (4) Conclusions: There are correlations between the use of CGA and evaluation of sarcopenia, sarcopenic dysphagia, and cachexia and nutritional goals.

Keywords: comprehensive geriatric assessment; multicomponent assessment; rehabilitation nutrition; sarcopenia; sarcopenic dysphagia

1. Introduction

The rapidly aging society warrants continuous advancements of the conventional medical care [1,2]. As frail older adults should have access to comprehensive medical and nursing care, provision of comprehensive care using multicomponent assessment is imperative [2]. The Comprehensive Geriatric Assessment (CGA) is a multidimensional, interdisciplinary diagnostic and treatment process that is designed to collect data about medical aspects of frail older adults [3,4]. The primary components of various models of the CGA comprise the coordinated multidisciplinary assessment, geriatric medicine expertise, determining medical, physical, social, and psychological problems, and the creation of a care plan involving appropriate rehabilitation [4]. Compared to typical medical care, the CGA implementation enhances the survival time of older adults, increases the duration during which they can live at home, and, perhaps, improves cognitive functions [1,4], improving their quality of life (QOL). Despite being recommended to be used in in the clinical practice, the CGA remains only partially utilized [5].

Sarcopenia, a key contributor of frailty [6], is a syndrome characterized by the presence of both the muscle mass and muscle function reduction due to aging, inactivity, malnutrition, and conditions such as cachexia [7]. Reportedly, sarcopenia is associated with an increased mortality and healthcare costs and declined QOL [8], and is considered as a severe public health-related concern [8,9]. Recently, some studies have described sarcopenic dysphagia (dysphagia due to sarcopenia in the whole body and swallowing-related muscles.) [10–14], which is occasionally detected in older adults and is related to physical deterioration, inadequate nutrition management, and cognitive decline [15]. Perhaps multicomponent assessment, such as the assessment of physical, social, and psychological problems, appropriate rehabilitation, and nutrition management could be necessary for the treatment [14,15], necessitating the early diagnosis of sarcopenia. In Nakahara et al. [16], we clarified the evaluation of sarcopenia and cachexia among different occupations, but when these items were evaluated remains unclear. In the rapidly aging society of Japan, the number of older adults with sarcopenia, nutritional deficiency, weakness, and disability are increasing at an alarming rate [17]. Therefore, it is important to assess physical functions and nutritional status as well as using CGA and to extract patients at risk early.

The usage of the multicomponent assessment is desirable to evaluate the elderly clinically and has been projected to attain a shared understanding of assessment and intervention goals. Besides the CGA, there are other multicomponent tools that clinically assess older adults such as the International Classification of Functioning, Disability, and Health (ICF) and the Kuchi–Kara Taberu Index (KT index) [18]. Wakabayashi et al. [11] advocates care that can maximize the physical function, physical activity, and social participation by assessing patients by ICF, including the nutritional status. Maeda et al. [18] recommended the multicomponent assessment and nutrition management for patients with eating and swallowing problems using the KT index. Recently, ICF-Dietetics [19] has been established as a systematically problem-solving method for ICF-related nutritional issues. The CGA usage mandates defining nutritional goals and controlling nutrition using nutritional problem-solving methods, such as the Nutrition Care Process (NCP) [20] and nutrition management, with a common understanding among healthcare workers in different occupations. Based on these, Wakabayashi [17] suggested providing high-quality nutritional care using the rehabilitation nutrition care process to people with disability and frailty. The rehabilitation nutrition care process assesses frailty, sarcopenia, dysphagia, and cachexia after using multicomponent assessment tools such as ICF or CGA and KT index. However, the rehabilitation nutrition care process has just begun, and the correlation between the CGA usage and the assessment of sarcopenia, cachexia, and sarcopenic dysphagia and defining nutritional goals using the NCP remain unclear. Moreover, the correlation between the CGA usage and the ICF usage and the KT index remains unknown.

In addition, a medical fee has been obtained since 2008 owing to the implementation of the CGA in Japan. Kihon Checklist [21] is an example of the CGA; although the assessment of frailty and assessment of muscle strength and physical functions are included in its components, the assessment of muscle mass and cachexia is not included.

Therefore, this study aims to elucidate the implementation rate and correlation between using the CGA and using nutrition-related assessment items, such as assessment of sarcopenia, cachexia, and sarcopenic dysphagia, NCP, defining nutritional goals, through a questionnaire-based survey. It also explains the implementation rate of CGA among different types of healthcare professionals and settings. Furthermore, this study intends to assess the correlation between the CGA usage and the use of other multicomponent tools, including the ICF and KT index.

2. Materials and Methods

2.1. Study Design and Setting

Between December 9, 2016, and January 16, 2017, we conducted a cross-sectional study using questionnaires. The questionnaire respondents were members of the Japanese Association of Rehabilitation Nutrition, which was established in 2011 and includes 5520 members from various medical and healthcare specialties. We conducted the survey online and anonymously to protect respondents' personal information and guarantee confidentiality.

2.2. Ethical Considerations

This study was performed following the ethical guidelines of the Declaration of Helsinki and was approved by the Ethics Committee of Suzuka General Hospital at Mie prefecture in Japan (No. 161). With answers to the questionnaire, we explained to the participants that they consented to the research and were given responses. For the protection of personal information in completed questionnaires, full confidentiality was given to respondents' data.

2.3. Participants

In this study, we enrolled respondents who provided consent to participate in the survey and responded to the questionnaire. Of note, those with missing data or duplications were excluded from the analysis.

2.4. Data Collection

We conducted the survey online, and it took approximately 5 min to complete the online questionnaire that comprised selective questions with dichotomous choice (yes/no). The consistency of the questionnaire content was evaluated by researchers. After several investigators conducted preliminary tests, the questionnaire content was enhanced regarding phrases, forms, length, consistency, and ease of answering, followed by converting into an actual survey. Table A1 lists the questions asked in the survey.

2.5. Parameters

In this study, we assessed parameters such as the standard implementation of the CGA, ICF, KT index, sarcopenia, sarcopenic dysphagia, cachexia, defining nutritional intervention goals, and the usage of NCP. The characterization of each evaluation item is in the Appendix (Table A2).

2.6. Statistical Analysis

Data analysis was performed on a sample size of >664 respondents, under the assumption of two-choice questions, and 50% selection with a 5% error based on 99% reliability. We expressed all categorical variables as the number of individuals and percentages. In addition, we performed a comparison of groups using the χ^2 test.

All quantitative variables were expressed as median (interquartile ranges). We used the Mann–Whitney U-test to compare values of the length of work experience. In addition, univariate and multivariate logistic regression analyses were performed to estimate the adjusted odds ratios (OR). Of note, the confounders were occupations, affiliations, and length of work experience. We performed all statistical procedures using EZR [22] software version 1.31, which was developed from the open-source statistical software R [23]. Furthermore, we considered $P < 0.05$ as statistically significant.

3. Results

Of 660 respondents, we excluded 8 (1.2%) from analyses because of incomprehensible answers. Consequently, the number of valid respondents was 652 (response rate, 12.0%). Table 1 summarizes the characteristics of the study cohort. The leading occupation of respondents was registered dietitian (28.2%), followed by a physical therapist (26.4%) and speech therapist (15.5%). Affiliations were with acute care (37.9%), convalescent rehabilitation (26.5%), nursing homes (10.4%), home care service (10.3%), long-term care (6.9%), and others (8%). Besides, the median work experience was 12 (range, 7–18) years.

Overall, 77 (11.8%) respondents were using the CGA in the general practice. The univariate analysis revealed that people using the CGA were more likely to assess sarcopenia ($P = 0.029$), sarcopenic dysphagia ($P = 0.001$), and define nutritional goals ($P < 0.001$). In contrast, using the ICF ($P = 0.051$), KT index ($P = 0.120$), and NCP ($P = 0.144$) and assessing cachexia ($P = 0.054$) was not significantly different (see Table 2).

The logistic regression analyses established a correlation between the CGA usage and several factors (see Table 3); these factors included using the ICF (adjusted OR, 3.01; 95% confidence interval [CI]: 1.63–3.57; $P < 0.001$), assessing sarcopenia (adjusted OR, 2.60; 95% CI: 1.50–4.50; $P = 0.001$), assessing sarcopenic dysphagia (adjusted OR, 1.86; 95% CI: 1.09–3.16; $P = 0.022$), assessing cachexia (adjusted OR, 1.86; 95% CI: 1.03–3.34; $P = 0.039$), and setting nutritional goals (adjusted OR, 2.79; 95% CI: 1.56–4.98; $P = 0.001$), which we observed with a statistical significance. Furthermore, the use of the KT index and NCP did not correlate with the CGA use.

Table 1. Demographic Characteristics of Participants.

Characteristics, n (%)	All	Usage of Comprehensive Geriatric Assessment		P-Value
		No	Yes	
Total Occupation	652 (100)	575 (88.2)	77 (11.8)	
Registered dietitian	184 (28.2)	162 (88.0)	22 (12.0)	0.01 [a]
Physical therapist	172 (26.4)	156 (90.7)	16 (9.3)	
Speech therapist	101 (15.5)	93 (92.1)	8 (7.9)	
Nurse	60 (9.2)	54 (90.0)	6 (10.0)	
Medical doctor	43 (6.6)	32 (74.4)	11 (25.6)	
Occupational therapist	36 (5.5)	33 (91.7)	3 (8.3)	
Dental hygienist	24 (3.7)	22 (91.7)	2 (8.3)	
Dentist	24 (3.7)	18 (75.0)	6 (25.0)	
Pharmacist	7 (1.1)	4 (57.1)	3 (42.9)	
Certified care worker	1 (0.1)	1 (100.0)	0 (0.0)	
Affiliation				
Acute care	247 (37.9)	231 (40.2)	16 (20.8)	0.02 [a]
Convalescent rehabilitation	173 (26.5)	149 (25.9)	24 (31.2)	
Nursing home	68 (10.4)	59 (10.3)	9 (11.7)	
Homecare service	67 (10.3)	53 (9.2)	14 (18.2)	
Medical care or long-term care	45 (6.9)	39 (6.8)	6 (7.8)	
Others	52 (8.0)	44 (7.7)	8 (10.4)	
Work experience				
Year(s), median (25–75%)	12 (7–18)	12 (7–18)	11 (7–20)	0.85 [b]

[a] Chi-square test; [b] Mann–Whitney U-test.

Table 2. Univariate Analysis of Factors Associated with Usage of Comprehensive Geriatric Assessment.

Factor, n (%)	All	Usage of Comprehensive Geriatric Assessment		P-Value
		No	Yes	
Using the ICF				
No	289 (44.3)	263 (45.7)	26 (33.8)	0.05
Yes	363 (55.7)	312 (54.3)	51 (66.2)	
Using the KT index				
No	557 (85.4)	496 (86.3)	61 (79.2)	0.12
Yes	95 (14.6)	79 (13.7)	16 (20.8)	
Assessing sarcopenia				
No	315 (48.3)	287 (49.9)	28 (36.4)	0.03
Yes	337 (51.7)	288 (50.1)	49 (63.6)	
Assessing sarcopenic dysphagia				
No	432 (66.3)	394 (68.5)	38 (49.4)	0.001
Yes	220 (33.7)	181 (31.5)	39 (50.6)	
Assessing cachexia				
No	478 (73.3)	429 (74.6)	49 (63.6)	0.05
Yes	174 (26.7)	146 (25.4)	28 (36.4)	
Setting nutritional goal				
No	359 (55.1)	333 (57.9)	26 (33.8)	<0.001
Yes	293 (44.9)	242 (42.1)	51 (66.2)	
Using Nutrition Care Process				
No	569 (87.3)	506 (88.0)	63 (81.8)	0.14
Yes	83 (12.7)	69 (12.0)	14 (18.2)	

Abbreviations: ICF, International Classification of Functioning, Disability and Health; KT index, Kuchi–Kara Taberu Index.

Table 3. Odds Ratio of Comprehensive Geriatric Assessment Usage in Uni- and Multi-Variate Logistic Regression Analyses.

Dependent Variables	Usage of Comprehensive Geriatric Assessment					
	Unadjusted OR	95% CI	P-Value	Adjusted OR	95% CI	P-Value
Using the ICF	1.65	0.98–2.84	0.05	3.01	1.63–5.57	<0.001
Using the KT index	1.66	0.84–3.07	0.12	1.76	0.91–3.43	0.10
Assessing sarcopenia	1.74	1.04–2.97	0.03	2.60	1.50–4.50	0.02
Assessing sarcopenic dysphagia	2.23	1.34–3.72	0.001	1.86	1.09–3.16	0.001
Assessing cachexia	1.68	0.98–2.84	0.05	1.86	1.03–3.34	0.04
Setting nutritional goal	2.70	1.60–4.64	<0.001	2.79	1.56–4.98	0.001
Using Nutrition Care Process	1.63	0.80–3.14	0.14	1.59	0.75–3.37	0.23

For each multivariate regression model, usage of CGA was adjusted by occupations, affiliations, and length of work experience. Abbreviations: ICF, International Classification of Functioning, Disability and Health; KT index, Kuchi–Kara Taberu Index; OR, odds ratio; 95% CI, 95% confidence interval.

4. Discussion

In brief, this study revealed three significant findings. First, it was suggested that participants using the CGA may have assessed sarcopenia or sarcopenic dysphagia more frequently in the daily clinical practice than those not using the CGA. Second, participants using the CGA defined nutritional goals more frequently; however, no significant difference was observed in using the NCP. Third, the percentage of people using the CGA was as low as 11.8%.

Participants using the CGA may have assessed sarcopenia or sarcopenic dysphagia more frequently in the daily clinical practice than those not using the CGA. Although there have been few studies on the relevance of assessing the CGA and sarcopenia. In recent studies, assessment of frailty was included as a component of CGA, but there was no sarcopenia [24]. Kihon Checklist [21] is a sample implementation of the CGA in Japan. It includes assessment of frailty, muscle strength, and physical functions in its components, and it has one aspect that motivates the assessment of sarcopenia. Sarcopenia is not only related to the physical activity and dysfunction [25,26] but also with several other factors, including independence [27,28] and cognitive function [29] of the daily life. In addition, sarcopenic dysphagia correlates with nutrition, activity (physical activity and swallowing), and cognitive function, which are causal factors of secondary sarcopenia [15]. Reportedly, the prevalence of sarcopenia among older adults is 1–29% in community dwellers, 14–33% in long-term care facilities, and 10–35% in acute-care hospitals [30,31]. Furthermore, it is a factor that predicts the life expectancy and disability. In fact, it is imperative to screen older adults who are susceptible to sarcopenia and sarcopenic dysphagia in the CGA and intervene at an early stage. As the CGA is the accepted gold standard for caring for frail older people in hospitals [24], it is essential to assess sarcopenia and sarcopenic dysphagia as a prolongation of the nutritional assessment and physical function evaluation of the CGA.

Participants using the CGA define nutritional goals more frequently; however, we observed no statistically significant difference in using the NCP. DiMaria-Ghalili et al. [32] reported that because all regions of the CGA and nutritional status were related, the nutritional assessment in the CGA facilitated the early recognition of nutritional risk factors or malnutrition, raising the possibility of a timely intervention. A study reported that it is crucial to illustrate the setting of nutritional goals at the time of the intervention after the nutrition assessment [33]. Although defining nutrition goals is encouraged for the NCP, a method of systematically solving nutrition-related problems, we observed no significant differences in using the NCP. Perhaps, participants related the nutritional assessment to the CGA, but the nutrition goal setting was implemented by methods other than the NCP. In Japan, NCP education has been initiated only recently for registered dietitians, and the NCP has not yet been applied in several occupations. In future, it will be crucial to define nutritional goals using nutrition-related problem-solving methods that could be shared among multiple occupations in Japan.

Among our study participants, the implementation rate of the CGA was as low as 11.8%, which was particularly low in acute-care hospitals. Apparently, the interdisciplinary work is necessary for the CGA implementation. We conjecture that the emergency departments of acute-care hospitals prioritize professional care over the CGA [5], or such an interdisciplinary working model has not been established [34]. Gladman et al. [5] reported that the CGA is challenging to comprehend and implement, even among those who care for the elderly. Li et al. [34] reported that even when the CGA was indicated, its implementation rate was as low as 20% because of inadequate education. In Japan, CGA education exists for medical doctors and dentists provided by gerontologists, but such an education is not provided for other medical professionals, although it is essential that all healthcare professionals should have access to adequate education. We need to clarify the reason why we are assessing sarcopenia and not using CGA, although we could not describe in this research. Thereby, we believe that the issue at the clinical practice will be highlighted.

This study has several limitations. First, based on the questionnaire response rate of only 12.0%, it is difficult to generalize our findings to the entire country. Second, it remains unclear how the questionnaire respondents diagnosed sarcopenia, sarcopenic dysphagia, and cachexia. When conducting similar research next time, it is necessary to describe diagnostic criteria of sarcopenia, sarcopenic dysphagia, and cachexia. If we clarify the reason why participants assess sarcopenia, sarcopenic dysphagia, cachexia, and the CGA, we can get more insights for clinical practice.

5. Conclusions

In conclusion, this study establishes correlations between the CGA usage and evaluation of sarcopenia, sarcopenic dysphagia, and cachexia and nutritional goals. In addition, those using the CGA are highly likely to assess older adults with a more multidimensional approach. However, the presence of few implementers is problematic. It is essential to extract older adults susceptible to sarcopenia at an early stage with an appropriate care plan, including the rehabilitation and nutrition management. Therefore, in the future it will be necessary to include items for the evaluation of sarcopenia, sarcopenic dysphagia, and cachexia in the CGA.

Author Contributions: J.U., concept and design, data acquisition, data interpretation, drafting the manuscript; K.M., H.W., S.N. (Shinta Nishioka), S.N. (Saori Nakahara), and Y.K., concept and design, data interpretation, critical revision of the manuscript. All the authors revised the manuscript critically for important intellectual content and approved the final version of the manuscript.

Appendix A

Table A1. Questionnaire contents.

Questions	Options
Q1. What is your occupation?	Registered dietitian Physical therapist Speech therapist Nurse Medical doctor Occupational therapist Dental hygienist Dentist Pharmacist Certified Care Worker
Q2. What is your sex?	Male Female
Q3. What is your affiliation?	Acute care Recovery rehabilitation Long-term care health facility Homecare service Medical care or long-term care Others
Q4. How long is your work experience?	
Q5. Do you use the CGA?	Yes/No
Q6. Do you assess sarcopenia?	Yes/No
Q7. Do you assess sarcopenic dysphagia?	Yes/No
Q8. Do you assess cachexia?	Yes/No
Q9. Do you set nutritional goals?	Yes/No
Q10. Do you use KT index?	Yes/No
Q11. Do you use the Nutrition Care Process?	Yes/No
Q12. Do you use the ICF?	Yes/No

Abbreviations: CGA, Comprehensive geriatric assessment; KT index, Kuchi–Kara Taberu Index; ICF, International Classification of Functioning, Disability and Health.

Table A2. The characterization of each evaluation items.

The ICF	The WHO framework for measuring health and disability at both individual and population levels. It is classified according to a combination of alphabet and number, and it consists of three factors, "physical and mental function/physical structure," "activity" and "participation," and influential factors, such as "environment" and "individual" [35].
The KT index	A simplified, validated tool that comprehensively assesses and intervenes in problems associated with eating and swallowing. The index comprises the following 13 items: (1) willingness to eat, (2) overall condition, (3) respiratory condition, (4) oral condition, (5) cognitive function while eating, (6) oral preparatory and propulsive phases, (7) severity of pharyngeal dysphagia, (8) position and endurance while eating, (9) eating behavior, (10) daily living activities, (11) food intake level, (12) food modification, and (13) nutritional status [18]. As each item is rated from 1 (worst) to 5 (best) points, the KT index ranges from 13 to 65 and is drawn with a radar chart that facilitates determining strong and weak items to ascertain items that caregivers need to emphasize and recognize the effect of an intervention by comparing before and after results.
The NCP	A systematic approach to provide high-quality nutritional care to patients/clients and is the unique function of nutrition in a standardized language through four related steps as follows: (1) nutrition assessment, (2) nutrition diagnosis, (3) nutrition management, and (4) nutrition monitoring and evaluation [20].

Abbreviations: WHO, World Health Organization; KT index, Kuchi–Kara Taberu Index; ICF, International Classification of Functioning, Disability and Health; NCP, Nutrition Care Process.

References

1. Ellis, G.; Whitehead, M.A.; Robinson, D.; O'Neill, D.; Langhorne, P. Comprehensive geriatric assessment for older adults admitted to hospital: Meta-analysis of randomized controlled trials. *BMJ* **2011**, *27*, 343. [CrossRef] [PubMed]
2. Arai, H.; Ouchi, Y.; Toba, K.; Endo, T.; Shimokado, K.; Tsubota, K.; Matsuo, S.; Mori, H.; Yumura, W.; Yokode, M.; et al. Japan as the front-runner of super-aged societies: Perspectives from medicine and medical care in Japan. *Geriatr. Gerontol. Int.* **2015**, *15*, 673–687. [CrossRef] [PubMed]
3. Rubenstein, L.Z.; Siu, A.L.; Wieland, D. Comprehensive geriatric assessment: Toward understanding its efficacy. *Aging* **1989**, *1*, 87–98. [CrossRef]
4. Ellis, G.; Whitehead, M.A.; O'Neill, D.; Langhorne, P.; Robinson, D. Comprehensive geriatric assessment for older adults admitted to hospital. *Cochrane Database Syst. Rev.* **2011**. [CrossRef]
5. Gladman, J.R.; Conroy, S.P.A.; Ranhoff, H.; Gordon, A.L. New horizons in the implementation and research of comprehensive geriatric assessment: Knowing, doing and the 'know-do' gap. *Age Ageing* **2016**, *45*, 194–200. [CrossRef]
6. Fried, L.P.; Tangen, C.M.; Walston, J.; Newman, A.B.; Hirsch, C.; Gottdiener, J.; Seeman, T.; Tracy, R.; Kop, W.J.; Burke, G.; et al. Frailty in older adults: Evidence for a phenotype. *J. Gerontol. A Biol. Sci. Med. Sci.* **2001**, *56*, M146–M156. [CrossRef]
7. Cruz-Jentoft, A.J.; Baeyens, J.P.; Bauer, J.M.; Boirie, Y.; Cederholm, T.; Landi, F.; Martin, F.C.; Michel, J.P.; Rolland, Y.; Schneider, S.M.; et al. Sarcopenia: European consensus on definition and diagnosis: Report of the European Working Group on Sarcopenia in Older People. *Age Ageing* **2010**, *39*, 412–423. [CrossRef]
8. Beaudart, C.; Rizzoli, R.; Bruyère, O.; Reginster, J.Y.; Biver, E. Sarcopenia: Burden and challenges for public health. *Arch. Public Health* **2014**, *72*, 45. [CrossRef]
9. Bruyère, O.; Beaudart, C.; Locquet, M.; Buckinx, F.; Petermans, J.; Reginster, J.-Y. Sarcopenia as a public health problem. *Eur. Geriatr. Med.* **2016**, *7*, 272–275. [CrossRef]
10. Fujishima, I.; Fujiu-Kurachi, M.; Arai, H.; Hyodo, M.; Kagaya, H.; Maeda, K.; Mori, T.; Nishioka, S.; Oshima, F.; Ogawa, S.; et al. Sarcopenia and dysphagia: Position paper by four professional organizations. *Geriatr. Gerontol. Int.* **2019**, *19*. [CrossRef]
11. Wakabayashi, H.; Sakuma, K. Rehabilitation nutrition for sarcopenia with disability: A combination of both rehabilitation and nutrition care management. *J. Cachexia Sarcopenia Muscle* **2014**, *5*, 269–277. [CrossRef] [PubMed]
12. Kuroda, Y.; Kuroda, R. Relationship between thinness and swallowing function in Japanese older adults: Implications for sarcopenic dysphagia. *J. Am. Geriatr. Soc.* **2012**, *60*, 1785–1786. [CrossRef]
13. Maeda, K.; Akagi, J. Sarcopenia is an independent risk factor of dysphagia in hospitalized older people. *Geriatr. Gerontol. Int.* **2016**, *16*, 515–521. [CrossRef] [PubMed]
14. Wakabayashi, H. Presbyphagia and sarcopenic dysphagia: Association between aging, sarcopenia, and deglutition disorders. *J. Frailty Aging* **2014**, *3*, 97–103.
15. Maeda, K.; Takaki, M.; Akagi, J. Decreased skeletal muscle mass and risk factors of sarcopenic dysphagia: A prospective observational cohort study. *J. Gerontol. A Biol. Sci. Med. Sci* **2017**, *72*, 1290–1294. [CrossRef] [PubMed]
16. Saori, N.; Hidetaka, W.; Keisuke, M.; Shinta, N.; Yoji, K. Sarcopenia and cachexia evaluation in different healthcare settings: A questionnaire survey of health professionals. *Asia Pac. J. Clin. Nutr.* **2018**, *27*, 167–175.
17. Wakabayashi, H. Rehabilitation nutrition in general and family medicine. *J. Gen. Fam. Med.* **2017**, *18*, 153–154. [CrossRef]
18. Maeda, K.; Shamoto, H.; Wakabayashi, H.; Enomoto, J.; Takeichi, M.; Koyama, T. Reliability and validity of a simplified comprehensive assessment tool for feeding support: Kuchi-KaraTaberu Index. *J. Am. Geriatr. Soc.* **2016**, *64*, e248–e252. [CrossRef]
19. Gäbler, G.; Coenen, M.C.; Bolleurs, C.; Visser, W.K.; Runia, S.; Heerkens, Y.F.; Stamm, T.A. Toward harmonization of the Nutrition Care Process terminology and the International Classification of Functioning, Disability and Health-Dietetics: Results of a mapping exercise and implications for nutrition and dietetics practice and research. *J. Acad. Nutr. Diet.* **2018**, *118*, 13–20. [CrossRef]
20. Writing Group of the Nutrition Care Process/Standardized Language Committee. Nutrition Care Process and Model Part I: The 2008 Update. *J. Am. Diet. Assoc.* **2008**, *108*, 1113–1117. [CrossRef]

21. Sewo Sampaio, P.Y.; Sampaio, R.A.; Yamada, M.; Arai, H. Systematic review of the Kihon Checklist: Is it a reliable assessment of frailty? *Geriatr. Gerontol. Int.* **2016**, *16*, 893–902. [CrossRef] [PubMed]

22. Kanda, Y. Investigation of the freely available easy-to-use software 'EZR' for medical statistics. *Bone Marrow Transpl.* **2013**, *48*, 452–458. [CrossRef] [PubMed]

23. Institute for Statistics and Mathematics of Wirtschaftsuniversität Wien. The Comprehensive R Archive Network. 2009. Available online: https://cran.r-project.org/ (accessed on 8 March 2017).

24. Parker, S.G.; McCue, P.; Phelps, K.; McCleod, A.; Arora, S.; Nockels, K.; Kennedy, S.; Roberts, H.; Conroy, S. What is Comprehensive Geriatric Assessment (CGA)? An umbrella review. *Age Ageing* **2018**, *47*, 149–155. [CrossRef] [PubMed]

25. Tanimoto, Y.; Watanabe, M.; Sun, W.; Sugiura, Y.; Tsuda, Y.; Kimura, M.; Hayashida, I.; Kusabiraki, T.; Kono, K. Association between sarcopenia and higher-level functional capacity in daily living in community-dwelling elderly subjects in Japan. *Arch. Gerontol. Geriatr.* **2012**, *55*, e9–e13. [CrossRef] [PubMed]

26. Guralnik, J.M.; Ferrucci, L.; Pieper, C.F.; Leveille, S.G.; Markides, K.S.; Ostir, G.V.; Studenski, S.; Berkman, L.F.; Wallace, R.B. Lower extremity function and subsequent disability: Consistency across studies, predictive models, and value of gait speed alone compared with the short physical performance battery. *J. Gerontol. A Biol. Sci. Med. Sci.* **2000**, *55*, M221–M231. [CrossRef]

27. Maeda, K.; Shamoto, H.; Wakabayashi, H.; Akagi, J. Sarcopenia is highly prevalent in older medical patients with mobility limitation. *Nutr. Clin. Pr.* **2017**, *32*, 110–115. [CrossRef]

28. Janssen, I.; Baumgartner, R.N.; Ross, R.; Rosenberg, I.H.; Roubenoff, R. Skeletal muscle cutpoints associated with elevated physical disability risk in older men and women. *Am. J. Epidemiol.* **2004**, *159*, 413–421. [CrossRef] [PubMed]

29. Maeda, K.; Akagi, J. Cognitive impairment is independently associated with definitive and possible sarcopenia in hospitalized older adults: The prevalence and impact of comorbidities. *Geriatr. Gerontol. Int.* **2017**, *17*, 1048–1056. [CrossRef]

30. Bianchi, L.; Abete, P.; Bellelli, G.; Bo, M.; Cherubini, A.; Corica, F.; Di Bari, M.; Maggio, M.; Manca, G.M.; Rizzo, M.R.; et al. Prevalence and clinical correlates of sarcopenia, identified according to the EWGSOP definition and diagnostic algorithm, in hospitalized older people: The GLISTEN Study. *J. Gerontol. A Biol. Sci. Med. Sci.* **2017**, *72*, 1575–1581. [CrossRef]

31. Cruz-Jentoft, A.J.; Landi, F.; Schneider, S.M.; Zúñiga, C.; Arai, H.; Boirie, Y.; Chen, L.K.; Fielding, R.A.; Martin, F.C.; Michel, J.P.; et al. Prevalence of and interventions for sarcopenia in ageing adults: A systematic review. Report of the International Sarcopenia Initiative (EWGSOP and IWGS). *Age Ageing* **2014**, *43*, 748–759. [CrossRef]

32. DiMaria-Ghalili, R.A. Integrating nutrition in the Comprehensive Geriatric Assessment. *Nutr. Clin. Pr.* **2014**, *29*, 420–427. [CrossRef] [PubMed]

33. Cederholm, T.; Barazzoni, R.; Austin, P.; Ballmer, P.; Biolo, G.; Bischoff, S.C.; Compher, C.; Correia, I.; Higashiguchi, T.; Holst, M.; et al. ESPEN guidelines on definitions and terminology of clinical nutrition. *Clin. Nutr.* **2017**, *36*, 49–64. [CrossRef] [PubMed]

34. Li, Y.; Wang, S.; Wang, L.X.; Meng, Z.M.; Li, J.; Dong, B.R. Is comprehensive geriatric assessment recognized and applied in Southwest China? A survey from Sichuan Association of Geriatrics. *J. Am. Med. Dir. Assoc.* **2013**, *14*, 775.e1–775.e3. [CrossRef] [PubMed]

35. World Health Organization. Available online: http://www.who.int/classifications/icf/en/ (accessed on 11 January 2019).

17

Thermal Sensation in Older People with and without Dementia Living in Residential Care: New Assessment Approaches to Thermal Comfort Using Infrared Thermography

Charmaine Childs [1,*], Jennifer Elliott [1], Khaled Khatab [1], Susan Hampshaw [2], Sally Fowler-Davis [1], Jon R. Willmott [3] and Ali Ali [4]

[1]   College of Health, Wellbeing and Life Sciences, Sheffield Hallam University, Sheffield S10 2BP, UK; jennifer@centralmedicalservices.co.uk (J.E.); k.khatab@shu.ac.uk (K.K.); s.fowler-davis@shu.ac.uk (S.F.-D.)

[2]   School of Health and Related Research (SCHARR), University of Sheffield, Sheffield S10 2TN, UK; s.hampshaw@sheffield.ac.uk

[3]   Electronic and Electrical Engineering Department, University of Sheffield, Sheffield S10 2TN, UK; j.r.willmott@sheffield.ac.uk

[4]   Sheffield Teaching Hospitals, National Institute for Health Research (NIHR), Biomedical Research Centre, Sheffield S10 2JF, UK; ali.ali@sheffield.ac.uk

*   Correspondence: c.childs@shu.ac.uk

Abstract: The temperature of the indoor environment is important for health and wellbeing, especially at the extremes of age. The study aim was to understand the relationship between self-reported thermal sensation and extremity skin temperature in care home residents with and without dementia. The Abbreviated Mental Test (AMT) was used to discriminate residents to two categories, those with, and those without, dementia. After residents settled and further explanation of the study given (approximately 15 min), measurements included: tympanic membrane temperature, thermal sensation rating and infrared thermal mapping of non-dominant hand and forearm. Sixty-nine afebrile adults (60–101 years of age) were studied in groups of two to five, in mean ambient temperatures of 21.4–26.6 °C (median 23.6 °C). Significant differences were observed between groups; thermal sensation rating ($p = 0.02$), tympanic temperature ($p = 0.01$), fingertip skin temperature ($p = 0.01$) and temperature gradients; fingertip-wrist $p = 0.001$ and fingertip-distal forearm, $p = 0.001$. Residents with dementia were in significantly lower air temperatures ($p = 0.001$). Although equal numbers of residents per group rated the environment as 'neutral' (comfortable), resident ratings for 'cool/cold' were more frequent amongst those with dementia compared with no dementia. In parallel, extremity (hand) thermograms revealed visual temperature demarcation, variously across fingertip, wrist, and forearm commensurate with peripheral vasoconstriction. Infrared thermography provided a quantitative and qualitative method to measure and observe hand skin temperature across multiple regions of interest alongside thermal sensation self-report. As an imaging modality, infrared thermography has potential as an additional assessment technology with clinical utility to identify vulnerable residents who may be unable to communicate verbally, or reliably, their satisfaction with indoor environmental conditions.

Keywords: infrared thermography; cutaneous temperature; skin blood flow; dementia; body temperature; thermal sensation; thermal comfort; imaging; mapping; environmental temperature; frailty

1. Introduction

To experience a thermally comfortable indoor environment, an older person living in residential care relies almost entirely upon decisions made by others. This is typically the care home staff who will regulate the temperature of the communal spaces and bedrooms. For those residents with dementia, simple interventions to adjust the physical stimuli of light, noise and temperature can improve a person's quality of life [1] experience [2] and behaviour [3]. Thermal comfort, therefore, becomes an important aspect of wellbeing and quality of life, which may require a different set of indoor thermal adjustments (including clothing) than required for active younger people.

A fundamental starting point is to understand the definition of thermal comfort; a condition of mind which expresses satisfaction with the immediate environment [4]. As a subjective experience, it may well differ amongst groups of people sharing the same environment at the same time.

The international standard, EN ISO 7730 [5] covering the evaluation of moderate thermal environments (developed in parallel with the revised American Society of Heating, Refrigerating and Air-Conditioning Engineers (ASHRAE, standard 55) specifies methods for measurement and evaluation of thermal environments. Thermal sensation is predominately related to heat balance and is influenced by physical activity, clothing and the indoor environmental factors of air temperature, mean radiant temperature, humidity and air velocity [5]. By seeking to provide a comfortable thermal environment for the majority, building and architectural sciences have led the way in finding solutions to achieve thermal comfort for the built environment. A subjective seven-point thermal sensation scale [4] developed originally from the work of Bedford [6] is completed by each individual. It is a scale widely used in thermal surveys and field trials [7] and forms the basis to calculate the average thermal sensation vote of large groups of individuals exposed to the same environment, along with an index of those dissatisfied i.e., people who vote feeling too hot, warm, cool or cold.

Whilst international standards are available, their use has largely been focused on determining thermal comfort of the workforce in offices and factories. Much less is known about thermal comfort in the old and very old living in residential care [8–10]. The need for new perspectives on thermal sensation and thermal comfort in older age is now appreciated [3,11–13] particularly given that the changes that occur in the nervous system associated with ageing leads to a decrease ('blunting') of thermal sensitivity and thermal perception [14] especially in response to cold stimuli [15] which is most pronounced at the extremities and follows a distal-proximal pattern [16]. Furthermore, due to a diminished cutaneous vasoconstrictor response to body cooling [17], older people may lose both their perception of the environment and their ability to conserve heat at the extremities. They may therefore (a) not perceive themselves as cold and (b) have a reduced physiological efficiency to conserve heat and are therefore at an increased risk of 'symptomless cooling' [14,18] putting the older person at greater risk of chilling or worse still, hypothermia [16].

As evidence emerges [11] that the existing analytical models for determination and interpretation of thermal comfort are not appropriate in older age, opportunities open up to investigate multidimensional approaches to thermal comfort, specifically of relevance to older people.

The aims of this study therefore, were to (i) identify the range of thermal sensation self-reports amongst groups of care-home residents, with and without dementia, sharing the same indoor environmental conditions (ii) use objective, long-wave infrared (LWIR) thermography to map extremity skin temperature and (iii) determine the correspondence between thermal sensation self-report and the extremity thermal map.

2. Materials and Methods

2.1. Study Design

Prospective observational feasibility investigation.
Inclusion Criteria: residents living in residential care aged 60 years or over.

Exclusion criteria: residents unable to communicate or lacking capacity to respond to simple questions.

2.2. Sample Size

As a feasibility study, the target population is 70 participants. Assuming attrition, the revised target is 60 participants. With this number, there will be 90% power, at significance level 0.05, to detect one value or unit ($^{\circ}$C) change in temperature with 1.4 SD difference between the two groups.

2.3. Participants

Adults living in residential care homes within the South Yorkshire and Derbyshire counties of the UK were recruited over 12 months.

2.4. Screening and Recruitment Pathway

Older adults were invited to give their written informed consent to participate in the study after first reading the participant information sheet. Screening for capacity was undertaken by research nurses of the clinical research network (CRN) for the Yorkshire-Humber and Derbyshire National Health Service (NHS regions). The manager of each residence was first contacted and information was provided verbally and via leaflets for the care home staff to retain. If the manager was interested in the objectives of the study, a researcher returned to the care home to discuss the specific details of the study. The care home manager identified those residents considered to have capacity to give their own informed consent as a study participant using a 'Noticeable Problems Checklist'. For those residents with a medical diagnosis of dementia, or those considered by the care staff to have fluctuating capacity, the relative (or independent clinician) was provided with study information, by letter, and asked to consider willingness to give their signed consent on behalf of the resident. Once consent had been obtained, a mutually convenient date for recruitment was made to obtain signed consent from the resident or appropriate authority.

2.5. Recruitment

On the day of study, and with consent obtained, a further screening for capacity was undertaken using the Abbreviated Mental Test (AMT) [19], a 10-point scale used as a guide to screening for dementia in those without a formal dementia diagnosis. A score below 8 indicates a level of cognitive impairment warranting 'assignment' to the dementia category (D). Residents with AMT score of ≥8 were assigned to a 'no dementia' category (ND).

2.6. Data Collection

2.6.1. Demographic Data

Demographic data was collected to include, age, gender, ethnicity, years in residence, 'handedness'.

2.6.2. Frailty Assessment

The level of clinical frailty was assessed on a seven-point, clinical frailty scale (version 2007–2009 Dalhousie University, Halifax, NS, Canada) [20].

2.6.3. Body Temperature Measurement

Body temperature was measured at the tympanum (T_{tymp}) using a Thermoscan device (Model LF 40, Braun, Lausanne, Switzerland) before thermography commenced.

2.6.4. Past Medical History (PMH) and Current Medications

For each older resident, a brief medical history was obtained along with co-morbid condition/s and medication history, including polypharmacy. Past medical history (PMH) and medication type may influence: (a) the individuals' thermal 'perception' and (b) heat distribution at the extremities; the former influencing feelings of thermal comfort and the latter, the appearance of the heat signature (i.e., the appearance of the thermal map).

PMH with potential to affect thermal comfort perception includes thyroid dysfunction, impaired neurological perception (e.g., learning difficulties, stroke, dementia, including Alzheimer's disease, peripheral neuropathy). A PMH likely to affect heat distribution at the extremities (and thus the thermal map) is linked to vascular compromise. Pre-existing conditions were documented and include all forms of diabetes, hypertension, vasculitis, peripheral vascular disease, heart failure and Raynaud's disease. Current medication/s and dose was also documented with drugs having potential thermoregulatory effects assigned to the following categories: (a) vasoconstrictor effects, (b) vasodilator effects, (c) neurological effects, (d) diuretic effects.

2.6.5. Indoor Environment

Residents were studied in groups of two or more sitting in their usual daytime communal room. Responses were sought under 'real world' conditions of the care home. The study was scheduled to commence at least one hour after breakfast. This gave sufficient time to complete imaging before lunch was served. Recommendations for measurement of ambient conditions (EN ISO 7730) [5] were made for air temperature, (T_a °C), relative humidity (RH%) and air velocity (m·s^{-1}) measured using a Kestrel environmental monitor (Kestrel 3000, Kestrel Instruments, Boothwyn, PA, USA).

2.6.6. Clothing

An approximation of clothing fabric insulation for each garment worn by the resident was made using available reference values [21]. Insulation of clothing is expressed as a 'Clo' unit. Clothing 'ensembles' were estimated from a weighted valuation:

$$0.676 \sum Icl,i + 0.117 \qquad (1)$$

where $\sum Icl$ refers to the sum of individual clothing items worn. A pragmatic approach to clothing category produced three groups: 0–0.50 Clo, 0.51–1.00 Clo, >1.0 Clo for light, medium and heavy clothing ensembles respectively. A Clo score of 0 corresponds to a person, nude. A Clo score of 1.0, the value of clothing insulation needed to maintain a person in comfort, sitting at 21 °C with air movement, 0.1 m·s^{-1}, relative humidity (RH) $\leq$ 50%, the example used being a person wearing a business suit [21].

2.6.7. Imaging-Long Wave Infrared (LWIR) Thermography

Infrared thermography was undertaken using an uncooled microbolometer detector, (model A-600 series, FLIR, Täby, Sweden) with image resolution 640 × 320 pixels, mounted on a tripod (Vanguard, Alta Pro 264AT, Dorset, UK) and connected to a laptop computer. The LWIR detector system was positioned such that the seated participants were comfortable. In the sitting position, acral region (both hands) were positioned, first with the dorsum followed by palmar surface upwards resting upon a paper 'hand template' (Figure 1) overlying an insulated tile.

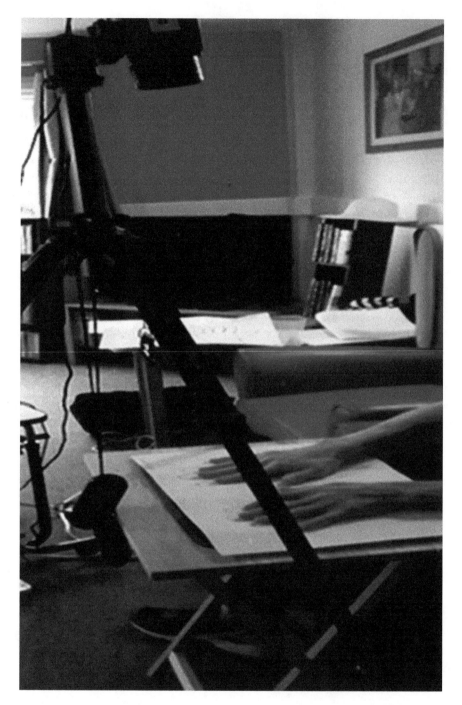

Figure 1. Long wave infrared imaging detector mounted on a tripod. The figure shows the participant during imaging with hands positioned upon a paper 'hand template' overlying an insulated tile. The portable table was used throughout the study to ensure consistency of the imaging set-up.

This provided visual orientation to the participants for the placement of fingers and hands in a consistent position and to obtain a clear field of view (FOV). After checking detector focus and distance, a maximum of three images were obtained. Colour thermal maps were obtained using a proprietary FLIR software (FLIR Systems AB, Täby, Sweden) and colour palette (see Figure 2).

In this paper, data were reported of the dorsum of the hand as this was the most comfortable position for older participants. The colour palette, with temperature key, shows darkest colours (indigo/blue) representing the lowest skin temperature and bright colour (white/yellow) highest temperatures (Figure 2).

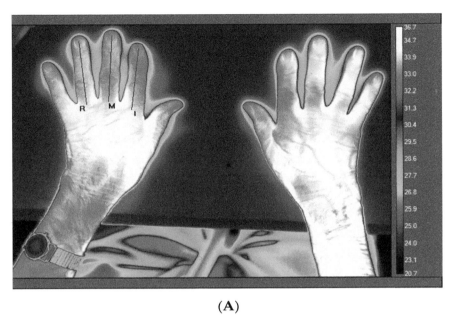

(A)

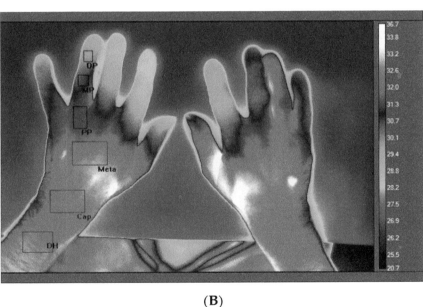

(B)

Figure 2. (**A**): Thermal map of left and right hand positioned upon an insulated tile. The region of interest (ROI, non-dominant hand) displayed as a vertical line constructed centrally for ring (R), middle (M) and index (I) fingers. Selection of the finger with greatest variability was used to construct six 'box' ROIs from which mean ROI values were obtained (B) and with data from the selected finger used in subsequent analyses. (**B**) shows anatomical ROI positions for temperature (°C) of distal phalange (T_{DP}), middle phalange (T_{Tmp}), proximal phalange (T_{PP}), metacarpal (T_{Meta}), capitate bones (T_{Cap}) and distal humerus (T_{DH}).

2.6.8. LWIR Region of Interest (ROI) and Image Processing

Emissivity was set to 0.98 for all images; temperature span 16 °C; range 20.7–36.7 °C. A 'first-pass' review of thermal maps for temperature variability across ring (R), middle (M) and index (I) finger was made. Thermograms showed that fingers typically appeared 'non-uniform' in temperature distribution. Thus, for each participant, a vertical 'line' ROI was constructed (Figure 2A) for each of R, M and I fingers. The finger with the greatest skin temperature value S.D (an indication of temperature variability) was used in subsequent analyses. For the selected finger, a series of six vertical 'box' ROIs (Figure 2B) were constructed (manually) traversing the centre of each finger of the non-dominant hand and using pre-defined dimensions; fingertip (distal phalange, T_{DP}), wrist (capitate bones, T_{Cap}) and forearm (distal humerus/ulnar T_{DH}). Thee ROI dimensions were used throughout the post-processing of LWIR images; T_{DP}, (280 pixels) T_{Cap}, (2436 pixels) and T_{DH}, (1900 pixels). On occasions, the anatomical ROI did not conform well to the finger (e.g., the hand was too slim for the size of the ROI or the hands were 'gnarled' by arthritis, preventing the 'flat' placement of the hands, so the ROI dimension was adjusted slightly to 'fit' ROI to finger anatomy. Mean temperature difference (°C) across the extremities were calculated as: $T_{DP} - T_{Cap}$ (ΔT_1) and $T_{DP} - T_{DH}$ (ΔT_2). The mean temperature difference between T_{DP} and tympanic temperature is given as ΔT_3.

2.6.9. Calibration

Calibration of the FLIR thermal camera was undertaken against a black-body source (P80P, Ametek-Land, Dronfield, UK) to determine temperature accuracy and thermal camera performance across a 20 °C environmental temperature range (20–40 °C).

2.6.10. Warmth Sensation Rating

After adjusting to the study environment, each participant was asked to rate their thermal sensation using the 7-point thermal sensation scale with options ranging from −3 (cold), −2 (cool), −1 (slightly cool), 0 (neutral), +1 (slightly warm), +2 (warm), +3 (hot) [4]. The McIntyre scale [22] for thermal preference (thermal vote, TV) was used to obtain a response to the question "I would like to be": options include (a) cooler (b) no change (c) warmer.

2.6.11. Statistical Analyses

All computations have been carries out with SPSS version 24 (IBM, Armonk, NY, USA). The associated factors analysed in participants over 60 years are presented as numbers, percentage, mean (standard deviation, SD), with p-value. Chi-Square tests were used for categorical data. Anova tests were performed for comparison of mean values of independent variables amongst the two participant groups: ND and D. ANOVA was used to determine whether there were any statistically significant differences between the means of two independent groups (Table 1).

Table 1. Characteristic of care home residents, clothing ensemble, ambient conditions and core and skin temperature values (°C) with temperature difference (ΔT). Table shows descriptive analysis that focused on associations between key variables.

Categorical Factor	Dementia Diagnosis/AMT < 8 Group D n = (%)		AMT 8–10 Group ND n = (%)		p Value
Male	10 (45.5)		12 (54.5)		0.43
Female	24 (51.5)		23 (48.9)		
Age: years					
60–70	2 (33.3)		4 (66.7)		
71–80	9 (69.2)		4 (30.8)		0.25
81–90	16 (51.6)		15 (48.4)		
Over 90	7 (36.8)		12 (63.2)		
Ethnicity					
White British	33 (50)		33 (50)		
White European	0		2 (100)		0.22
White	1 (100)		0		
Frailty Score					
Well	0		1(100)		
Managing Well	6 (75)		2 (25)		
Vulnerable	1 (10)		9 (90)		
Mildly Frail	1 (50)		1 (50)		0.028
Moderately Frail	9 (40.9)		13 (59.1)		
Severely Frail	17 (65.4)		9 (34.6)		
Dominant Hand					
Right	31 (49.2)		32 (50.8)		
Left	3 (60)		2 (40)		0.4
Ambidextrous	0		1 (100)		
Finger with greatest SD					
Left ring	11 (68.8)		5 (31.2)		
Left middle	5 (38.5)		8 (61.5)		
Left index	14 (43.8)		18 (56.2)		
Right ring	1 (100		0		0.34
Right middle	0		1 (100)		
Right index	2 (40)		3 (60)		
Clothing ensemble (Clo unit)					
Light	6 (30)		14 (70)		
Medium	26 (55.3)		21 (44.7)		0.05
Heavy	2 (100)		0		
Thermal sensation rating					
−2	1 (100)		0		
−1	10 (76.9)		3 (23.1)		
0	21 (48.8)		22 (51.2)		
1	0		7 (100)		0.02
1.5	1 (100)		0		
2	1 (33.3)		2 (66.7)		
Thermal Vote					
Cooler	1 (16)		5 (84)		
No change	27 (49.1)		28 (50.9)		0.09
Warmer	6 (75)		2 (25)		
Temperature	n = (%)	Mean (SD)	n = (%)	Mean (SD)	
Air temperature (°C)	34 (49.3)	23.1 (0.2)	35 (50.7)	24.1 (0.17)	0.001
Relative Humidity (%RH)	34 (49.3)	49 (1.1)	35 (50.7)	52.1 (1.6)	0.2
ROI: mean DP (°C)	33 (48.5)	30.0 (0.46)	35 (51.5)	31.6 (0.4)	0.01
ROI: mean Cap (°C)	33 (48.5)	31.7 (0.25)	35 (51.5)	32.0 (0.25)	0.4
ROI: mean DH (°C)	33 (48.5)	31.9 (0.19)	35 (51.5)	32.0 (0.24)	0.1
ΔT_1 (mean DP- mean CAP) °C	33 (48.5)	−1.7 (0.29)	35 (51.5)	−0.43 (0.24)	0.001
ΔT_2 (mean DP-mean DH) °C	33 (48.5)	−1.8 (0.34)	35 (51.5)	−0.39 (0.26)	0.001
Tympanic temperature (°C)	34 (50)	36.6 (0.07)	34 (50)	36.8 (0.6)	0.01

ROI—region of interest; DP—distal phalange; CAP—capitate bones; DH—distal humerus.

2.7. Ethics Approval, Screening and Recruitment

All subjects gave their informed consent for inclusion before they participated in the study. The study was conducted in accordance with the Declaration of Helsinki, and the protocol was approved by the East Midlands (Derby, UK) research ethics committee and Health Research Authority (HRA) (16/EM/0483).

3. Results

3.1. Characteristics of Older Adults Living in Residential Care

Seventy-three residents gave their consent to the study. Data was analysed from 69 people aged 60–101 (mean 84) years; 47 were female. Participants were recruited from 15 English residences. All were white British, Irish or European. Sixty residents had mild, moderate, or severe frailty. Nine residents only, were 'well' or 'managing well' on the frailty score. There was a significant difference concerning frailty with more residents in the dementia (D) group being severely frail ($p = 0.028$) (Table 1).

AMT ranged from 0–10 (median 8). Thirty-four residents were assigned to 'dementia' category, (D) and 35 residents, (ND) (Table 1). Residents were studied in groups of two to five at each imaging session (median three residents per session) in still air (<0.1 m·sec^{-1}) T_a 21.4–26.6 °C (mean 23.6 °C) RH 32–78% (mean 51%). Under these indoor ambient conditions, a variety of clothing ensembles were worn (Clo range 0.26–1.54, mean 0.61 Clo) corresponding to light ($n = 20$) medium ($n = 47$) heavy ($n = 2$) clothing ensembles respectively.

3.2. Thermal Sensation (TS) Self-Rating

Of the 68 of 69 participants who provided a TS self-report, the majority rated the environment 'comfortable' (TS score 0, $n = 43$, 63%). For the remainder, responses raged from +2 ($n = 3$), +1 ($n = 7$), −1 ($n = 13$), −2 ($n = 1$) corresponding to 'warm', 'slightly warm', 'slightly cool', 'cool' respectively with a range of different TS ratings between residents across individual care homes (Table 2). None of the residents rated −3 (cold) or +3 (hot). Overall, 92% of residents rated TS −1 to +1. Most residents ($n = 55$, 80%) on providing a TV did not wish to change the temperature of the environment whereas eight (11%) would have preferred a warmer temperature and six (9%) a lower air temperature.

Table 2. Individual thermal sensation ratings reported by residents sharing the same environmental conditions at each imaging session in groups of two to five. Study undertaken over a period of 12 calendar months at 15 residential care sites. Residents with dementia who participated in the imaging sessions are identified by highlighted and emboldened text. Four residential care sites (6,9,11,12) were visited twice.

Site ID	Month/Day of Study	Mean T_a (°C)	Mean RH %	Thermal Sensation Rating				
				Resident 1	Resident 2	Resident 3	Resident 4	Resident 5
1	7 June	24.3	60	**0**	missing	0		
2	13 July	24.0	47	0	0	0	−1	
3	12 July	24.3	56	0	1	1	1	
4	28 July	22.5	54	0	0			
5	6 September	24.6	60	0	0	0		
6	28 September	25.8	52	0	1	1	0	
6	6 October	23.6	38	0	−1	0	**0**	
7	12 October	23.1	57	**2**	**0**			
8	20 October	24.2	60	0	1	0	0	
9	7 November	22.0	53	**−1**	**−1**			
9	8 December	24.0	32	1	0			
10	11 April	22.0	55	**0**	1.5			
11	17 April	24.5	48	−1	0	**0**		
11	24 April	21.8	44	**0**	**0**	−1		
12	11 May	25.3	37	−1	0			
13	16 May	22.6	45	**0**	**0**	**0**	0	
14	18 May	24.2	46	**0**	**0**	0		
12	21 May	22.7	50	−1	0	0	**−1**	**−1**
11	12 June	22.0	53	**−1**	0	0		
15	14 June	23.6	54	**0**	−2	−1	0	2
11	19 June	22.1	54	**0**	**−1**	0		
6	19 June	24.0	58	0	2			

RH—relative humidity, emboldened text within highlighted cells indicates the residents with a confirmed diagnosis of dementia or Abbreviated Mental Test (AMT) < 8.

3.3. Thermal Sensation Ratings and Clothing Insulation

When sharing the same room (and thus same T_a), differences in TS rating and TV were reported. A significant difference in TS rating was noted between residents (D vs. ND) ($p = 0.02$, Table 1). Residents (D) more frequently expressed feeling 'slightly cool' or 'cool' ($n = 11$) compared with ND residents ($n = 3$; Table 1). By contrast, residents without dementia more frequently expressed feelings of being 'slightly warm' or 'warm' ($n = 9$) compared to those with dementia ($n = 2$). Throughout the months during which the study was conducted, clothing worn by the majority of residents (Table 1) provided light to medium insulation; differences in clothing insulation tending towards medium to heavy Clo units for residents with dementia (borderline significance, $p = 0.05$).

3.4. Core (Tympanic) Temperature

Residents were afebrile, T_{tymp} 35.5–37.5 °C (mean 36.7 °C). A statistical but not clinically significant difference was observed between ND vs. D groups ($p = 0.01$, Table 1). Differences ($T_{DP} - T_{tymp}$) were consistently negative for all older adults; ΔT_3 range −12.5 °C to −2.3 °C.

3.5. Skin Extremity Temperature

Right hand was dominant in 63 of 69 residents (91%). Thermal mapping and data analysis of 'non-dominant' finger/hand ROIs were therefore performed predominately for left hand. Individual extremity skin temperature values for T_{DP}, T_{Cap}, T_{DH} for all residents are lowest for T_{DP}. Mean vales for T_{DP}, T_{Cap}, T_{DH} were 30.9 °C (2.6 °C), 31.9 °C (1.5 °C), 31.9 °C (1.3 °C) respectively. Mean T_{DP} was significantly lower ($p = 0.01$) for residents with dementia compared to ND (Table 1; Figure 3).

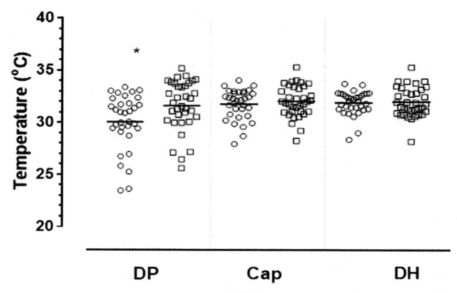

Figure 3. Mean skin temperature at each of three ROI regions represented by finger-tip (distal phalange, T_{DP}), capitate bones (T_{Cap}) and forearm at distal humerus/ulner (T_{DH}) of residents with dementia/AMT < 8 (D) (open circles, O) and residents without a confirmed diagnosis of dementia/AMT ≥ 8 (ND) (open square □). * Significant difference between mean temperature for T_{DP} of residents D vs. ND group ($p = 0.01$). Horizonal bars represent mean values.

3.6. Comparisons Between Groups

D vs. ND: Air, extremity skin and tympanic temperature: T_a of the communal rooms where residents were sitting was, on average, 1.0 °C lower ($p = 0.001$) in D compared to the ND group (Table 1; Figure 4).

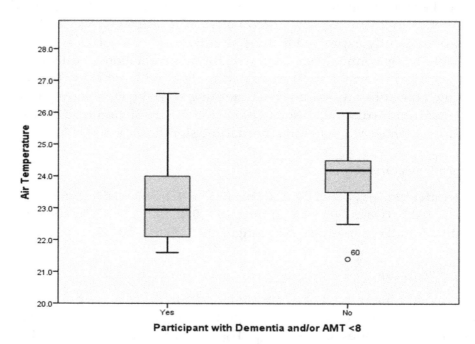

Figure 4. Distribution of air temperature (°C) within care homes by group: dementia or an AMT < 8 (yes/no) showing median, lower and upper quartiles, and lower and upper extremes of air temperature. Outlier: participant studied at lowest T_a, 21.4 °C.

A wide range of ROI temperature differences were recorded at each ROI (Figure 5) and from these values the temperature gradient, delta T (ΔT) calculated for ΔT_1 ($T_{DP} - T_{Cap}$) and ΔT_2 ($T_{DP} - T_{DH}$)

with respect to TS rating. Figure 6 shows the mean temperature (°C) at each of the three ROIs with respect to each residents' reported TS rating.

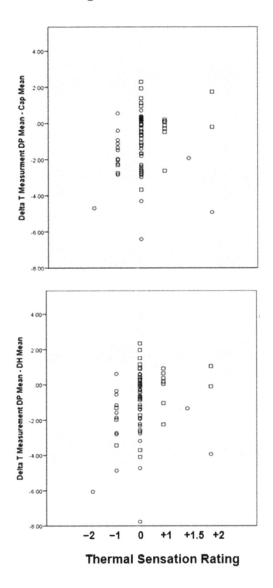

Figure 5.   Upper panel: extremity temperature difference between fingertip to wrist ΔT_1 (mean T_{DP}- mean T_{Cap}) and lower panel: fingertip to forearm, ΔT_2 (mean T_{DP} − T_{DH}) by group and TS ratings; dementia (O); no dementia (ND).

For ΔT_1, mean difference, 0.43 °C (0.24) (ND) vs. −1.7 °C (0.29 °C) (D) $p = 0.001$. For ΔT_2, mean difference, 0.39 °C (0.26 °C) (ND) vs. −1.8 °C (−0.34 °C) (D) $p = 0.001$ (Table 1) The range of temperature differences, ΔT_1 for residents with dementia ranged from −6.4 °C to −1.5 °C and for residents without dementia, −3.7 °C to 2.3 °C. The range of temperature differences, ΔT_2, −7.7 °C to 0.6 °C and −4.1 °C to 2.3 °C for D vs. ND respectively. A significant difference (mean 0.2 °C) for tympanic temperature ($p = 0.01$) was observed between groups ND and D.

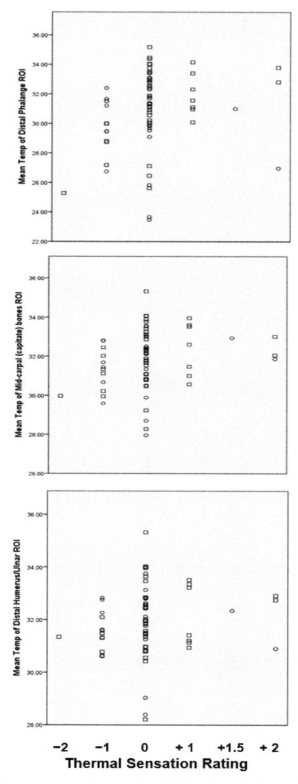

Figure 6. Mean extremity temperature values at three ROIs; distal phalange T_{DP} (upper panel); capitate bones, T_{Cap} (middle); distal humerus, T_{DH} (lower) by group and TS rating. dementia (O), no□ dementia (□) for each reported thermal sensation rating.

3.7. Extremity Temperature Values and Thermal Sensation Rating

On further exploration of thermal sensation for T_{DP}, residents who were dissatisfied with the environment provided ratings of −2 and −1 (slightly cool, cool, respectively), 11 were residents with dementia (D) and 4 did not have dementia (ND). Eleven residents (9 ND, 2 D) were also dissatisfied with the environment perceiving it as slightly warm (+1, +1.5) or warm (+2).

3.8. Thermal Mapping of Extremities: Correspondence Between the Thermal Map and Thermal Sensation Report

Qualitative review of hand thermograms, showed the visual appearance of skin temperature for ΔT_1 and ΔT_2 of all residents in the environment of their cluster groups:

(A) 'Cold hands': LWIR thermogram appearance was not consistent with thermal sensation report. Thirteen residents (9 in D category) showed the visible appearance of 'cold hands' mean $T_{DP} < 30\,°C$ (range 23.5–29.9 °C; median 26.5 °C) in air temperatures ranging from 21.4 °C to 25.6 °C (median 23.5 °C) (Figure 7). Thermal sensation ratings were variable ranging from −2 (cool $n = 1$), −1 (slightly cool, $n = 3$), 0 (comfortable/neutral, $n = 8$) to +2 (warm $n = 1$). For cold hands, the temperature difference for ΔT_1 ranged from −6.4 °C to −2.0 °C (median −2.8 °C) and for ΔT_2 −7.8 °C to −1.3 °C (median −3.8 °C). A clear demarcation in temperature across the hands was observed such that areas were 'invisible' against ambient temperature on the thermal map. 'Thermal amputation' was evident visually for the digits in 4 residents with (D) where ΔT_1 was −6.4 °C, −4.7 °C, −4.3 °C ($n = 1$ data missing).

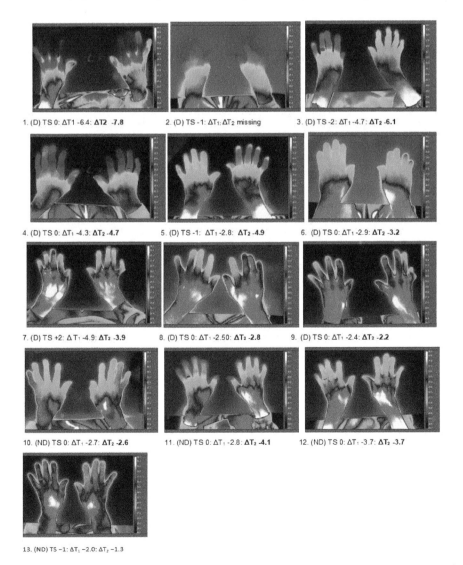

1. (D) TS 0: ΔT1 -6.4: **ΔT2 -7.8** 2. (D) TS -1: ΔT1: ΔT2 missing 3. (D) TS -2: ΔT1 -4.7: **ΔT2 -6.1**

4. (D) TS 0: ΔT1 -4.3: **ΔT2 -4.7** 5. (D) TS -1: ΔT1 -2.8: **ΔT2 -4.9** 6. (D) TS 0: ΔT1 -2.9: **ΔT2 -3.2**

7. (D) TS +2: ΔT1 -4.9: **ΔT2 -3.9** 8. (D) TS 0: ΔT1 -2.50: **ΔT2 -2.8** 9. (D) TS 0: ΔT1 -2.4: **ΔT2 -2.2**

10. (ND) TS 0: ΔT1 -2.7: **ΔT2 -2.6** 11. (ND) TS 0: ΔT1 -2.8: **ΔT2 -4.1** 12. (ND) TS 0: ΔT1 -3.7: **ΔT2 -3.7**

13. (ND) TS -1: ΔT1 -2.0: ΔT2 -1.3

Figure 7. Thermal maps of hand and forearm of 13 residents with the visual appearance of 'cold' hands. Figure shows the study group; dementia (D) or no dementia (ND), thermal sensation (TS) rating and the individual temperature difference (°C) for ΔT_1 and for ΔT_2.

(B) 'Warm hands': By contrast (Figure 8) the brightest colour appearance visually on thermograms corresponded with highest hand temperatures in 10 residents (5 D; 5 ND) (mean T_{DP} 31.7–35.2 °C; median 33.7 °C) across air temperature of 21.9 °C to 25.3 °C (median 22.9 °C) i.e., similar air temperature to those with cold hands. Individual thermal sensation ratings for this group were: −1 (slightly cool, $n = 1$); 0 (comfortable/neutral, $n = 7$), 1 (slightly warm, $n = 1$) and 2 (warm, $n = 1$). Temperature difference across the hands for ΔT_1 ranged from −1.1 °C to +1.9 °C (median 0.3 °C). Similarly, for ΔT_2, mean temperature differences between ROIs was small: range −1.2 °C to +2.34 °C (median 0.45 °C).

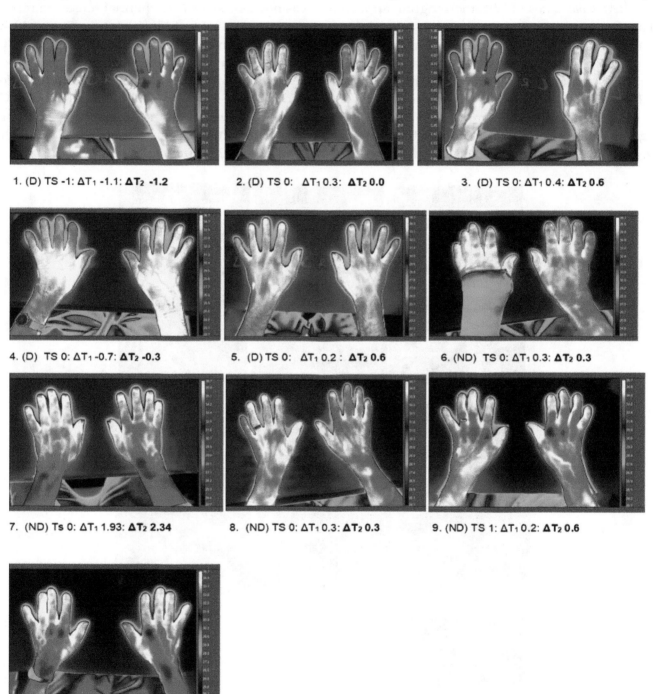

1. (D) TS -1: ΔT_1 -1.1: ΔT_2 -1.2

2. (D) TS 0: ΔT_1 0.3: ΔT_2 0.0

3. (D) TS 0: ΔT_1 0.4: ΔT_2 0.6

4. (D) TS 0: ΔT_1 -0.7: ΔT_2 -0.3

5. (D) TS 0: ΔT_1 0.2 : ΔT_2 0.6

6. (ND) TS 0: ΔT_1 0.3: ΔT_2 0.3

7. (ND) Ts 0: ΔT_1 1.93: ΔT_2 2.34

8. (ND) TS 0: ΔT_1 0.3: ΔT_2 0.3

9. (ND) TS 1: ΔT_1 0.2: ΔT_2 0.6

10. (ND) TS 2: ΔT_1 1.7: ΔT_2 1.0

Figure 8. Thermal maps of hand and forearm of 10 residents with the visual appearance of 'warm' hands. Figure shows the study group; dementia (D) or no dementia (ND), thermal sensation (TS) rating and temperature difference (°C) for ΔT_1 and for ΔT_2.

3.9. Medical History and Medications with Potential Influence on Perception of Temperature and Thermal Appearance

None of the residents had a past medical history of Raynaud's disease. There was however, a significant difference in the number of current medications between the residents with and without dementia ($p = 0.001$). However, with respect to medication with known vasoconstrictor or vasodilator effects which might be expected to have an effect on the distribution of blood flow (and temperature) at the extremities, there was no significant difference between the groups, neither were there significant difference in the medications given with known effects on neurological function known to impact on perception of thermal comfort. No other significant difference in medication type was noted for the remaining classes of prescribed drugs.

4. Discussion

The majority of care home residents in this study were in the older-old age group; 27% aged 90 years or more and with approximately half of the group with cognitive deficits. Studies of thermal comfort are typically performed under controlled conditions of a climate chamber e.g., [13,23]. Whilst Soebarto et al. [24] did undertake studies (of young and old people) in a climate chamber in both young and older people, the authors comment that this is not practical for the very old and frail. Undertaking the current study under the 'real-world' conditions of the care home provides a true representation of an individual's day to day indoor environment and associated thermoregulatory responses. In seeking to understand the responses of older people to their environment, we recognise that identifying those with cognitive deficits (vascular cognitive impairment, Alzheimer's prodrome) often falls short of an exact medical diagnosis [25]. This makes disease classification for research [26] to two binary groups ('dementia' vs. 'no dementia') rather more 'nuanced' because age-related cognitive decline follows a continuum across the boundary between normal cognition to the severely demented [26]. It was therefore not possible to assign residents accurately to two groups based on diagnostic differentiation using neuropathology or amyloid biomarkers [27] so the AMT score was used as a pragmatic alternative in the absence of a confirmed diagnosis.

Conducted across 15 English residential care homes, the overarching finding was that older people exposed to the same environmental conditions sense thermal comfort quite differently from one another and this carriers an important message for their carers, alerting them to the potential that residents will experience both satisfaction and dissatisfaction under the same indoor conditions.

Thermal comfort is just one aspect of the environment that exerts an effect on older people [11,28] especially those with dementia [29]. It is clear from the work of Walker et al. [10] that during cold weather, carers and managers are concerned about keeping residents warm and comfortable but see this as challenging due to the diversity of co-morbid conditions, frailty, and different levels of activity of people who live together. The same concerns hold for keeping residents cool in hot weather [3]. However, in the absence of any established method or consensus on how best to provide thermal comfort for the majority, it is likely that those residents in thermal discomfort (whether too cold or too hot) will be overlooked, especially if they are unable to communicate effectively.

Many researchers [30–33] have explored skin temperature (the physiological interface with the environment) as a predictor of thermal comfort. For example Wu et al. [34] investigated upper skin extremity temperature (finger, wrist, hand, forearm) and the conditions required for indoor thermal comfort in an office environment using the same 7-point thermal sensation scale as for the current study. In mean air temperature of 26.8 °C, 60% of adults rated thermal sensation 0 ('neutral') and 90%, rated TS from −1 to +1 (slightly cool, neutral, slightly warm). Similar results were observed in the older aged residents in this study, 63% and 92% rating TS 0 (neutral) and −1 to +1 respectively, albeit in mean air temperature 2 °C lower than the office-based adults. As for upper extremity temperatures in the older residents, mean finger-tip (30.9 °C), wrist (31.9 °C) and forearm (31.9 °C) temperatures were 2 °C lower than reported by Wu et al. [34] where corresponding regions (fingertip, wrist, forearm temperatures) were 33.4 °C 33.7 °C and 33.7 °C respectively. Of interest therefore is that whilst older adults had lower mean skin temperatures and were in lower indoor temperatures, a comparable percentage of residents were satisfied with the environment and rated their TS as 0 (neutral/comfortable). The possibility that the older person's thermal perception of the environment is 'blunted' is consistent with the biological consequences of ageing on thermogenesis and decline in thermosensitivity [35]. This blunting of thermal sensation can occur similarly as in other types of sensory perception loss with age [36]; hearing, vision, taste and smell being additional examples. We have observed features of thermal blunting in the older residents, particularly those with dementia where we observed residents with low extremity (digit) temperatures corresponding to 'cold hands' reporting thermal sensation as neutral (or comfortable) even with obvious visual 'thermal amputation' on the thermal map and even where environmental temperature was within the thermoneutral range [37,38].

In the thermoneutral zone, skin blood flow in the hands is tonically active and vasomotor tone of skin capillaries operates as the primary 'controller' of deep body temperature. Hands (and feet) represent 'radiator' organs [39] losing heat to the environment as well as retaining and conserving body heat. Skin temperature therefore varies with changes in vasomotor tone. Capillaries of non-glabrous skin, along with arterio-venous anastomoses (AVAs) of glabrous (hairless) skin of hands and feet are continuously adjusting (cycling) blood flow to extremity skin to balance heat loss with heat retention [38,40]. These physiological measures, independent of an individual's TS perception may provide a more robust indicator of temperature derangement than achieved through thermal comfort scales, especially under conditions where there is a risk of 'symptomless cooling' [14,18]. If it is possible to measure and/or 'see' the consequences of marked vasoconstriction (or vasodilation) at the extremities this may provide a more reliable indicator of thermal risk; 'cooling without noticing'. We have shown previously [8], as have others [41], that the feeling of being chilled tends to start in the hands or feet. Harazin et al. [42] report finger skin temperature (at a 'cut-off' temperature below 29 °C) in adults (with vibrotactile perception disorders consequent on peripheral neuropathy) as a characteristic of 'cold hands' even in air temperature above 21 °C.

In addition, Pathak et al. [23] have shown that skin temperature gradients are significantly related to resting metabolic rate such that air temperature of 25 °C may serve as an objective measure for the conditions to maintain homeothermy. Looking further at both extremity skin temperature, Wu et al. [34] report finger temperature above 30 °C (and finger-forearm temperature gradients close to 0 °C) to represent a significant threshold for an overall sensation of thermal comfort. Furthermore, at mean air temperature of 26.8 °C, Wu et al. [34] report temperature gradients between fingertip to wrist and fingertip to forearm ranging from −3.5 to 0.3 °C and −4.0 °C to −0.3 °C respectively; the negative temperature gradient serving as an indicator of a 'cool' TS response.

In the current study, older adults showed peripheral vasoconstriction as evidenced by the temperature gradients across the extremities; more intense in those with D than ND for both fingertip to wrist (ΔT_1) and fingertip to distal forearm (ΔT_2). At mean air temperature of 23 °C (Group D) and 24 °C (group ND) this air temperature is within the thermoneutral (comfort) zone (23–27 °C) for light to moderately clothed adults [23] yet older residents show evidence of extremes of thermoregulation as evidenced by both marked peripheral vasoconstriction and vasodilation in hand ROIs observable on the thermal maps.

Being able to take temperature measurements using conventional thermometry and across multiple areas of the skin surface in the setting of care homes presents a significant challenge in routine care. However, with infrared thermography, a quick visual assessment of the physiological response to the environment can be made by imaging of the extremities. Heat maps reflect the net effect of changes in vasomotor tone on skin temperature. As far as it is possible to tell, this is the first report of an independent imaging technology to map 'what we see' on LWIR thermography with 'what people say' about their thermal comfort. In other words, can we 'see' signs of thermal discomfort using thermal imaging and is there a potential benefit in doing so? Although other techniques; laser Doppler imaging [43], laser speckle imaging [44] or venous occlusion plethysmography [45] are available, they are rather less practical for the conditions of the care home whereas LWIR thermography offers an 'at a glance' imaging solution about thermal conditions of the 'radiator' organs, the most obvious exposed skin site being the hands. What we see on thermal imaging is the distribution of heat at the extremities which, at least for digit skin temperature (where metabolically active tissue is minimal) is entirely due to blood flow.

On qualitative review of thermal maps, the appearance of 'cold' and 'warm' hands emerged based on colour coding across a temperature span of 16 °C. For residents with 'cold hands', fingertip temperature (T_{DP}) was, in all cases <30 °C with fingertips consistently colder than wrist and forearm and with a wide (negative) skin temperature gradients for ΔT_1 and ΔT_2 irrespective of TS rating. These results support the work of both Pathak and Wu [23,34] (albeit studying younger, healthy adults) that fingertip temperature below a cut-off, together with wide (negative) temperature gradient (fingertip-wrist and fingertip-forearm) occur across the thermoneutral range. As we have observed, on review of the hand thermograms, this powerful vasoconstrictor response, which can decrease skin blood essentially to zero [46], is not always accompanied by a sensation equivalent to thermal discomfort.

Whilst commonly used models for thermal comfort are based on Fanger's work [47], such models were developed from studies in young, healthy adults in the workplace. That these models are inappropriate for older people is now recognized because changes in the structure of the nervous system as people age means that thermal sensitivity and perception decreases [14]. In the older group of residents, we have seen how varied the thermal comfort responses of older people are, even under the same environmental temperature. Shahzad et al. [48] have shown that neutral thermal sensation does not guarantee thermal comfort; 36% of participants in their study did not want to feel 'neutral' as their comfort condition, preferring a non-neutral thermal sensation. This finding supports the work of de Dear [49] in differentiating thermal 'pleasure' from thermal 'neutrality'; some people finding a cool environment more 'pleasing' than a neutral position which, apart from personal preference may also be influenced by cultural and social factors. For example, Florez-Duquet et al. [50] showed that older subjects generally did not report, or complain, of cold even during an entire cold exposure test whereas young adults did. Taylor et al. [15] showed that older people require a more intense stimulus, starting at the extremities before they 'feel' cold. Consequently, older people are being exposed to intense thermoregulatory challenges that will go unnoticed under the 'normal' indoor temperatures of the care home.

As the focus for long-term care has shifted from processes of care (safety, medical concerns) towards improving outcomes for residents [1] opportunities arise to meet this new challenge; to improve quality of life through considerations of the care home environment [51].

Whilst the majority of residents (both groups), expressed satisfaction with the environment by rating 0 on the thermal sensation scale, many did not; rating the environment too cool or even too warm. The first impression therefore, would be that residents were not in their comfort zone even in warm conditions but is this truly a measure of true satisfaction with the environment? Further evidence of the validity of the thermal sensation report can be explored by investigating concomitant changes in physiological factors, notably the degree of peripheral skin vasomotor tone.

Finally, of importance, in the context of determining the health and thermal comfort of older people in residential care, is not only in the ability to spot the vulnerable person at risk of chilling (or overheating) but in finding a practical solution to the variability in thermal sensation responses to the indoor environment in this older population, many of whom are immobile. Personal thermal comfort approaches could include 'smart' garments and local climate 'bubbles'. Our next step will be in tackling the best approaches to determine a range of approaches that are practical and feasible within the care home. What is clear, due to the COVID-19 pandemic, is that assessing residents by touch will now be excluded for any thermal comfort assessment for the near future.

5. Conclusions

What we have observed by undertaking this feasibility study, perhaps more useful to those involved in the care of older people than relying on a persons reported thermal sensation rating, is in being able to 'see' the physiological responses to the environment in which they live. It is recognised that in older age, cultural factors as well as decline in neurosensory function can have an impact on sensory perception such that these senses may be blunted. This further confounds the value of thermal comfort rating scales in older people. The quick, relatively inexpensive, technique of thermal imaging, allows an immediate assessment of 'live' efferent thermoregulatory activity without the need for absolute measurements per se, so providing a new aspect of multi-dimensional thermal assessment. Thus, from the physiological 'first responders' of thermoregulation: skin extremity temperature (and concomitant extremity skin perfusion), the technique of infrared thermography could, in the future, provide technology-driven approaches to thermal assessment. Thermographic mapping of extremities as a prodromal thermal signature of incipient chilling (or overheating) could offer a better biomarker of thermal satisfaction and temperature safety within the environment than an older person's own temperature sensibility. The future for this challenging field of health care will be in designing solutions to promote personalised thermal comfort involving interdisciplinary collaborations across medical, engineering, design and the built environment.

Author Contributions: Conceptualization, C.C.; data curation, J.E., C.C. and K.K.; formal analysis, C.C. and K.K.; funding acquisition, Principal Investigator C.C.; investigation, C.C., J.E., S.F.-D., J.R.W. and A.A.; methodology, C.C., K.K. and A.A.; project administration, J.E.; visualization, C.C., S.H.; writing—original draft, C.C.; review & editing, K.K., S.H., S.F.-D., J.R.W. and A.A. All authors have read and agreed to the published version of the manuscript.

Acknowledgments: We would also like to express our sincere thanks to the Trustees of the Dunhill Medical Trust for funding the study. Their support has been invaluable to the delivery of this work. We also thank The Dowager Countess Eleanor Peel Trust for the purchase of an infrared thermal imaging detector. We also thank the managers and care staff of the many residences we visited. They generously gave of their time to assist and support the study. We acknowledge the support of the Clinical Research Networks, who provided assistance in screening participants, especially the significant contribution of Graham Spencer, Derbyshire CRN. Our thanks also go to our colleagues Lee Pearse and Andrew Pearse of Heeley City Farm, Sheffield for their support, advice and experience of dementia care in the community. Finally, our thanks go to the residents who participated in the study, without whom this study would not have been possible.

Abbreviations

AMT	Abbreviated Mental Test
ASHRAE	American Society of Heating, Refrigerating and Air-Conditioning Engineers
CIT	Cold induced thermogenesis
Clo	clothing insulation unit
CRN	clinical research network
Icl	overall insulation of assembly in Clo units (Clo)
FOV	field of view
LWIR	long wave infrared thermography
PMH	past medical history
RH	relative humidity
ROI	region of interest
SD	standard deviation
T_a	air temperature
T_r	rectal temperature
T_{DP}	distal phalange skin temperature
T_{CAP}	capitate bones skin temperature
T_{DH}	distal humerus/ulnar skin temperature
T_{tymp}	tympanic membrane temperature
TV	thermal vote
Δ	delta
ΔT	temperature difference
UK	United Kingdom of Great Britain and Northern Ireland
TC	thermal comfort
TS	thermal sensation

References

1. Garre-Olmo, J.; Lopez-Pousa, S.; Turon-Estrada, A.; Juvinya, D.; Ballester, D.; Vilalta-Franch, J. Environmental determinants of quality of life in nursing home residents with severe dementia. *J. Am. Geriatr. Soc.* **2012**, *60*, 1230–1236. [CrossRef] [PubMed]
2. Bills, R.; Soebarto, V.; Williamson, T. Thermal experiences of older people during hot conditions in Adelaide. In *Fifty Years Later: Revisiting the Role of Architectural Science in Design and Practice: 50th International Conference of the Architectural Science Association, Adelaide, Australia, 6–9 December 2016*; School of Architecture and Built Environment, The University of Adelaide: Adelaide, Australia, 2016; pp. 657–664.
3. Van Hoof, J.H.B.; Hansen, A.; Kazak, J.K.; Soebarto, V. The living environment and thermal behaviours of older south Australians. *Int. J. Environ. Public Health Res.* **2019**, *16*, 935. [CrossRef] [PubMed]
4. ASHRAE: Standard 55-2013. *Thermal Environmental Conditions for Human Occupancy*; The American Society of Heating, Refrigerating and Air-Conditioning Engineers: Atlanta, GA, USA, 2013.
5. International Standards Organisation (ISO). *Ergonomics of the Thermal Environment–Analytical Determination and Interpretation of Thermal Comfort Using Calculation of the PMV And PPD Indices and Local Thermal Comfort Criteria*; ISO 7730; ISO Standardization: Geneva, Switzerland, 2015.
6. Bedford, T. The Warmth Factor in Comfort at Work. In *A Physiological Study of Heating and Ventilation*; H.M.S.O.: London, UK, 1936.
7. Parsons, K.C. Human response to thermal environments Principles and methods. In *Evaluation of Human Work*; Wilson, J.R., Corlett, E.N., Eds.; Taylor and Francis: London, UK, 1990.
8. Childs, C.; Gwilt, A.; Sherriff, G.; Homer, C. Old and Cold: Challenges in the Design of Personalised Thermal Comfort at Home. In Proceedings of the 3rd European Conference on Design4Health, Sheffield, UK, 13–16 July 2015; ISBN 978-1-84387-385-3.
9. Cleary, M.; Raeburn, T.; West, S.; Childs, C. The environmental temperature of the residential care home: Role in thermal comfort and mental health. *Contemp. Nurse* **2019**, *55*, 38–46. [CrossRef] [PubMed]
10. Walker, G.; Brown, S.; Neven, L. Thermal comfort in care homes: Vulnerability, responsibility and 'thermal care'. *Build. Res. Inf.* **2016**, *44*, 135–146. [CrossRef]
11. Van Hoof, J.; Schellen, L.; Soebarto, V.; Wong, J.K.W.; Kazak, J.K. Ten questions concerning thermal comfort and ageing. *Build. Environ.* **2017**, *120*, 123–133. [CrossRef]
12. Iommi, M.; Barbera, E. Thermal Comfort for older adults. An experimental study on the thermal requirements for older adults. In Proceedings of the CISBAT Conference, Lausanne, Switzerland, 9–11 September 2015; pp. 357–362.
13. Schellen, L.; van Marken Lichtenbelt, W.; Loomans, M.G.L.C.; Frijns, A.; Toftum, J.; deWit, M. Thermal comfort physiological responses and performance of elderly during exposure to a moderate temperature drift. In Proceedings of the 9th International Conference and Exhibition on Healthy Buildings 2009 (HB09), Syracuse, NY, USA, 13–17 September 2009.
14. Szekely, M.; Garai, J. Thermoregulation and age. In *Handbook of Clinical Neurology; Thermoregulation: From basic Neuroscience to Clinical Neurology Part 1*; Romanovsky, A., Ed.; Elsevier B.V.: Amsterdam, The Netherlands, 2018; Volume 156, pp. 715–725.
15. Taylor, N.A.S.; Allsopp, N.K.; Parkes, D.G. Preferred Room Temperature of Young vs. Aged Males: The Influence of Thermal Sensation, Thermal Comfort, and Affect. *J. Gerontol. Ser. A* **1995**, *50*, M216–M221. [CrossRef]
16. Blatteis, C.M. Age-dependent changes in temperature regulation—A mini review. *Gerontology* **2012**, *58*, 289–295. [CrossRef]
17. Holowatz, L.A.; Thompson-Torgerson, C.; Kenney, W.L. Aging and the control of human skin blood flow. *Front. Biosci.* **2010**, *15*, 718–739. [CrossRef]
18. Lloyd, E.L. *Hypothermia and Cold Stress*; Croom Helm: London, UK, 1986.
19. Hodkinson, H.M. Evaluation of a mental test score for assessment of mental impairment in the elderly. *Age Ageing* **1972**, *1*, 233–238. [CrossRef]
20. Rockwood, K.; Song, X.; MacKnight, C.; Bergman, H.; Hogan, D.B.; McDowell, I.; Mitnitski, A. A global clinical measure of fitness and frailty in elderly people. *CMAJ* **2005**, *173*, 489–495. [CrossRef]
21. Parsons, K. The thermal properties of clothing. In *Human Thermal Environments*; CRC Press: London, UK, 2014.

22.   McIntyre, D.A. Thermal sensation. A comparison of rating scales and cross modality matching. *Int. J. Biometeorol.* **1976**, *20*, 295. [CrossRef] [PubMed]

23.   Pathak, K.; Calton, E.K.; Soares, M.J.; Zhao, Y.; James, A.P.; Keane, K.; Newsholme, P. Forearm to fingertip skin temperature gradients in the thermoneutral zone were significantly related to resting metabolic rate: Potential implications for nutrition research. *Eur. J. Clin. Nutr.* **2017**, *71*, 1074–1079. [CrossRef] [PubMed]

24.   Soebarto, V.; Zhang, H.; Schiavon, S. A thermal comfort environmental chamber study of older and younger people. *Build. Environ.* **2019**, *155*, 1–14. [CrossRef]

25.   Stephan, B.C.; Matthews, F.E.; Khaw, K.T.; Dufouil, C.; Brayne, C. Beyond mild cognitive impairment: Vascular cognitive impairment, no dementia (VCIND). *Alzheimer's Res. Ther.* **2009**, *1*, 1–9. [CrossRef]

26.   Vos, S.J.; Verhey, F.; Frölich, L.; Kornhuber, J.; Wiltfang, J.; Maier, W.; Peters, O.; Rüther, E.; Nobili, F.; Morbelli, S.; et al. Prevalence and prognosis of Alzheimer's disease at the mild cognitive impairment stage. *Brain* **2015**, *138*, 1327–1338. [CrossRef]

27.   Blennow, K.; Zetterberg, H. Biomarkers for Alzheimer's disease: Current status and prospects for the future. *J. Intern. Med.* **2018**, *284*, 643–663. [CrossRef]

28.   Tartarini, F.; Cooper, P.; Fleming, R.; Batterham, M. Indoor air temperature and agitation of nursing home residents with dementia. *Am. J. Alzheimer's Dis. Dement.* **2017**, *32*, 272–281. [CrossRef]

29.   Day, K.; Carreon, D.; Stump, C. The Therapeutic Design of Environments for People with Dementia: A Review of the Empirical Research. *Gerontology* **2000**, *40*, 397–416.

30.   Wang, Z.; He, Y.; Hou, J.; Jiang, L. Human skin temperature and thermal responses in asymmetrical cold radiation environments. *Build. Environ.* **2013**, *67*, 217–223. [CrossRef]

31.   Liu, W.; Lian, Z.; Deng, Q. Use of mean skin temperature in evaluation of individual thermal comfort for a person in a sleeping posture under steady thermal environment. *Indoor Built Environ.* **2014**, *24*, 489–499. [CrossRef]

32.   Sakoi, T.; Tsuzuki, K.; Kato, S.; Ooka, R.; Song, D.; Zhu, S. Thermal comfort, skin temperature distribution, and sensible heat loss distribution in the sitting posture in various asymmetric radiant fields. *Build. Environ.* **2007**, *42*, 3984–3999. [CrossRef]

33.   Wang, D.; Zhang, H.; Arens, E.; Huizenga, C. Observations of upper-extremity skin temperature corresponding overall-body thermal sensations and comfort. *Build. Environ.* **2007**, *42*, 3933–3943. [CrossRef]

34.   Wu, Z.; Li, N.; Cui, H.; Peng, J.; Chen, H.; Liu, P. Using Upper Extremity Skin Temperatures to Assess Thermal Comfort in Office Buildings in Changsha, China. *Int. J. Environ. Res. Public Health* **2017**, *14*, 1092.

35.   Horvath, S.; Radcliffe, C.E.; Hutt, B.K.; Spurr, G.B. Metabolic response of old people to a cold environment. *J. Appl. Physiol.* **1955**, *8*, 45–148. [CrossRef] [PubMed]

36.   Cavazzana, A.; Röhrborn, A.; Garthus-Niegel, S.; Larsson, M.; Hummel, T.; Croy, I. Sensory-specific impairment among older people. An investigation using both sensory thresholds and subjective measures across the five senses. *PLoS ONE* **2018**, *13*, e0202969. [CrossRef]

37.   Savage, M.V.; Brengelmann, G.L. Control of skin blood flow in the neutral zone of human body temperature regulation. *J. Appl. Physiol. (1985)* **1996**, *80*, 1249–1257. [CrossRef]

38.   Walløe, L. Arterio-venous anastomoses in the human skin and their role in temperature control. *Temperature* **2016**, *3*, 92–103. [CrossRef]

39.   Romanovsky, A.A. The thermoregulation system and how it works. *Handb. Clin. Neurol.* **2018**, *156*, 3–43.

40.   Wilson, T.E.; Zhang, R.; Levine, B.D.; Crandall, C.D. Dynamic autoregulation of cutaneous circulation: Differential control in glabrous versus nonglabrous skin. *Heart Circ. Physiol.* **2005**, *289*, H385–H391. [CrossRef]

41.   Cheung, S.S. Responses of the hands and feet to cold exposure. *Temperature* **2005**, *2*, 105–120. [CrossRef]

42.   Harazin, B.; Harazin-Lechowska, A.; Kalamarz, J. Effect of individual finger skin temperature on vibrotactile perception threshold. *Int. J. Occup. Med. Environ. Health* **2013**, *26*, 930–939. [CrossRef] [PubMed]

43.   Murray, A.K.; Herrick, A.L.; King, T.A. Laser Doppler imaging: A developing technique for application in the rheumatic diseases. *Rheumatology* **2004**, *43*, 1210–1218. [CrossRef] [PubMed]

44.   Wilkinson, J.D.; Leggett, S.A.; Marjanovic, E.J.; Moore, T.L.; Allen, J.; Anderson, M.E.; Britton, J.; Buch, M.H.; Del Galdo, F.; Denton, C.P.; et al. A Multicenter Study of the Validity and Reliability of Responses to Hand Cold Challenge as Measured by Laser Speckle Contrast Imaging and Thermography: Outcome Measures for Systemic Sclerosis-Related Raynaud's Phenomenon. *Arthritis Rheumatol.* **2018**, *70*, 903–911. [CrossRef] [PubMed]

45. Mathiassen, O.N.; Buus, N.H.; Olsen, H.W.; Larsen, M.L.; Mulvany, M.J.; Christensen, K.L. Forearm plethysmography in the assessment of vascular tone and resistance vasculature design: New methodological insights. *Acta Physiol.* **2006**, *188*, 91–101. [CrossRef]

46. Charkoudian, N. Skin blood flow in adult human thermoregulation: How it works, when it does not, and why. *Mayo Clin. Proc.* **2003**, *78*, 603–612. [CrossRef]

47. Fanger, P.O. Assessment of man's thermal comfort in practice. *Br. J. Ind. Med.* **1973**, *30*, 313–324. [CrossRef]

48. Shahzad, S.; Brennan, J.; Theodossopoulos, D.; Calautit, J.K.; Hughes, B. Does a neutral thermal sensation determine thermal comfort? *Build. Serv. Eng. Res. Technol.* **2018**, *39*, 183–195. [CrossRef]

49. De Dear, R. Revisiting an old hypothesis of human thermal perception: Alliesthesia. *Build. Res. Inf.* **2011**, *39*, 108–117. [CrossRef]

50. Florez-Duquet, M.; McDonald, R.B. Cold-induced thermogenesis and biological aging. *Physiol. Rev.* **1998**, *78*, 339–358. [CrossRef]

51. White-Chu, E.F.; Graves, W.J.; Godfrey, S.M.; Bonner, A.; Sloane, P. Beyond the medical model: The culture change revolution in long-term care. *J. Am. Med Dir. Assoc.* **2009**, *10*, 370–378. [CrossRef]

18

Geriatric Resource Teams: Equipping Primary Care Practices to Meet the Complex Care Needs of Older Adults

Gwendolen Buhr [1,*], Carrissa Dixon [2], Jan Dillard [3,4], Elissa Nickolopoulos [3,4], Lynn Bowlby [3], Holly Canupp [3,5], Loretta Matters [6], Thomas Konrad [7], Laura Previll [1,8], Mitchell Heflin [1,8] and Eleanor McConnell [1,6,8]

[1] Duke Center for the Study of Aging and Human Development, Durham, NC 27710, USA; laura.previll@duke.edu (L.P.); mitchell.heflin@duke.edu (M.H.); eleanor.mcconnell@duke.edu (E.M.)

[2] Duke Office of Clinical Research, Durham, NC 27710, USA; carrissa.dixon@duke.edu

[3] Duke Outpatient Clinic, Durham, NC 27704, USA; janice.dillard@duke.edu (J.D.); elissa.rumer@duke.edu (E.N.); lynn.bowlby@duke.edu (L.B.); holly.causey@duke.edu (H.C.)

[4] Department of Case Management and Clinical Social Work, Duke University Medical Center, Durham, NC 27710, USA

[5] Department of Pharmacy, Duke University Medical Center, Durham, NC 27710, USA

[6] Duke University School of Nursing, Durham, NC 27710, USA; loretta.matters@duke.edu

[7] Cecil G. Sheps Center for Health Services Research at University of North Carolina, Chapel Hill, NC 27516, USA; bobkonrad@gmail.com

[8] Durham VA Geriatric Research, Education and Clinical Center, Durham, NC 27705, USA

* Correspondence: gwendolen.buhr@duke.edu

Abstract: Primary care practices lack the time, expertise, and resources to perform traditional comprehensive geriatric assessment. In particular, they need methods to improve their capacity to identify and care for older adults with complex care needs, such as cognitive impairment. As the US population ages, discovering strategies to address these complex care needs within primary care are urgently needed. This article describes the development of an innovative, team-based model to improve the diagnosis and care of older adults with cognitive impairment in primary care practices. This model was developed through a mentoring process from a team with expertise in geriatrics and quality improvement. Refinement of the existing assessment process performed during routine care allowed patients with cognitive impairment to be identified. The practice team then used a collaborative workflow to connect patients with appropriate community resources. Utilization of these processes led to reduced referrals to the geriatrics specialty clinic, fewer patients presenting in a crisis to the social worker, and greater collaboration and self-efficacy for care of those with cognitive impairment within the practice. Although the model was initially developed to address cognitive impairment, the impact has been applied more broadly to improve the care of older adults with multimorbidity.

Keywords: geriatrics; collaborative practice; geriatric workforce enhancement program; primary care

1. Introduction

The limitations of primary care practices' capacity to care for older adults have been underscored by the Institute of Medicine, which recommended a workforce with enhanced geriatric competence and reimbursement policies that would reward effective models of care for older adults [1]. Further, the World Health Organization has advocated for the development of age friendly primary health centers accessible to older adults, employing healthcare workers well versed in geriatric syndromes and knowledgeable about community resources [2]. More recently, the Institute for Healthcare Improvement (IHI) proposed that all care for older adults be age-friendly, which they have defined as utilizing the 4Ms—What Matters, Medication, Mentation, and Mobility—to make the complex care of older adults more manageable [3].

Diagnosing dementia presents challenges for primary care practices who lack the expertise, time, and resources to perform traditional comprehensive geriatric assessment. Yet, primary care practices are caring for an increasingly older and more complex older adult patient population. In particular, 20% of those older than 65 years have mild cognitive impairment and 14% over 70 years have dementia, yet cognitive impairment is markedly underdiagnosed in primary care [4]. In its traditional form, comprehensive geriatric assessment is an interprofessional and multidimensional process that utilizes the expertise of nurses, physicians, social workers, and other health professionals to evaluate not only physical illness, but also functional status and environmental and social issues, so as to create a plan to optimize wellbeing [5]. Comprehensive geriatric assessment is the ideal process for the diagnosis and care of patients with cognitive impairment. However, it is challenging for most busy primary care practices that care for older people with multimorbidity to employ such a model.

A systematic review of the barriers primary care practices face when diagnosing and managing patients with dementia found that the barriers could be grouped into patient factors, provider factors, and system factors [6]. In particular, the studies found that primary care practices lacked essential support services, including limited access to and knowledge of community resources, lack of access to an interprofessional team to enhance management, and lack of caregiver education and support. In addition, the research found that primary care practices lacked time and sufficient reimbursement to adequately diagnose and manage patients with dementia, as well as a lack of training undermined providers' confidence in making the diagnosis and managing subsequent care. The patient factors included stigma attached to receiving a diagnosis of dementia and delayed presentation of the patient to primary care for memory complaints. This article will describe a process by which an exemplary primary care practice developed an interprofessional and multidimensional process for the care of the older adults with mentoring from a team of geriatric experts. In particular, the practice focused on developing a method to more effectively identify and care for older adults with cognitive impairment.

2. Materials and Methods

The Duke Geriatric Workforce Enhancement Program (Duke-GWEP) was established to develop a healthcare workforce that maximizes patient and family engagement and improves health outcomes for older adults by integrating geriatrics with primary care [7]. To achieve this goal, we recruited primary care practices, and worked with them to create interprofessional geriatric resource teams (GRT) that could serve as a source of expertise in geriatrics and quality improvement (QI) within the practice. Each GRT was unique to the practice, but contained diverse professionals working within the practice—i.e., physicians, nurses, social worker, physician assistants, nurse practitioner, pharmacist, etc. We provided the GRTs a curriculum focused on team building, geriatric knowledge and skills, QI methods, and access to expert consultation and community resources using a hybrid learning model (Figure 1).

Previously, we found that before expecting teams to carry out QI projects, they need to establish a foundation of interprofessional collaborative practice. Therefore, GRT training began with a workshop on interprofessional collaborative practice, based on the Interprofessional Education Collaborative four core competency domains of values and ethics, roles and responsibilities, communication, and teamwork [8]. We emphasized the importance of engaging all team members in shared vision and problem solving using flexible role definitions and encouraging all team members to work at the top of their scope of practice.

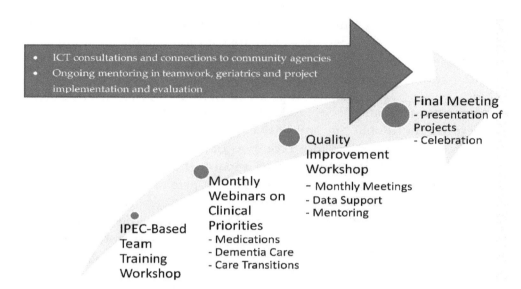

Figure 1. Geriatric Workforce Enhancement Program Primary Care Geriatric Resource Team Training: a year-long commitment to educational programs and process improvement activities. Abbreviations: ICT: Interagency Care Team; IPEC: Interprofessional Education Collaborative.

Throughout the academic year, we held monthly webinars that focused on three clinical priorities specified by the GWEP funding—dementia, medication management, and care transitions—and highlighted local community resources and agencies to help address these issues (Table 1). The webinars were recorded and provided continuing education credit. The GRTs were assigned mentors from the Duke-GWEP team who guided them in choosing QI topics prior to a QI workshop that was held midway through the academic year. We encouraged practices to implement a practice improvement project focused on one of the three priority topics. The QI workshop is based on the IHI model for improvement [9]. We also provided data support and mentoring. We encouraged practices to hold monthly GRT meetings with the GRT members, the Duke-GWEP mentors, and a data support specialist. The data support specialist had expertise in public health research, health communication, project management, IT/data management, and community engagement. At the end of the year all of the GRTs gathered together to present their QI projects.

Table 1. Geriatric resource teams (GRT) webinar topics.

Title	Objectives
Deprescribing	• Explain the process of deprescribing • Assess a patient's need for deprescribing • List at least two services provided by Senior PharmAssist, a community resource that provides financial assistance, medication management, community referrals, and Medicare insurance counseling
Improving Care Transitions	• Define the core principles of high-quality transitions of care • Describe a model for improving transitions in primary care practice • Identify community resources to improve transitions of care
Improving Skilled Nursing Facility (SNF) to Home Care Transitions	• Define the core principles of high-quality transitions of care from SNF to home • Describe a process and model for improving SNF to home transitions that engages teams from facility, health system, community, and primary care practices • Identify a role for options counselors in aiding the transitions process

Table 1. *Cont.*

Title	Objectives
Dementia: Recognition and Initial Assessment	• Describe the scope and impact of dementia • Develop a strategy for improving case recognition of cognitive impairment using questionnaires, structured assessments and specialty referrals • Communicate effectively with older adults and families with suspected cognitive disorders • Identify resources to help seniors and families cope with cognitive problems
Living with Dementia: Safety, Security, and Staying at Home	• Describe the balance between autonomy and safety in caring for people with dementia • List methods for improving safe management of finances and medications • Develop a plan for maintaining home safety • Implement measures to reduce falls among people with dementia
Medication Safety: Preventing Adverse Drug Events and Improving Transition of Care	• Define and classify medication errors and preventable medication related harms • Identify medication related quality measures for various care providers and settings • Identify opportunities to engage community pharmacists in healthcare improvement • Explain the difference between medication therapy management and medication management • List at least 3 community resources for medication management
Accounting for Health Literacy in Primary Care of Older Adults	• Acknowledge that healthcare is complex and problems with understanding and adherence are universal • Describe the association of low health literacy with poor health outcomes • Identify strategies for enhancing communication in practice to optimize a personal experience and outcomes

The Duke-GWEP also offered GRTs access to an Interagency Care Team (ICT): a team of geriatricians, nurse practitioners, and community partners, including clinical pharmacists and social workers who provided virtual consultations via the Electronic Health Record (EHR) for older adults with complex care needs residing in the community. This Duke-GWEP-ICT contacted the patient and family member, did a chart review, and met together to discuss the case and identify resources to help the patient remain at home. A recommendation was subsequently made to the patient and family member and to the providers at the practice.

3. Results

The Duke-GWEP recruited 13 practices in total over the three years, four in year 1, three in year 2, and six in year 3. To illustrate how comprehensive geriatric assessment principles are implemented in primary care, we present as a case one of the primary care practices from the first of three GRT cohorts.

Example GRT at the Duke Outpatient Clinic (DOC)

The DOC is the major internal medicine resident teaching clinic for Duke University Medical Center, where the physician faculty and interprofessional staff recognized the challenge of caring for older adults. The clinic serves a medically and socially complex group of 4500 patients, with an average age of 62 years, many of whom are under- or uninsured. The clinic employs an interprofessional team including a licensed clinical social worker who also functions as a behavioral health specialist, a Clinical Pharmacist Practitioner, registered nurses, certified medical assistants (CMA), attending physicians, and more than 70 internal medicine residents. The DOC GRT members included the licensed clinical social worker, behavioral health specialist, Clinical Pharmacist Practitioner, attending physician and clinic medical director, and a registered nurse.

Prior to forming the GRT, there was neither a systematic approach to identify patients with cognitive impairment nor a routine process to connect patients with dementia and their caregivers to needed community resources. Barriers identified by clinic staff included a lack of expertise in the diagnosis and management of patients with cognitive impairment and a lack of time. Consequently, the evaluation of cognitive impairment often did not happen until a crisis occurred, and the default response was to refer to the geriatric specialty clinic for comprehensive geriatric assessment. Timely access to this resource was hampered by a wait time of several months to obtain an appointment, and the need to visit the large medical center across town, which resulted in missed appointments. Because many patient and family crises involved an immediate need for placement, this sometimes resulted in a hospital admission for the patient.

During the workshops, the DOC team developed both a formal vision statement and QI aim. Vision statement: "Partner with the Duke-GWEP to foster educational initiatives, interdisciplinary care teams, and collaboration with community resources to improve the care of older adult patients and their loved ones-with a specific focus on cognitive impairment." QI project aim: "Develop and implement an interdisciplinary approach to improve care of patients and families affected by cognitive impairment."

After developing the vision and aim statements, the clinic's first step was workflow development, so as to screen for and diagnose cognitive impairment and clarify a process for caring for the patient once cognitive impairment was recognized. The GRT met monthly with their interprofessional team and Duke-GWEP mentors to systematically work through developing care processes to support the workflow, identify gaps, and provide additional training. The initial screening was incorporated into an ongoing project to screen for problems of social determinants of health. The team added a question to the existing screening form—"In the last two months, have you or your family had concerns about your memory or thinking?" In response to a positive answer, cognitive evaluation was then initiated using the Mini-Cog [10] performed by the CMA or the Montreal Cognitive Assessment tool (MoCA) [11] performed by the social worker, as well as for patients with concerns identified by the medical team. As the project continued, requests for cognitive evaluation began to increase from once every few months to a few times a week as providers became more aware of the clinical indicators of cognitive impairment.

The GRT developed a second workflow to guide the next steps after cognitive impairment was identified. The team obtained collateral history, performed further medical work up and treatment, documented cognitive impairment on the problem list within the EHR, and then counselled the patient and family on the diagnosis and treatment plan. An important aspect of the treatment plan was linking the patient and their caregivers to the appropriate community resources such as caregiver support programs. As cognitive impairment is now being identified earlier in the trajectory of illness, and not necessarily in conjunction with a crisis, there has been a resultant dramatic decrease in both requests for emergency placement for patients and referrals to the geriatric specialty clinic (Figure 2). The clinic is now only referring their most complex patients who can be seen more promptly since the less complex patients are managed within the primary care practice.

As part of their new process for screening, assessing, and providing care for patients with cognitive impairment, the clinic created a patient list of those with identified cognitive impairment to ensure that some of the most vulnerable patients received the services they needed. For example, they used that list to take a more proactive role in reviewing the advance care planning (ACP) needs and prioritizing these patients for ACP visits [12].

Although the model was developed to address cognitive impairment, the impact has been greater, expanding to focus on older adults with multimorbidity. The model continues to evolve and grow as other needs are uncovered. Beginning in quarter 3 of 2018, the team implemented an internal process for interdisciplinary review of complex patients, using a population health approach in which patients were identified for review by the clinical social workers based on presence of dementia and multimorbidity. The GRT modeled their processes after the Duke-GWEP's ICT and received consultation from the Duke-GWEP nurse practitioner who developed the ICT systems. Specifically, the clinical social worker and clinical pharmacist practitioner completed a thorough review of issues regarding cognition, medication access, medication management, disease management, advance care planning, social determinants of health, labs, behavioral health/social isolation, personal/home safety, insurance/access to care, and transitions of care. The review was documented in the EHR and reviewed with the entire team including physicians and geriatrics consultants at monthly meetings.

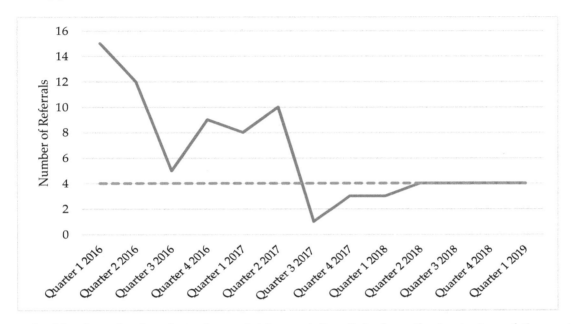

Figure 2. Number of referrals to the geriatric specialty clinic from the beginning of the project. The orange dotted line indicates the median.

Case Studies

The following case studies serve to illustrate how developing a GRT in a primary care practice enhances the capacity for conducting comprehensive geriatric assessment within primary care.

Case 1: An 88-year-old female with multiple medical problems, including recurrent GI bleeding, COPD, glaucoma, cachexia, and osteoarthritis, was abruptly left without a caregiver when her son unexpectedly died. She experienced worsening mental status and mood in the last year of her life, including an episode of delirium. Prior to establishing the GRT, this type of patient would have received a referral to the geriatrics clinic for comprehensive geriatric assessment. Instead, the primary care practice was able to manage the patient's complex needs without a geriatrics referral. The GRT's enhanced expertise in evaluation of her cognitive disturbance, enhanced teamwork processes, and awareness of community resources led to a timely referral to adult protective services and establishment of a new healthcare power of attorney (HCPOA) to replace her son who had recently died. Soon after, the patient experienced a serious health crisis. Her HCPOA was able to advocate effectively due to the work that had been done, and the patient was transferred to an inpatient hospice, where she died while receiving comfort care, in accordance with her wishes.

Case 2: At an acute care visit, a 63-year-old patient complained of word-finding and trouble remembering her medications. Prior to forming a GRT, the provider would have noted the concerns and advised that the patient follow-up with her primary care provider (PCP), and if the complaint persisted, a referral to the geriatrics specialty clinic would have occurred. Instead, the provider referred the patient to the GRT social worker, who was already embedded in the clinic, and able to administer the MoCA. The patient's score was 22 out of 30; however, most of the points missed were in executive function, not memory or attention. So, the social worker, recognizing that depression can present atypically in older adults, administered a depression screen. The patient tearfully reported that her mother had died 3 years ago last week, and admitted that she has not slept well since her mother passed away, getting on average about 3 h of sleep a night. The PHQ-9 results were 19 out of 26, and after declining counseling, the patient accepted pharmacotherapy for her depression. Even though the primary diagnosis was depression, not dementia, the presence of the GRT and related protocols for cognitive impairment improved teamwork and access to staff with geriatrics expertise that, in turn, supported the diagnosis and treatment of depression which had previously been undetected.

4. Discussion

The barriers to the diagnosis of dementia in primary care are myriad and include provider factors, patient factors, and system factors. The GRT effectively addressed most of these barriers. Specifically, the practice was provided with training and mentorship to increase the knowledge of the providers in the identification, evaluation and management of cognitive impairment. In addition, much attention was given to linking patients and their families to community resources to support them in their homes. Further, patients were universally screened for memory concerns, addressing the barrier of delayed presentation. The time constraints and reimbursement issues remain challenging [13], but the team is better positioned to utilize all members of the interprofessional team to address some of these barriers. The GRT example and case studies illustrate effective collaborative care for patients with complex care needs, including dementia, in primary care. The members of the GRT engaged in shared problem solving; rather than a workflow that relied on one profession to identify and care for the older adult, flexible role definitions were developed that allow each profession to work at the top of their scope of practice (Figure 3).

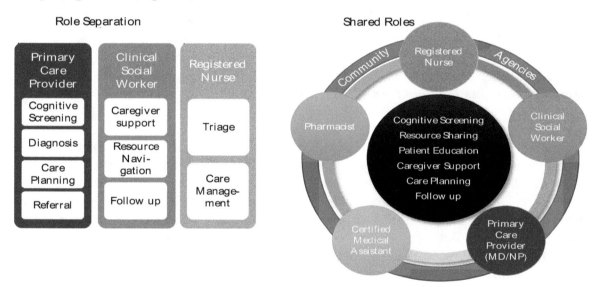

Figure 3. Redefining Roles and Workflow in Geriatric Primary Care before and after the establishment of a GRT.

Although not all of the team members received GRT training, the effects spread to all team members. As a result of the Duke-GWEP, the CMAs received additional geriatric training from the Duke Nurses Improving Care for Healthsystem Elders (Duke-NICHE) program [14], and for subsequent GRTs similar training was offered upfront. The Duke-GWEP training resulted in enhanced trust and confidence especially between the physicians and non-physician team members to identify and address geriatric issues. The social worker previously was brought in only during a crisis and the pharmacist was not involved. Now the pharmacist is involved in deprescribing and the social worker helps when mild cognitive impairment is identified, and an EHR-based patient list for all patients in the practice with cognitive impairment has been established so that their care needs can be anticipated and managed proactively. The CMAs are now more often included in the team discussions regarding patients and are viewed by the providers as key members of the team, resulting in empowerment and a greater sense of purpose or meaning. The practice learned from the Duke-GWEP virtual consultations performed by the ICT and was able to adopt these strategies for resource referrals to help other patients with similar problems—fall prevention, medication recommendations, and community resources.

Many programs strive to improve the care of older adults in primary care with system changes or processes with variable degrees of success [15,16]. The GRT program was unique in that there was an emphasis on team formation and webinars on geriatric principles and community resources coupled with mentoring by geriatric experts.

This example GRT from the DOC has applicability to teaching clinics in other academic health centers. As trainees rotate through these clinics that model interprofessional collaborative practice and team-based care, we expect to see improved uptake of processes that expand capacity through more effective teamwork. Team-based care that includes a variety of disciplines working to the top of their scope of practice and with expanded geriatric competency can achieve improved care of older adults without higher costs [17]. Furthermore, we believe that with the current structure of Medicare reimbursement, mentored comprehensive geriatric assessment is possible within primary care practices. Recognizing changes in cognition is a required part of the Medicare Annual Wellness Visit (G0438, G0439). As of January of 2018, Medicare provides reimbursement to providers for a comprehensive clinical visit for patients with dementia, resulting in a written care plan (CPT code 99483). This code requires an independent historian; a multidimensional assessment that includes cognition, function, and safety; evaluation of neuropsychiatric and behavioral symptoms; review and reconciliation of medications; and assessment of the needs of the patient's caregiver. These additional billing codes provide reimbursement for practitioners for the additional time that is required in the care of these patients.

The model of shared roles allows for flexibility in the role definitions. The key is to engage all team members in shared problem solving and to make sure all of the team members are working at the top of their scope of practice. In addition, linkages with community resources are critical, as well as enhanced training in geriatrics. This example GRT illustrates sustainability since the initial training occurred over three years ago, and the practice has developed systems to sustain the program despite only one year of intensive support from the Duke-GWEP. By focusing on team formation and interprofessional collaborative practice, the teams were equipped to continue their work. We are investigating models to continue to support primary care practices in their care of older adults. This can occur through the accountable care organization or through various e-consult or telehealth programs. Without GWEP funding, teams can obtain training on geriatric care principles, QI, and interprofessional collaborative practice through a variety of professional development opportunities and organizations, such as IPEC, American Geriatric Society, and the IHI age-friendly health systems resources.

Author Contributions: Conceptualization, E.M., J.D., H.C., L.B., and C.D.; methodology, T.K., G.B., E.M., and M.H.; formal analysis, C.D. and G.B.; investigation, J.D., H.C., E.N., L.B., E.M., and C.D.; data curation, C.D.; writing—original draft preparation, G.B.; writing—review and editing, L.B., J.D., G.B., C.D., E.N., H.C., and T.K., L.P., E.M., M.H.; visualization, L.P., G.B., C.D., M.H., and E.M.; supervision, M.H., G.B.; funding acquisition, E.M., M.H., and L.M.

References

1. Institute of Medicine (IOM). *Retooling for an Aging America: Building the Health Care Workforce*; The National Academies Press: Washington, DC, USA, 2008.
2. World Health Organization. Age-friendly Primary Health Care Centres Toolkit. 2008. Available online: https://www.who.int/ageing/publications/AF_PHC_Centretoolkit.pdf (accessed on 12 July 2019).
3. Age-Friendly Health Systems: Guide to Using the 4Ms in the Care of Older Adults. April 2019. Available online: http://www.ihi.org/Engage/Initiatives/Age-Friendly-Health-Systems/Documents/IHIAgeFriendlyHealthSystems_GuidetoUsing4MsCare.pdf (accessed on 12 July 2019).

4.   Alzheimer's Association. 2019 Alzheimer's Disease Facts and Figures. *Alzheimers Dement.* **2019**, *15*, 321–387. [CrossRef]

5.   Rubenstein, L.Z.; Stuck, A.E.; Siu, A.L.; Wieland, D. Impacts of Geriatric Evaluation and Management Programs on defined Outcomes: Overview of the Evidence. *J. Am. Geriat. Soc.* **1991**, *39*, 8S–16S. [CrossRef] [PubMed]

6.   Koch, T.; Iliffe, S.; EVIDEM-ED Project. Rapid appraisal of barriers to the diagnosis and management of patients with dementia in primary care: A systematic review. *BMC Fam. Pract.* **2010**, *11*, 52. [CrossRef] [PubMed]

7.   Health Resources and Services Administration. Geriatric Workforce Enhancement Program. 8 November 2018. Available online: https://bhw.hrsa.gov/fundingopportunities/default.aspx?id=4c8ee9ff-617a-495e-ae78-917847db86a9 (accessed on 21 September 2019).

8.   Interprofessional Education Collaborative Expert Panel. *Core Competencies for Interprofessional Collaborative Practice: Report of an Expert Panel*; Interprofessional Education Collaborative: Washington, DC, USA, 2011.

9.   Ogrinc, G.S.; Headrick, L.A.; Moore, S.M.; Barton, A.J.; Dolansky, M.A.; Madigosky, W.S. *Fundamentals of Health Care Improvement: A Guide to Improving Your Patients' Care*, 2nd ed.; The Joint Commission and the Institute for Healthcare Improvement: Oakbrook Terrace, IL, USA, 2012.

10. Borson, S.; Scanlan, J.; Brush, M.; Vitaliano, P.; Dokmak, A. The Mini-Cog: A cognitive 'vital signs' measure for dementia screening in multi-lingual elderly. *Int. J. Geriatr. Psychiatry* **2000**, *15*, 1021–1027. [CrossRef]

11. Razak, M.A.; Ahmad, N.A.; Chan, Y.Y.; Kasim, N.M.; Yusof, M.; Ghani, M.A.; Omar, M.; Abd Aziz, F.A.; Jamaluddin, R. Validity of screening tools for dementia and mild cognitive impairment among the elderly in primary health care: A systematic review. *Public Health* **2019**, *169*, 84–92. [CrossRef] [PubMed]

12. Frequently Asked Questions about Billing the Physician Fee Schedule for Advance Care Planning Services. July 2016. Available online: https://www.cms.gov/Medicare/Medicare-Fee-for-Service-Payment/PhysicianFeeSched/Downloads/FAQ-Advance-Care-Planning.pdf (accessed on 3 August 2019).

13. Boustani, M.; Alder, C.A.; Solid, C.A.; Reuben, D. An Alternative Payment Model to Support Widespread Use of Collaborative Dementia Care Models. *Health Aff.* **2019**, *38*, 54–59. [CrossRef] [PubMed]

14. Hendrix, C.C.; Matters, L.; West, Y.; Stewart, B.; McConnell, E.S. The Duke-NICHE program: An academic-practice collaboration to enhance geriatric nursing care. *Nurs. Outlook* **2011**, *59*, 149–157. [CrossRef] [PubMed]

15. Giuliante, M.M.; Greenberg, S.A.; McDonald, M.V.; Squires, A.; Moore, R.; Cortes, T.A. Geriatric Interdisciplinary Team Training 2.0: A collaborative team-based approach to delivering care. *J. Interprof. Care* **2018**, *32*, 629–633. [CrossRef] [PubMed]

16. Elliott, J.; Stolee, P.; Boscart, V.; Giangregorio, L.; Heckman, G. Coordinating care for older adults in primary care settings: Understanding the current context. *BMC Fam. Pract.* **2018**, *19*, 137. [CrossRef] [PubMed]

17. Kunik, M.E.; Mills, W.L.; Amspoker, A.B.; Cully, J.A.; Kraus-Schuman, C.; Stanley, M.; Wilson, N.L. Expanding the geriatric mental health workforce through utilization of non-licensed providers. *Aging Ment. Health* **2017**, *21*, 954–960. [CrossRef] [PubMed]

19

Comprehensive Geriatric Assessment as a Versatile Tool to Enhance the Care of the Older Person Diagnosed with Cancer

Janine Overcash [1],*, Nikki Ford [2], Elizabeth Kress [2], Caitlin Ubbing [2] and Nicole Williams [2]

[1]   The College of Nursing, The Ohio State University, 1585 Neil Ave, Newton Hall, Columbus, OH 43201, USA
[2]   Stephanie Spielman Comprehensive Breast Center, The Ohio State University, 1145 Olentangy River Road, Columbus, OH 43121, USA; Nikki.Ford@osumc.edu (N.F.); Eizabeth.Kress@osumc.edu (E.K.); Caitlin.Ubbing@osumc.edu (C.U.); Nicole.Williams@osumc.edu (N.W.)
*   Correspondence: Overcash.1@osu.edu

Abstract: The comprehensive geriatric assessment (CGA) is a versatile tool for the care of the older person diagnosed with cancer. The purpose of this article is to detail how a CGA can be tailored to Ambulatory Geriatric Oncology Programs (AGOPs) in academic cancer centers and to community oncology practices with varying levels of resources. The Society for International Oncology in Geriatrics (SIOG) recommends CGA as a foundation for treatment planning and decision-making for the older person receiving care for a malignancy. A CGA is often administered by a multidisciplinary team (MDT) composed of professionals who provide geriatric-focused cancer care. CGA can be used as a one-time consult for surgery, chemotherapy, or radiation therapy providers to predict treatment tolerance or as an ongoing part of patient care to manage malignant and non-malignant issues. Administrative support and proactive infrastructure planning to address scheduling, referrals, and provider communication are critical to the effectiveness of the CGA.

Keywords: comprehensive geriatric assessment; CGA; multidisciplinary team; senior adult; cancer

Caring for the older adult who is diagnosed with cancer can be a complex orchestration of managing existing comorbid conditions, cancer care, caregiver concerns, while maintaining quality of life [1–4]. Older people have unique healthcare needs compared to younger adults who may not have challenges regarding comorbidities [4–7], functional ability [8], transportation and social support [9]. Many academic and community cancer centers establish some type of multidisciplinary geriatric oncology program to meet the needs of the older person [10–15]. The central element associated with a geriatric oncology program is a comprehensive geriatric assessment (CGA). Despite the evidence showing the benefits of CGA, only 9% and 8% of Phase II and Phase III clinical trials use CGA [16]. Many healthcare settings do not use CGA also because of time constraints, availability of a multidisciplinary team, and lack of professionals trained in geriatrics/gerontology. Conducting a CGA is feasible in ambulatory geriatric oncology programs (AGOPs) [10,17] including radiation therapy and surgical oncology [18–20]. There are strategies to reduce the time and resources often required to conduct a CGA. The purpose of this article is to illustrate how CGA can be used in different types of AGOPs and is a feasible option despite limited time and personnel. A review of the classic and current literature was conducted using the Ohio State University (OSU) Health Sciences Library (HSL) including PubMed and Cumulative Index to Nursing and Allied Health Literature (CINAHL) to support this article.

1. Defining a Comprehensive Geriatric Assessment

A CGA is a battery of screening tools necessary to uncover actual and potential limitations that can compromise cancer diagnosis and treatment [21]. The Society for International Oncology in

Geriatrics (SIOG) recommends a CGA be administered to older patients who are receiving cancer care [22,23]. Benefits of a CGA are prolonged survival [24], prediction of those who may not benefit from treatment [25], prediction of mortality [26], of cancer treatment tolerance [27], of chemotherapy toxicities [28], of surgical complications [29], and aid in decision-making to help avoid over- and undertreatment of cancer [30]. The battery of screening tools is generally assembled to address common problems associated with aging; however, any number of valid and reliable clinical instruments can be included, depending on the resources. Some cancer centers may be able to conduct large-scale CGA with a robust multidisciplinary team (MDT), and others may limit assessment instruments and MDT members.

The comprehensive character of geriatric assessment allows clinicians to gain perspective beyond the traditional oncology-related history and physical exam [31]. A CGA can detect previously unidentified problems in approximately 70% of patients [32], which can impact cancer treatment [19] and provide the foundation for a treatment plan to address malignant and nonmalignant conditions [33]. CGA is used to develop and refine a cancer management plan specific to the needs of the person diagnosed with cancer [20]. A prime goal of geriatric oncology is helping an older person achieve the best health possible while receiving cancer care to maintain independence [4].

2. Instruments Included in a Comprehensive Geriatric Assessment

Generally, screening tools to detect depression [34], comorbidity [35], cognitive impairment [36], functional status [37,38], risk for falls [39], and nutritional status [40] are commonly included in a CGA. The CGA is multidimensional in that many types of screening instruments can be included to meet the needs of people who are diagnosed with cancer or who are receiving end-of-life care [41], caregivers [42], and providers [43]. SIOG recommends a variety of instruments that can be tailored to any patient population [44].

When choosing instruments to include in a CGA, consider that there are performance-based evaluations and self-report measures. Performance-based evaluations provide a depiction of a person's capability using tools such as the Timed Up and Go Test (TUAGT) [45], balance testing [46], grip strength [47], sit-to-stand test [48], cognitive screening using the Clock Drawing Test [49], and other empirically measured tests. Self-report measures are also commonly included in the CGA, such as the Geriatric Depression Scale (GDS) [34], Activities of Daily Living Scale [37], Instrumental Activities of Daily Living [38], quality-of-life measures [50], and nutritional assessment [40]. Self-report measures tend to be rather easy to use and have validity and reliability metrics for clinical and research use. Including both self-report and performance-based evaluations provides patient perception of functioning at home in conjunction with an objective assessment. Some patients may tend to over-estimate their functional ability, and the empirical observation of task performance may help providers develop realistic management plans.

Supporting the caregiver is also important to the health of the person with cancer [51]. The Modified Caregiver Strain Index [52,53] is a 13-item tool that measures the financial, psychological, personal, physical, and social domains of caregiving which can be incorporated into a CGA. Caregivers of people diagnosed with cancer who have functional impairment [54] and have increased comorbidity [55] report greater strain and burden. CGA can stratify people with cancer into levels of caregiver burden risk so that clinicians can recognize caregivers who may need help [42]. Caregivers of people with advanced cancer often neglect their own health and wellness and report high levels of depression and anxiety [56]. Depression is not rare among caregivers (42%), and clinicians must support and encourage health maintenance and wellness [57]. If caregiver health is not maintained and perceptions of strain and burden exist, the individual with cancer is at risk for re-hospitalization [58] and increased morbidity/mortality [59]. Help for caregivers navigating community resources, Medicare, insurance, and cancer treatment can be very welcomed [60]. Cancer can be overwhelming and expensive, and providing psychosocial support can reduce caregiver stress associated with financial toxicity [61], address depression, and establish coping strategies [62]. No matter the scale of the CGA, caregiver support is important to geriatric oncology.

3. Multidisciplinary Team

A MDT has historically been used in geriatrics to administer the CGA and manage the many interwoven concerns that can affect older people [63,64]. An MDT can be composed of physicians, social workers, pharmacists, nurses, nurse practitioners, dietitians, physical therapists, and other types of healthcare professionals. Not every clinic may have access to a variety of specialists, and it is important to remember that geriatric care and screening can be provided by physicians, nurse practitioners, and nurses. An MDT may simply include a physician and a nurse who are trained in geriatrics. Administering and coordinating a CGA is well within the scope of practice of nursing and can be central to the effectiveness of the MDT [65].

Whatever the size, an MDT functions symbiotically to assess, manage, and monitor many limitations and complications associated with aging and deconditioning [66]. Geriatric oncology has adopted the MDT approach to improve or maintain independence [67] and to provide CGA by which to impact the cancer management plan [20]. Key to an effective MDT are communication, collaboration, and coordination [68]. A social worker, nurse practitioner, and dietitian can evaluate a patient simultaneously and hear the responses from individual assessments, so that questions are not duplicated. This method requires a cohesive teamwork, does save some time, and enhances communication within the MDT. An MDT with a perception of cohesive teamwork provides higher quality of care and less attrition in the nursing staff [69]. Communication with primary care providers and other specialists is critical to geriatric oncology and successful interventions [70]. When primary care providers and oncology providers agree on recommendations, adherence to CGA recommendations is more likely to occur [71].

For providers who lack a MDT, nurse-conducted CGA is a viable option. Nurses and/or advanced practice nurses often function in the role of coordinator, provider, communicator, and organizer. Awareness of the current knowledge in normative aging, geriatric syndromes, wellness, and prevention are components of nursing best practices [72]. Best practices in geriatric/gerontological competencies are provided by the American Association of Colleges of Nursing (AACN) for advanced practice and baccalaureate nurses and largely guide curriculum development for colleges of nursing throughout the United States [73,74]. However, geriatric training is often lacking in nursing schools throughout the country [75], and geriatric education is often received outside of the academic curriculum. The National Hartford Center of Gerontological Nursing Excellence (NHCGNE) aims to enhance gerontological education among nurses in the academic and clinical workforce [76]. The NHCGNE recognizes gerontological nurse educators as *Distinguished Educators in Gerontological Nursing Program* for working with faculty to enhance university and college curricula, educate nursing students at all levels, and work with other providers to better care for the older person [77]. It is important that nurses are educated in gerontology/geriatrics so they are prepared to assess and contribute to the care of the older person who is diagnosed with cancer [78].

4. Management of Problems Detected by Comprehensive Geriatric Assessment

Geriatric syndromes (poor functional status, cognitive impairment, frailty), life expectancy, and comorbidity are realities that oncology providers must consider when caring for older individuals. The mean number of geriatric syndromes is 2.9 in community-dwelling older people [79] and when uncontrolled, may interfere with cancer treatment. Complex problems associated with geriatric syndromes often cannot be addressed in one clinic visit or with a single medication or intervention. For frailer people, determining the cause of a problem may require an MDT-administered CGA and several clinic visits to detect and manage complex problems [80]. Good general health and absence of severe comorbidity allow older people to be considered for surgical [81] and other types of standard treatments [82].

People who have well-managed comorbidities may not have any deterioration in their functional status or life expectancy. In non-metastatic prostate cancer patients receiving treatment, 10-year life expectancy was not impacted by comorbid conditions nor age [83]. However, data show that for every chronic condition, life expectancy decreases 1.8 years [61]. Life expectancy, comorbid conditions, and functional status are sentinel factors in geriatric oncology [84]. Functional status and not chronological age is an important consideration in cancer treatment planning for the older adult [28,85].

Initiating a CGA requires a process to manage the limitations uncovered by the evaluation, and providers should be trained on how to incorporate the MDT recommendations in the decision-making process [86]. The mean number of CGA recommendations to address the uncovered limitations ranges from seven [87] to two [88], depending on the type of patient (frail, vulnerable, or fit) [89]. A CGA performed upon an initial oncology encounter can render three interventions [90]. Patients are most likely to adhere to four or less recommendations unless they present cognitive decline, in which case adherence is lower [87].

Follow-up care is important to determine adherence to recommendations and to reassess the issues that were previously detected [91]. The problems detected in the CGA should be managed or referred and detailed in the medical record [92,93]. How often to administer the CGA depends on the degree of fitness or frailty of the patient. A primary care nurse who is trained in geriatrics can be effective in coordinating the recommendations [94].

5. Comprehensive Geriatric Assessment with Limited Resources

A CGA conducted by an MDT can require an hour or more to administer; however, there are strategies to conduct CGA in a timely and efficient manner. Targeting the person who would most likely benefit from the CGA with a prescreening instrument can help preserve the resources of clinical time and personnel and reduce the respondent burden (Figure 1).

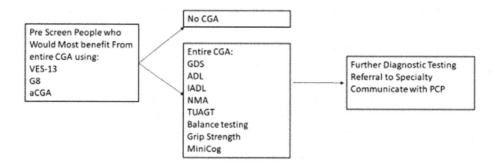

Figure 1. Prescreening using CGA to Determine Further Treatment or Diagnostics.

Prescreens have been developed, such as the abbreviated CGA [95], the G8 [96], and the Vulnerable Elders Survey-13 [97]. SIOG recommends several valid and reliable pre-screen tools [1]. The purpose of pre-screen tools is to target those who most benefit from conducting the entire CGA, rather than to replace a CGA. People who have functional decline and a higher risk of mortality and of cancer treatment complications tend to benefit from the CGA [98,99]. For those people who are independent and with minimal comorbid conditions, a CGA may not be as beneficial [100].

Depending on resources and type of healthcare setting, a CGA can be fashioned to include only several instruments rather than an exhaustive battery of tools requiring hours of clinic encounter time. Creating a smaller version of CGA which can include two or three screening instruments (GDS, Mini-Cog, TUAGT) will allow time to gain experience administering the instrument and managing the limitations. Using only two or three screening instruments has reasonable benefit to people who are diagnosed with cancer and to their families. The detection and management of depression can contribute to better cancer treatment outcomes, particularly with adherence to recommendations [101]. Benefits of screening for cognitive limitations are inconclusive [102]; however, other considerations such as planning, awareness of limitations, preparation for future and other important tasks can be very helpful for patients and families. Screening using the TUAGT can lead to physical therapy consults [88] to enhance lower extremity strength and to provide falls education and proactive planning should a fall occur (determining how to get help, keeping a phone on the bathroom floor near the bathing area). The use of three tools can provide the opportunity to address common problems that can be associated with aging without requiring the time to conduct a more robust CGA (Figure 2).

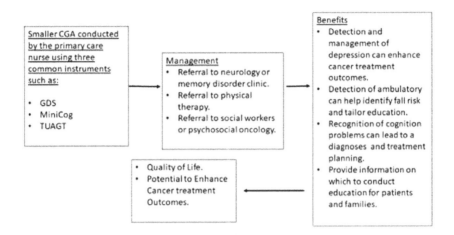

Figure 2. Smaller CGA to Determine Further Treatment or Diagnostics.

The use of pre-screens and a smaller battery of assessment instruments is a viable option when using CGA with limited clinical resources. Understanding the versatility of CGA may motivate more clinicians to employ best practices in geriatric assessment.

Cost and resources are a factor when establishing a geriatric oncology program; however, not all data indicate that CGA is cost-prohibitive when looking at long-term expenses and hospital stay. The SIOG suggests that CGA is cost-effective and reduces hospitalizations [103]. CGA in people who experience a hip fracture reduces hospital costs and hospital length of stay and improves health outcomes [104]. However, for those people admitted to the hospital for nonmalignant conditions, CGA is thought to slightly increase costs [105]. A Swedish study found ambulatory oncology CGA to have increased costs due to the number of interventions and increased survival [25]. Another Swedish study found ambulatory CGA to increase survival in frail people, with fewer hospital days and without higher costs [106]. In the United States, the cost savings or expenses may be different, however, people tend to benefit from CGA [85,107].

6. Models of Geriatric Oncology Programs Using CGA

AGOPs often include regular CGAs and manage a patient throughout cancer care. There are different types of AGOPs, such as those that provide ongoing geriatric oncology management, one-time consult programs, site specific programs, and programs that address patients according to age and not a particular tumor type. Scale also varies among AGOPs, with some using large MDTs and others consisting of an oncologist and a geriatric trained nurse. Regardless of the structure, AGOPs can provide CGA and offer management strategies to enhance the care of the older person diagnosed with cancer.

The CGA can be administered by a nurse or nurse practitioner, and scores on the measures can be shared with the entire MDT, so that more in-depth screening can be conducted by the appropriate specialists. In some situations, the MDT members individually screen new patients to establish a baseline condition prior to cancer treatment. The MDT members can then evaluate the patient as needed throughout cancer treatment. Established patients who have received a baseline CGA can receive regular geriatric assessment screening every 6 months or every year. No data exist on how often to conduct a CGA; however, frail or vulnerable patients may require more frequent screening. The National Comprehensive Cancer Network (NCCN) has established guidelines for using CGA when caring for the older adult [108]. A pre-cancer treatment decision tree addresses how and when to use a prescreening and an entire CGA and how CGA can impact treatment decisions for the patient, family, and provider [108].

Scheduling new and established patients visits for any type of AGOP requires planning for extra time to conduct the CGA. For AGOPs conducting the entire CGA with an MDT in addition to establishing a cancer management plan, a new patient visit may require two hours. For those AGOPs using limited measures in the CGA and a limited MDT, perhaps a 30 min visit is appropriate. One-time CGA consults can be easier to schedule in that all patients tend to receive the same screening instruments and assessment from the MDT. Generally, the consult can be conducted in approximately 1.5 to 2 h per patient. Depending on the physical environment of the clinic, three patients can be scheduled every 2–2.5 hour and be accommodated with rotating members of the team conducting the assessments.

An AGOP one-time CGA consult functions to provide recommendations for cancer treatment, identifies comorbid conditions, and addresses actual and potential risk factors that can affect health and independence. A one-time CGA consult can be helpful to surgical teams to predict complications [109] and post-surgical delirium when administered prior to surgery [110]. A one-time CGA conducted by a geriatrician prior to emergency surgery reduces hospital length of stay by 55 days [111]. Despite the positive contributions of CGA, many surgeons and other providers fail to consult geriatric services [112]. Education on the benefits of CGA in cancer treatment decision-making is critical for all cancer specialties and providers.

Conducting a CGA and incorporating an MDT require infrastructures and administrative support to lay the foundation for a sustainable geriatric oncology. Often, facilities and providers have difficulty launching and maintaining senior adult programs, for many reasons [113]. Patient scheduling to accommodate longer visit times [114], avenues of referral when limitations are found, adapting the medical record to accommodate scores and recommendations are important tasks to address before initiating geriatric assessment [13]. AGOPs require continued evaluation and maintenance to ensure the process of clinic is working well and the MDT is functioning effectively and productively. Regular team meetings can be helpful to discuss assessment process, patients, and research activities. Regular meetings should include administration, office staff who schedule patient visits, as well as people who work with medical records, who can be helpful in establishing highly functioning clinics, especially in big medical centers. MDT meetings prior to geriatric oncology clinic are very useful to review new and established patients.

A prime component of infrastructure is communication with other providers, which is key to the effectiveness of AGOPs. Many providers feel under-utilized in the development of cancer management plans, and communication is often poor between oncologists and primary care providers [94]. Proactive planning to establish avenues of communication to coordinate the CGA recommendations can reduce redundant assessments and increase effectiveness. Follow-up care and adherence to recommendations are likely to be improved with better communication between geriatric MDTs and other providers and typically require organizational modifications for adequate transfer of patient information [115].

Patient referral to an AGOP is also a consideration when establishing a clinic or a process for other oncology providers to refer patients for a one-time CGA consult or ongoing management. Awareness of the AGOP should be created within the organization and the community. Often, community members are not aware of geriatric oncology services, and providing educational symposiums or brief presentations at various sites common to potential patients and families can offer the opportunity to receive a CGA and cancer care.

An AGOP can provide valuable clinical data to enhance the care of the older person diagnosed with cancer. Establishing a research protocol incorporating CGA data can help improve the science of geriatric oncology and establish a foundation for future funding. Select CGA instruments can be useful clinically as well as appropriate for research. Dissemination is critical to geriatric oncology and helps address the importance of CGA in the care of the older person diagnosed with cancer.

7. Conclusions

CGA is a versatile tool that can be integrated into various oncology clinics and specialties to provide the best care for the older person. Integrating a CGA does require administrative support, infrastructure for patient scheduling, MDT involvement, and a great deal of planning. The importance of understanding the needs of older people with cancer and of their caregivers underscores the significance of CGA and inspires a comprehensive view, helpful to make treatment decisions. CGA is the central element of geriatric oncology and the gold standard of practice to meet the needs of older people.

Author Contributions: Individual contributions are as follows: conceptualization, writing original—draft preparation, writing- review and editing draft preparation was performed by J.O., conceptualization writing—review and editing draft preparation was completed by E.K., N.F., C.U. and N.W.

Acknowledgments: We would like to thank the Stephanie Spielman Comprehensive Breast Cancer for continued support of geriatric oncology and our Senior Adult Oncology Program.

References

1. Rocque, G.; Azuero, A.; Halilova, K.; Williams, C.; Kenzik, K.; Yagnik, S.K.; Pisu, M. Most Impactful Factors on the Health-Related Quality of Life of a Geriatric Population with Cancer (S769). *J. Pain Symptom Manag.* **2018**, *55*, 694–695. [CrossRef]

2. Hurria, A. Management of Elderly Patients With Cancer. *J. Natl. Compr. Cancer Netw.* **2013**, *11*, 698–701. [CrossRef]

3. Vallet-Regí, M.; Manzano, M.; López, M.C.; Aapro, M.; Barbacid, M.; Guise, T.A.; Balducci, L.; Mena, A.C.; Romero, P.L.O.; Orellana, M.R.; et al. Management of Cancer in the Older Age Person: An Approach to Complex Medical Decisions. *Oncol.* **2017**, *22*, 335–342. [CrossRef] [PubMed]

4. Balducci, L. Treatment of Breast Cancer in Women Older Than 80 Years Is a Complex Task. *J. Oncol. Pr.* **2016**, *12*, 133–134. [CrossRef] [PubMed]

5. Williams, G.R.; Deal, A.M.; Lund, J.L.; Chang, Y.; Muss, H.B.; Pergolotti, M.; Guerard, E.J.; Shachar, S.S.; Wang, Y.; Kenzik, K.; et al. Patient-Reported Comorbidity and Survival in Older Adults with Cancer. *Oncologist* **2018**, *23*, 433–439. [CrossRef]

6. Klepin, H.D.; Pitcher, B.N.; Ballman, K.V.; Kornblith, A.B.; Hurria, A.; Winer, E.P.; Hudis, C.; Cohen, H.J.; Muss, H.B.; Kimmick, G.G.; et al. Comorbidity, Chemotherapy Toxicity, and Outcomes Among Older Women Receiving Adjuvant Chemotherapy for Breast Cancer on a Clinical Trial: CALGB 49907 and CALGB 361004 (Alliance). *J. Oncol. Pr.* **2014**, *10*, e285–e292. [CrossRef] [PubMed]

7. Kim, K.H.; Lee, J.J.; Kim, J.; Zhou, J.-M.; Gomes, F.; Sehovic, M.; Extermann, M. Association of multidimensional comorbidities with survival, toxicity, and unplanned hospitalizations in older adults with metastatic colorectal cancer treated with chemotherapy. *J. Geriatr. Oncol.* **2019**. [CrossRef]

8. Mariano, C.; Williams, G.; Deal, A.; Alston, S.; Bryant, A.L.; Jolly, T.; Muss, H.B. Geriatric Assessment of Older Adults With Cancer During Unplanned Hospitalizations: An Opportunity in Disguise. *Oncol.* **2015**, *20*, 767–772. [CrossRef]

9. Tjong, M.C.; Menjak, I.; Trudeau, M.; Mehta, R.; Wright, F.; Leahey, A.; Ellis, J.; Gallagher, D.; Gibson, L.; Bristow, B.; et al. Perceptions and Expectations of Older Women in the Establishment of the Senior Women's Breast Cancer Clinic (SWBCC): A Needs Assessment Study. *J. Cancer Educ.* **2017**, *32*, 850–857. [CrossRef]

10. Magnuson, A.; Dale, W.; Mohile, S. Models of Care in Geriatric Oncology. *Curr. Geriatr. Rep.* **2014**, *3*, 182–189. [CrossRef]

11. O'Donovan, A.; Leech, M.; Mohile, S. Expert consensus panel guidelines on geriatric assessment in oncology. *Eur. J. Cancer Care* **2015**, *24*, 574–589. [CrossRef] [PubMed]

12.   Burhenn, P.S.; Perrin, S.; McCarthy, A.L.; Information, P.E.K.F.C. Models of Care in Geriatric Oncology Nursing. *Semin. Oncol. Nurs.* **2016**, *32*, 24–32. [CrossRef] [PubMed]

13.   Overcash, J. Integrating Geriatrics Into Oncology Ambulatory Care Clinics. *Clin. J. Oncol. Nurs.* **2015**, *19*, E80–E86. [CrossRef] [PubMed]

14.   Goede, V.; Stauder, R. Multidisciplinary care in the hematology clinic: Implementation of geriatric oncology. *J. Geriatr. Oncol.* **2018**, *10*, 497–503. [CrossRef] [PubMed]

15.   Chapman, A.E.; Swartz, K.; Schoppe, J.; Arenson, C. Development of a comprehensive multidisciplinary geriatric oncology center, the Thomas Jefferson University Experience. *J. Geriatr. Oncol.* **2014**, *5*, 164–170. [CrossRef]

16.   Le Saux, O.; Falandry, C.; Gan, H.K.; You, B.; Freyer, G.; Péron, J. Changes in the Use of Comprehensive Geriatric Assessment in Clinical Trials for Older Patients with Cancer over Time. *Oncol.* **2019**. [CrossRef] [PubMed]

17.   Puts, M.T.E.; Hardt, J.; Monette, J.; Girre, V.; Springall, E.; Alibhai, S.M.H. Use of Geriatric Assessment for Older Adults in the Oncology Setting: A Systematic Review. *J. Natl. Cancer Inst.* **2012**, *104*, 1134–1164. [CrossRef] [PubMed]

18.   Szumacher, E.; Sattar, S.; Neve, M.; Do, K.; Ayala, A.; Gray, M.; Lee, J.; Alibhai, S.; Puts, M. Use of Comprehensive Geriatric Assessment and Geriatric Screening for Older Adults in the Radiation Oncology Setting: A Systematic Review. *Clin. Oncol.* **2018**, *30*, 578–588. [CrossRef]

19.   Alibhai, S.M.; Jin, R.; Loucks, A.; Yokom, D.W.; Watt, S.; Puts, M.; Timilshina, N.; Berger, A. Beyond the black box of geriatric assessment: Understanding enhancements to care by the geriatric oncology clinic. *J. Geriatr. Oncol.* **2018**, *9*, 679–682. [CrossRef]

20.   Festen, S.; Kok, M.; Hopstaken, J.S.; van der Wal-Huisman, H.; van der Leest, A.; Reyners, A.K.L.; de Bock, G.H.; de Graeff, P.; van Leeuwen, B.L. How to incorporate geriatric assessment in clinical decision-making for older patients with cancer. An implementation study. *J. Geriatr. Oncol.* **2019**. [CrossRef]

21.   Solomon, D. National Institutes of Health Consensus Development Conference Statement: Geriatric Assessment Methods for Clinical Decision-Making. *Am. Geriatr. Soc.* **1988**, *36*, 342–437.

22.   Wildiers, H.; Heeren, P.; Puts, M.; Topinkova, E.; Janssen-Heijnen, M.L.; Extermann, M.; Falandry, C.; Artz, A.; Brain, E.; Colloca, G.; et al. International Society of Geriatric Oncology Consensus on Geriatric Assessment in Older Patients With Cancer. *J. Clin. Oncol.* **2014**, *32*, 2595–2603. [CrossRef] [PubMed]

23.   Mohile, S.G.; Velarde, C.; Hurria, A.; Magnuson, A.; Lowenstein, L.; Pandya, C.; O'Donovan, A.; Gorawara-Bhat, R.; Dale, W. Geriatric Assessment-Guided Care Processes for Older Adults: A Delphi Consensus of Geriatric Oncology Experts. *J. Natl. Compr. Cancer Netw.* **2015**, *13*, 1120–1130. [CrossRef]

24.   Kenis, C.; Baitar, A.; DeCoster, L.; De Grève, J.; Lobelle, J.-P.; Flamaing, J.; Milisen, K.; Wildiers, H. The added value of geriatric screening and assessment for predicting overall survival in older patients with cancer. *Cancer* **2018**, *124*, 3753–3763. [CrossRef] [PubMed]

25.   Lundqvist, M.; Alwin, J.; Henriksson, M.; Husberg, M.; Carlsson, P.; Ekdahl, A.W. Cost-effectiveness of comprehensive geriatric assessment at an ambulatory geriatric unit based on the AGe-FIT trial. *BMC Geriatr.* **2018**, *18*, 32. [CrossRef] [PubMed]

26.   Hamaker, M.E.; Vos, A.G.; Smorenburg, C.H.; De Rooij, S.E.; Van Munster, B.C. The Value of Geriatric Assessments in Predicting Treatment Tolerance and All-Cause Mortality in Older Patients With Cancer. *Oncol.* **2012**, *17*, 1439–1449. [CrossRef] [PubMed]

27.   Freyer, G.; Geay, J.-F.; Touzet, S.; Provencal, J.; Weber, B.; Jacquin, J.-P.; Ganem, G.; Mathieu, N.T.; Gisserot, O.; Pujade-Lauraine, E. Comprehensive geriatric assessment predicts tolerance to chemotherapy and survival in elderly patients with advanced ovarian carcinoma: A GINECO study. *Ann. Oncol.* **2005**, *16*, 1795–1800. [CrossRef] [PubMed]

28.   Soto-Perez-De-Celis, E.; Li, D.; Yuan, Y.; Lau, Y.M.; Hurria, A. Functional versus chronological age: Geriatric assessments to guide decision making in older patients with cancer. *Lancet Oncol.* **2018**, *19*, e305–e316. [CrossRef]

29.   Kristjansson, S.R.; Nesbakken, A.; Jordhøy, M.S.; Skovlund, E.; Audisio, R.A.; Johannessen, H.-O.; Bakka, A.; Wyller, T.B. Comprehensive geriatric assessment can predict complications in elderly patients after elective surgery for colorectal cancer: A prospective observational cohort study. *Crit. Rev. Oncol.* **2010**, *76*, 208–217. [CrossRef]

30. Schiphorst, A.H.; Ten Bokkel Huinink, D.; Breumelhof, R.; Burgmans, J.P.; Pronk, A.; Hamaker, M.E. Geriatric consultation can aid in complex treatment decisions for elderly cancer patients. *Eur. J. Cancer Care (Engl.)* **2016**, *25*, 365–370. [CrossRef]

31. Caillet, P.; Laurent, M.; Bastuji-Garin, S.; Liuu, E.; Culine, S.; Lagrange, J.-L.; Canoui-Poitrine, F.; Paillaud, E. Optimal management of elderly cancer patients: Usefulness of the Comprehensive Geriatric Assessment. *Clin. Interv. Aging* **2014**, *9*, 1645–1660. [PubMed]

32. Horgan, A.M.; Leighl, N.B.; Coate, L.; Liu, G.; Palepu, P.; Knox, J.J.; Perera, N.; Emami, M.; Alibhai, S.M. Impact and feasibility of a comprehensive geriatric assessment in the oncology setting: A pilot study. *Am. J. Clin. Oncol.* **2012**, *35*, 322–328. [CrossRef] [PubMed]

33. Hamaker, M.E.; Molder, M.T.; Thielen, N.; Van Munster, B.C.; Schiphorst, A.H.; Van Huis, L.H. The effect of a geriatric evaluation on treatment decisions and outcome for older cancer patients – A systematic review. *J. Geriatr. Oncol.* **2018**, *9*, 430–440. [CrossRef] [PubMed]

34. Yesavage, J.A.; Brink, T.; Rose, T.L.; Lum, O.; Huang, V.; Adey, M.; Leirer, V.O. Development and validation of a geriatric depression screening scale: A preliminary report. *J. Psychiatr. Res.* **1982**, *17*, 37–49. [CrossRef]

35. Charlson, M.E.; Pompei, P.; Ales, K.L.; MacKenzie, C. A new method of classifying prognostic comorbidity in longitudinal studies: Development and validation. *J. Chronic Dis.* **1987**, *40*, 373–383. [CrossRef]

36. Borson, S.; Scanlan, J.; Brush, M.; Vitaliano, P.; Dokmak, A. The Mini-Cog: A cognitive "vital signs" measure for dementia screening in multi-lingual elderly. *Int. J. Geriatr. Psychiatry* **2000**, *15*, 1021–1027. [CrossRef]

37. Katz, S.; Grotz, R.C.; Downs, T.D.; Cash, H.R. Progress in Development of the Index of ADL. *Gerontol.* **1970**, *10*, 20–30. [CrossRef] [PubMed]

38. Lawton, M.P.; Brody, E.M. Assessment of Older People: Self-Maintaining and Instrumental Activities of Daily Living. *Gerontol.* **1969**, *9*, 179–186. [CrossRef]

39. Kellogg International Work Group. A report of the Kellogg International Work Group on the Prevention of Falls by the Elderly. *Dan. Med. Bull.* **1987**, *34* (Suppl. 4), 1–24.

40. Vellas, B.; Guigoz, Y.; Garry, P.J.; Nourhashemi, F.; Bennahum, D.; Lauque, S.; Albarède, J.-L. The mini nutritional assessment (MNA) and its use in grading the nutritional state of elderly patients. *Nutr.* **1999**, *15*, 116–122. [CrossRef]

41. Baronner, A.; MacKenzie, A. Using Geriatric Assessment Strategies to Lead End-of-Life Care Discussions. *Curr. Oncol. Rep.* **2017**, *19*. [CrossRef] [PubMed]

42. Rajasekaran, T.; Tan, T.; Ong, W.S.; Koo, K.N.; Chan, L.; Poon, D.; Chowdhury, A.R.; Krishna, L.; Kanesvaran, R.; Information, P.E.K.F.C. Comprehensive Geriatric Assessment (CGA) based risk factors for increased caregiver burden among elderly Asian patients with cancer. *J. Geriatr. Oncol.* **2016**, *7*, 211–218. [CrossRef] [PubMed]

43. Hamaker, M.; Seynaeve, C.; Wymenga, A.; Van Tinteren, H.; Nortier, J.; Maartense, E.; De Graaf, H.; De Jongh, F.; Braun, J.; Los, M.; et al. Baseline comprehensive geriatric assessment is associated with toxicity and survival in elderly metastatic breast cancer patients receiving single-agent chemotherapy: Results from the OMEGA study of the Dutch Breast Cancer Trialists' Group. *Breast* **2014**, *23*, 81–87. [CrossRef] [PubMed]

44. International Society of Oncology Geraitrics. Comprehensive Geraitric Assessment of the Older Person with Cancer. 2015. Available online: http://www.siog.org/content/comprehensive-geriatric-assessment-cga-older-patient-cancer (accessed on 11 June 2019).

45. Podsiadlo, D.; Richardson, S. The Timed "Up & Go": A Test of Basic Functional Mobility for Frail Elderly Persons. *J. Am. Geriatr. Soc.* **1991**, *39*, 142–148. [PubMed]

46. Berg, K.O.; Wood-Dauphinee, S.L.; Williams, J.I.; Maki, B. Measuring balance in the elderly: Validation of an instrument. *Can. J. Public Heal.* **1992**, *83*, S7–S11.

47. Mathiowetz, V.; Weber, K.; Volland, G.; Kashman, N. Reliability and validity of grip and pinch strength evaluations. *J. Hand Surg.* **1984**, *9*, 222–226. [CrossRef]

48. Jones, C.J.; Rikli, R.E.; Beam, W.C. A 30-s Chair-Stand Test as a Measure of Lower Body Strength in Community-Residing Older Adults. *Res. Q. Exerc. Sport* **1999**, *70*, 113–119. [CrossRef]

49. Borson, S.; Brush, M.; Gil, E.; Scanlan, J.; Vitaliano, P.; Chen, J.; Cashman, J.; Maria, M.M.S.; Barnhart, R.; Roques, J. The Clock Drawing Test: Utility for Dementia Detection in Multiethnic Elders. *Journals Gerontol. Ser. A: Boil. Sci. Med Sci.* **1999**, *54*, M534–M540. [CrossRef]

50. Cella, D.F.; Tulsky, D.S.; Gray, G.; Sarafian, B.; Linn, E.; Bonomi, A.; Silberman, M.; Yellen, S.B.; Winicour, P.; Brannon, J. The Functional Assessment of Cancer Therapy scale: Development and validation of the general measure. *J. Clin. Oncol.* **1993**, *11*, 570–579. [CrossRef]

51. Sakurai, R.; Kawai, H.; Suzuki, H.; Kim, H.; Watanabe, Y.; Hirano, H.; Ihara, K.; Obuchi, S.; Fujiwara, Y. Poor Social Network, Not Living Alone, Is Associated With Incidence of Adverse Health Outcomes in Older Adults. *J. Am. Med Dir. Assoc.* **2019**. [CrossRef]

52. Thornton, M.; Travis, S.S. Analysis of the Reliability of the Modified Caregiver Strain Index. *Journals Gerontol. Ser. B* **2003**, *58*, S127–S132. [CrossRef] [PubMed]

53. Robinson, B.C. Validation of a Caregiver Strain Index. *J. Gerontol.* **1983**, *38*, 344–348. [CrossRef] [PubMed]

54. Bień-Barkowska, K.; Doroszkiewicz, H.; Bień, B. Silent strain of caregiving: Exploring the best predictors of distress in family carers of geriatric patients. *Clin. Interv. Aging* **2017**, *12*, 263–274. [CrossRef] [PubMed]

55. Dauphinot, V.; Ravier, A.; Novais, T.; Delphin-Combe, F.; Moutet, C.; Xie, J.; Mouchoux, C.; Krolak-Salmon, P.; Information, P.E.K.F.C. Relationship Between Comorbidities in Patients With Cognitive Complaint and Caregiver Burden: A Cross-Sectional Study. *J. Am. Med Dir. Assoc.* **2016**, *17*, 232–237. [CrossRef]

56. Dionne-Odom, J.N.; Demark-Wahnefried, W.; Taylor, R.A.; Rocque, G.B.; Azuero, A.; Acemgil, A.; Martin, M.Y.; Astin, M.; Ejem, D.; Kvale, E.; et al. The Self-Care Practices of Family Caregivers of Persons with Poor Prognosis Cancer: Differences by Varying Levels of Caregiver Well-being and Preparedness. *Support. Care Cancer* **2017**, *25*, 2437–2444. [CrossRef] [PubMed]

57. Geng, H.M.; Chuang, D.M.; Yang, F.; Yang, Y.; Liu, W.M.; Liu, L.H.; Tian, H.M. Prevalence and determinants of depression in caregivers of cancer patients: A systematic review and meta-analysis. *Medicine (Baltimore)* **2018**, *97*, e11863. [CrossRef]

58. Bonin-Guillaume, S.; Durand, A.-C.; Yahi, F.; Curiel-Berruyer, M.; Lacroix, O.; Cretel, E.; Alazia, M.; Sambuc, R.; Gentile, S. Predictive factors for early unplanned rehospitalization of older adults after an ED visit: Role of the caregiver burden. *Aging Clin. Exp. Res.* **2015**, *27*, 883–891. [CrossRef] [PubMed]

59. Aggarwal, B.; Liao, M.; Christian, A.; Mosca, L. Influence of caregiving on lifestyle and psychosocial risk factors among family members of patients hospitalized with cardiovascular disease. *J. Gen. Intern. Med.* **2009**, *24*, 93–98. [CrossRef]

60. Lawn, S.; Westwood, T.; Jordans, S.; O'Connor, J. Support workers as agents for health behavior change: An Australian study of the perceptions of clients with complex needs, support workers, and care coordinators. *Gerontol. Geriatr. Educ.* **2017**, *38*, 496–516. [CrossRef]

61. DuGoff, E.H.; Canudas-Romo, V.; Buttorff, C.; Leff, B.; Anderson, G.F. Multiple chronic conditions and life expectancy: A life table analysis. *Med. Care* **2014**, *52*, 688–694. [CrossRef]

62. Nelson, C.J.; Saracino, R.M.; Roth, A.J.; Harvey, E.; Martin, A.; Moore, M.; Marcone, D.; Poppito, S.R.; Holland, J. Cancer and Aging: Reflections for Elders (CARE): A pilot randomized controlled trial of a psychotherapy intervention for older adults with cancer. *Psychooncology* **2019**, *28*, 39–47. [CrossRef] [PubMed]

63. Rubenstein, L.Z.; Josephson, K.R.; Wieland, G.D.; English, P.A.; Sayre, J.A.; Kane, R.L. Effectiveness of a Geriatric Evaluation Unit. *New Engl. J. Med.* **1984**, *311*, 1664–1670. [CrossRef] [PubMed]

64. Warren, M.W. Care of Chronic Sick. *Br. Med. J.* **1943**, *2*, 822–823. [CrossRef] [PubMed]

65. Trotta, R.L.; Rao, A.D.; Hermann, R.M.; Boltz, M.P. Development of a Comprehensive Geriatric Assessment Led by Geriatric Nurse Consultants: A Feasibility Study. *J. Gerontol. Nurs.* **2018**, *44*, 25–34. [CrossRef] [PubMed]

66. Flood, K.L.; Booth, K.; Vickers, J.; Simmons, E.; James, D.H.; Biswal, S.; Deaver, J.; White, M.L.; Bowman, E.H. Acute Care for Elders (ACE) Team Model of Care: A Clinical Overview. *Geriatr.* **2018**, *3*, 50. [CrossRef] [PubMed]

67. Balducci, L.; Yates, J. General guidelines for the management of older patients with cancer. *Oncol. (Williston Park. N.Y.)* **2000**, *14*, 221–227.

68. Karnakis, T.; Gattas-Vernaglia, I.F.; Saraiva, M.D.; Gil-Junior, L.A.; Kanaji, A.L.; Jacob-Filho, W. The geriatrician's perspective on practical aspects of the multidisciplinary care of older adults with cancer. *J. Geriatr. Oncol.* **2016**, *7*, 341–345. [CrossRef] [PubMed]

69. Piers, R.D.; Versluys, K.; Devoghel, J.; Vyt, A.; Noortgate, N.V.D. Interprofessional teamwork, quality of care and turnover intention in geriatric care: A cross-sectional study in 55 acute geriatric units. *Int. J. Nurs. Stud.* **2019**, *91*, 94–100. [CrossRef]

70. Nazir, A.; Unroe, K.; Tegeler, M.; Khan, B.; Azar, J.; Boustani, M. Systematic Review of Interdisciplinary Interventions in Nursing Homes. *J. Am. Med Dir. Assoc.* **2013**, *14*, 471–478. [CrossRef]

71. Maly, R.C.; Leake, B.; Frank, J.C.; DiMatteo, M.R.; Reuben, D.B. Implementation of consultative geriatric recommendations: The role of patient-primary care physician concordance. *J. Am. Geriatr. Soc.* **2002**, *50*, 1372–1380. [CrossRef]

72. McConnell, E.S.; Lekan, D.; Bunn, M.; Egerton, E.; Corazzini, K.N.; Hendrix, C.D.; E Bailey, D. Teaching evidence-based nursing practice in geriatric care settings: The geriatric nursing innovations through education institute. *J. Gerontol. Nurs.* **2009**, *35*, 26–33. [PubMed]

73. American Assocaition of Colleges of Nursing. Adult Gerontology Acute Care and Primary Care Competencies. 2016. Available online: http://www.aacnnursing.org/Portals/42/AcademicNursing/pdf/Adult-Gero-NP-Comp-2016.pdf (accessed on 20 June 2019).

74. American Nurses Credentialing Center. Gerontological Nursing Certification. 2018. Available online: https://www.nursingworld.org/our-certifications/gerontological-nurse/ (accessed on 20 June 2019).

75. Gilje, F.; Lacey, L.; Moore, C. Gerontology and Geriatric Issues and Trends in U.S. Nursing Programs: A National Survey. *J. Prof. Nurs.* **2007**, *23*, 21–29. [CrossRef] [PubMed]

76. Bednash, G.; Mezey, M.; Tagliareni, E. The Hartford Geriatric Nursing Initiative experience in geriatric nursing education: Looking back, looking forward. *Nurs. Outlook* **2011**, *59*, 228–235. [CrossRef] [PubMed]

77. National Hartford Center of Nursing Excellence. Distinguished Educator in Gerontological Nursing. 2018. Available online: https://www.nhcgne.org/leadership-development/distinguished-educator-in-gerontological-nursing-program (accessed on 18 May 2019).

78. Burhenn, P.S.; McCarthy, A.L.; Begue, A.; Nightingale, G.; Cheng, K.; Kenis, C. Geriatric assessment in daily oncology practice for nurses and allied health care professionals: Opinion paper of the Nursing and Allied Health Interest Group of the International Society of Geriatric Oncology (SIOG). *J. Geriatr. Oncol.* **2016**, *7*, 315–324. [CrossRef] [PubMed]

79. Tkacheva, O.N.; Runikhina, N.K.; Ostapenko, V.S.; Sharashkina, N.V.; A Mkhitaryan, E.; Onuchina, J.S.; Lysenkov, S.N.; Yakhno, N.N.; Press, Y. Prevalence of geriatric syndromes among people aged 65 years and older at four community clinics in Moscow. *Clin. Interv. Aging* **2018**, *13*, 251–259. [CrossRef] [PubMed]

80. Overcash, J.; Cope, D.G.; Van Cleave, J.H. Frailty in Older Adults: Assessment, Support, and Treatment Implications in Patients With Cancer. *Clin. J. Oncol. Nurs.* **2018**, *22*, 8–18.

81. Banysch, M.; Akkaya, T.; Gurenko, P.; Papadakis, M.; Heuer, T.; Kasim, E.; Tavarajah, S.S.; Kaiser, G.M. Surgery for colorectal cancer in elderly patients: Is there such a thing as being too old? *G Chir* **2018**, *39*, 355–362.

82. Vitale, S.G.; Capriglione, S.; Zito, G.; Lopez, S.; Gulino, F.A.; Di Guardo, F.; Vitagliano, A.; Noventa, M.; La Rosa, V.L.; Sapia, F.; et al. Management of endometrial, ovarian and cervical cancer in the elderly: Current approach to a challenging condition. *Arch. Gynecol. Obstet.* **2019**, *299*, 299–315. [CrossRef]

83. Boehm, K.; Dell'Oglio, P.; Tian, Z.; Capitanio, U.; Chun, F.K.H.; Tilki, D.; Haferkamp, A.; Saad, F.; Montorsi, F.; Graefen, M.; et al. Comorbidity and age cannot explain variation in life expectancy associated with treatment of non-metastatic prostate cancer. *World J. Urol.* **2017**, *35*, 1031–1036. [CrossRef]

84. Shachar, S.S.; Hurria, A.; Muss, H.B. Breast Cancer in Women Older Than 80 Years. *J. Oncol. Pr.* **2016**, *12*, 123–132. [CrossRef]

85. Droz, J.-P.; Boyle, H.; Albrand, G.; Mottet, N.; Puts, M. Role of Geriatric Oncologists in Optimizing Care of Urological Oncology Patients. *Eur. Urol. Focus* **2017**, *3*, 385–394. [CrossRef] [PubMed]

86. Sarrió, R.G.; On behalf of the Spanish Working Group on Geriatric Oncology of the Spanish Society of Medical Oncology (SEOM); Rebollo, M.A.; Garrido, M.J.M.; Guillen-Ponce, C.; Blanco, R.; Flores, E.G.; Saldaña, J. General recommendations paper on the management of older patients with cancer: The SEOM geriatric oncology task force's position statement. *Clin. Transl. Oncol.* **2018**, *20*, 1246–1251.

87. Morin, T.; Lanièce, I.; Desbois, A.; Amiard, S.; Gavazzi, G.; Couturier, P. Evaluation of adherence to recommendations within 3 months after comprehensive geriatric assessment by an inpatient geriatric consultation team. *Geriatr Psychol Neuropsychiatr Vieil* **2012**, *10*, 285–293. [PubMed]

88. Overcash, J. Comprehensive Geriatric Assessment: Interprofessional Team Recommendations for Older Adult Women With Breast Cancer. *Clin. J. Oncol. Nurs.* **2018**, *22*, 304–315. [CrossRef] [PubMed]

89. Balducci, L. Frailty: A Common Pathway in Aging and Cancer. *Primate Reproductive Aging* **2013**, *38*, 61–72.

90. Boulahssass, R.; Gonfrier, S.; Champigny, N.; Lassalle, S.; François, E.; Hofman, P.; Guerin, O. The Desire to Better Understand Older Adults with Solid Tumors to Improve Management: Assessment and Guided Interventions—The French PACA EST Cohort Experience. *Cancers* **2019**, *11*, 192. [CrossRef] [PubMed]

91. Extermann, M.; Aapro, M.; Bernabei, R.; Cohen, H.J.; Droz, J.P.; Lichtman, S.; Topinkova, E. Use of comprehensive geriatric assessment in older cancer patients: Recommendations from the task force on CGA of the International Society of Geriatric Oncology (SIOG). *Crit. Rev. Oncol. Hematol.* **2005**, *55*, 241–252. [CrossRef]

92. Mohile, S.G.; Dale, W.; Somerfield, M.R.; Schonberg, M.A.; Boyd, C.M.; Burhenn, P.S.; Canin, B.; Cohen, H.J.; Holmes, H.M.; Hopkins, J.O.; et al. Practical Assessment and Management of Vulnerabilities in Older Patients Receiving Chemotherapy: ASCO Guideline for Geriatric Oncology. *J. Clin. Oncol.* **2018**, *36*, 2326–2347. [CrossRef]

93. Verweij, N.M.; Souwer, E.T.D.; Schiphorst, A.H.W.; Maas, H.A.; Portielje, J.E.A.; Pronk, A.; Bos, F.V.D.; Hamaker, M.E. The effect of a geriatric evaluation on treatment decisions for older patients with colorectal cancer. *Int. J. Color. Dis.* **2017**, *32*, 1625–1629. [CrossRef]

94. Puts, M.T.; Strohschein, F.J.; Del Giudice, M.E.; Jin, R.; Loucks, A.; Ayala, A.P.; Alibhai, S.H. Role of the geriatrician, primary care practitioner, nurses, and collaboration with oncologists during cancer treatment delivery for older adults: A narrative review of the literature. *J. Geriatr. Oncol.* **2018**, *9*, 398–404. [CrossRef]

95. Overcash, J.A.; Beckstead, J.; Extermann, M.; Cobb, S. The abbreviated comprehensive geriatric assessment (aCGA): A retrospective analysis. *Crit. Rev. Oncol.* **2005**, *54*, 129–136. [CrossRef]

96. Soubeyran, P.-L.; Bellera, C.; Goyard, J.; Heitz, D.; Curé, H.; Rousselot, H.; Albrand, G.; Servent, V.; Jean, O.S.; Van Praagh, I.; et al. Screening for Vulnerability in Older Cancer Patients: The ONCODAGE Prospective Multicenter Cohort Study. *PLOS ONE* **2014**, *9*, 115060. [CrossRef] [PubMed]

97. Mohile, S.G.; Bylow, K.; Dale, W.; Dignam, J.; Martin, K.; Petrylak, D.P.; Stadler, W.M.; Rodin, M. A pilot study of the vulnerable elders survey-13 compared with the comprehensive geriatric assessment for identifying disability in older patients with prostate cancer who receive androgen ablation. *Cancer* **2007**, *109*, 802–810. [CrossRef] [PubMed]

98. Torres, C.H.; Hsu, T. Comprehensive Geriatric Assessment in the Older Adult with Cancer: A Review. *Eur. Urol. Focus* **2017**, *3*, 330–339. [CrossRef] [PubMed]

99. Locher, C.; Pourel, N.; Le Caer, H.; Bérard, H.; Auliac, J.-B.; Monnet, I.; Descourt, R.; Vergnenègre, A.; Lafay, I.M.; Greillier, L.; et al. Impact of a comprehensive geriatric assessment to manage elderly patients with locally advanced non-small–cell lung cancers: An open phase II study using concurrent cisplatin–oral vinorelbine and radiotherapy (GFPC 08-06). *Lung Cancer* **2018**, *121*, 25–29. [CrossRef]

100. Palmer, K.; Onder, G. Comprehensive geriatric assessment: Benefits and limitations. *Eur. J. Intern. Med.* **2018**, *54*, e8–e9. [CrossRef] [PubMed]

101. Decker, V.; Sikorskii, A.; Given, C.W.; Given, B.A.; Vachon, E.; Krauss, J.C. Effects of depressive symptomatology on cancer-related symptoms during oral oncolytic treatment. *Psychooncology* **2019**, *28*, 99–106. [CrossRef]

102. Moyer, V.A.; Force, U.P.S.T. Screening for cognitive impairment in older adults: U.S. Preventive Services Task Force recommendation statement. *Ann. Intern. Med.* **2014**, *160*, 791–797. [CrossRef]

103. Extermann, M. Geriatric Assessment with Focus on Instrument Selectivity for Outcomes. *Cancer J.* **2005**, *11*, 474–480. [CrossRef]

104. Eamer, G.; Saravana-Bawan, B.; Van Der Westhuizen, B.; Chambers, T.; Ohinmaa, A.; Khadaroo, R.G. Economic evaluations of comprehensive geriatric assessment in surgical patients: A systematic review. *J. Surg. Res.* **2017**, *218*, 9–17. [CrossRef]

105. Gardner, M.; Tsiachristas, A.; Langhorne, P.; Burke, O.; Harwood, R.H.; Conroy, S.P.; Kircher, T.; Somme, D.; Saltvedt, I.; Wald, H.; et al. Comprehensive geriatric assessment for older adults admitted to hospital. *Cochrane Database Syst. Rev.* **2017**, *2017*, CD006211.

106. Ekdahl, A.W.; Alwin, J.; Eckerblad, J.; Husberg, M.; Jaarsma, T.; Mazya, A.L.; Milberg, A.; Krevers, B.; Unosson, M.; Wiklund, R.; et al. Long-Term Evaluation of the Ambulatory Geriatric Assessment: A Frailty Intervention Trial (AGe-FIT): Clinical Outcomes and Total Costs After 36 Months. *J. Am. Med. Dir. Assoc.* **2016**, *17*, 263–268. [CrossRef] [PubMed]

107. Bhatt, V.R. Personalizing therapy for older adults with acute myeloid leukemia: Role of geriatric assessment and genetic profiling. *Cancer Treat. Rev.* **2019**, *75*, 52–61. [CrossRef]

108. NCCN. *Clinical Practice Guidelines in Oncology: Older Adult Oncology*; NCCN: Plymouth Meeting, PA, USA, 2019.

109. Xue, D.-D.; Cheng, Y.; Wu, M.; Zhang, Y. Comprehensive geriatric assessment prediction of postoperative complications in gastrointestinal cancer patients: A meta-analysis. *Clin. Interv. Aging* **2018**, *13*, 723–736. [CrossRef] [PubMed]

110. Maekawa, Y.; Sugimoto, K.; Yamasaki, M.; Takeya, Y.; Yamamoto, K.; Ohishi, M.; Ogihara, T.; Shintani, A.; Doki, Y.; Mori, M.; et al. Comprehensive Geriatric Assessment is a useful predictive tool for postoperative delirium after gastrointestinal surgery in old-old adults. *Geriatr. Gerontol. Int.* **2016**, *16*, 1036–1042. [CrossRef] [PubMed]

111. Mason, M.C.; Crees, A.L.; Dean, M.R.; Bashir, N. Establishing a proactive geriatrician led comprehensive geriatric assessment in older emergency surgery patients: Outcomes of a pilot study. *Int. J. Clin. Pr.* **2018**, *72*, e13096. [CrossRef] [PubMed]

112. Ghignone, F.; Van Leeuwen, B.; Montroni, I.; Huisman, M.; Somasundar, P.; Cheung, K.; Audisio, R.; Ugolini, G. The assessment and management of older cancer patients: A SIOG surgical task force survey on surgeons' attitudes. *Eur. J. Surg. Oncol. (EJSO)* **2016**, *42*, 297–302. [CrossRef]

113. To, T.H.M.; Soo, W.K.; Lane, H.; Khattak, A.; Steer, C.; Devitt, B.; Dhillon, H.M.; Booms, A.; Phillips, J. Utilization of geriatric assessment in oncology—A survey of Australian medical oncologists. *J. Geriatr. Oncol.* **2019**, *10*, 216–221. [CrossRef]

114. Koneru, R.; Freedman, O.; Lemonde, M.; Froese, J. Evaluation of a comprehensive geriatric assessment tool in geriatric cancer patients undergoing adjuvant chemotherapy: A pilot study. *Support. Care Cancer* **2019**, *27*, 1871–1877. [CrossRef]

115. Kagan, E.; Freud, T.; Punchik, B.; Barzak, A.; Peleg, R.; Press, Y.A. Comparative Study of Models of Geriatric Assessment and the Implementation of Recommendations by Primary Care Physicians. *Rejuvenation Res.* **2017**, *20*, 278–285. [CrossRef]

Permissions

List of Contributors

Hiroyuki Shimada, Takehiko Doi, Kota Tsutsumimoto, Sangyoon Lee and Seongryu Bae
Center for Gerontology and Social Science, National Center for Geriatrics and Gerontology, 7-430 Moriokacho, Obu City, Aichi Prefecture 474-8511, Japan

Hidenori Arai
National Center for Geriatrics and Gerontology, 7-430 Morioka-cho, Obu City, Aichi Prefecture 474-8511, Japan

Yoshiaki Nomura, Ayako Okada, Ryoko Otsuka and Nobuhiro Hanada
Department of Translational Research, School of Dental Medicine, Tsurumi University, Yokohama 230-8501, Japan

Mieko Shimada
Department of Dental Hygiene, Chiba Prefectural University of Health Sciences, Chiba 261-0014, Japan

Erika Kakuta
Department of Oral Bacteriology, School of Dental Medicine, Tsurumi University, Yokohama 230-8501, Japan

Yasuko Tomizawa
Department of Cardiovascular Surgery, Tokyo Women's Medical University, Tokyo 162-8666, Japan

Chieko Taguchi and Kazumune Arikawa
Department of Preventive and Public Oral Health, School of Dentistry at Matsudo, Nihon University, Matsudo 470-2101, Japan

Hideki Daikoku and Tamotsu Sato
Iwate Dental Association, Morioka 020-0045, Japan

Katherine T. Ward, Mailee Hess and Shirley Wu
Section of Geriatrics, Division of General Internal Medicine, Department of Medicine, Harbor-UCLA Medical Center, Torrance, CA 90509, USA
David Geffen School of Medicine at UCLA, Los Angeles, CA 90095, USA

Ian T. Zajac, Danielle Herreen, Kathryn Bastiaans, Varinderpal S. Dhillon and Michael Fenech
Health & Biosecurity, Commonwealth Scientific and Industrial Research Organisation (CSIRO), 5000 Adelaide, South Australia, Australia

Theresa Westgård and Synneve Dahlin-Ivanoff
Department of Health and Rehabilitation, Institute of Neuroscience and Physiology, The Sahlgrenska Academy, University of Gothenburg, 40530 Gothenburg, Sweden
Centre of Aging and Health-AGECAP, University of Gothenburg, 40530 Gothenburg, Sweden

Isabelle Ottenvall Hammar
Department of Health and Rehabilitation, Institute of Neuroscience and Physiology, The Sahlgrenska Academy, University of Gothenburg, 40530 Gothenburg, Sweden
Centre of Aging and Health-AGECAP, University of Gothenburg, 40530 Gothenburg, Sweden
Department of Occupational Therapy and Physiotherapy, The Sahlgrenska University Hospital, 40530 Gothenburg, Sweden

Andrea de la Garza Puentes
Department of Nutrition, Food Sciences and Gastronomy, Faculty of Pharmacy and Food Sciences, University of Barcelona, 08028 Barcelona, Spain
Institut de Recerca en Nutrició i Seguretat Alimentària UB (INSA-UB), 08921 Barcelona, Spain
Teaching, Research & Innovation Unit, Parc Sanitari Sant Joan de Déu, 08830 Sant Boi, Spain
Department of Nutrition, Food Sciences and Gastronomy, Faculty of Pharmacy and Food Sciences, University of Barcelona, Av. Joan XXIII 27-31, E-08028 Barcelona, Spain
Parc Sanitari Sant Joan de Déu, Fundació Sant Joan de Déu, Institut de Recerca Sant Joan de Déu, 08830 Sant Boi de Llobregat, Spain

Adrià Martí Alemany
Department of Nutrition, Food Sciences and Gastronomy, Faculty of Pharmacy and Food Sciences, University of Barcelona, 08028 Barcelona, Spain

Aida Maribel Chisaguano
Nutrition, Faculty of Health Sciences, University of San Francisco de Quito, 170157 Quito, Ecuador

Rosa Montes Goyanes
Food Research and Analysis Institute, University of Santiago de Compostela, 15705 Santiago de Compostela, Spain

Ana I. Castellote and M. Carmen López-Sabater
Department of Nutrition, Food Sciences and Gastronomy, Faculty of Pharmacy and Food Sciences, University of Barcelona, Av. Joan XXIII 27-31, E-08028 Barcelona, Spain
Institut de Recerca en Nutrició i Seguretat Alimentària de la UB (INSA-UB), 08921 Barcelona, Spain
CIBER Physiopathology of Obesity and Nutrition CIBERobn, Institute of Health Carlos III, 28029 Madrid, Spain
Department of Nutrition, Food Sciences and Gastronomy, Faculty of Pharmacy and Food Sciences, University of Barcelona, 08028 Barcelona, Spain

Franscisco J. Torres-Espínola, Luz García-Valdés, Mireia Escudero-Marín and Maria Teresa Segura
Centre of Excellence for Paediatric Research EURISTIKOS, University of Granada, 18071 Granada, Spain
Department of Paediatrics, University of Granada, 18071 Granada, Spain

Cristina Campoy
Centre of Excellence for Paediatric Research EURISTIKOS, University of Granada, 18071 Granada, Spain
Department of Paediatrics, University of Granada, 18071 Granada, Spain
CIBER Epidemiology and Public Health CIBEResp, Institute of Health Carlos III, 28029 Madrid, Spain

Rebekah L. Young
Newham University Hospital, Bart's Health NHS Trust, London E13 8SL, UK

David G. Smithard
Queen Elizabeth Hospital, Lewisham and Greenwich NHS Trust, London SE18 4QH, UK
Department of Sports Science, University of Greenwich, London SE10 9BD, UK

Mariane Lutz
Thematic Task Force on Healthy Aging, CUECH Research Network, Viña del Mar 2520000, Chile
Interdisciplinary Center for Health Studies, CIESAL, Faculty of Medicine, Universidad de Valparaíso, Angamos 655, Reñaca, Viña del Mar 2520000, Chile

Guillermo Petzold
Thematic Task Force on Healthy Aging, CUECH Research Network, Viña del Mar 2520000, Chile
Department of Food Engineering, Universidad del Bio-Bio, Andrés Bello 720, Casilla 447, Chillán 3780000, Chile

Cecilia Albala
Thematic Task Force on Healthy Aging, CUECH Research Network, Viña del Mar 2520000, Chile
Institute of Nutrition and Food Technology, INTA, Universidad de Chile, El Líbano 5524, Macul, Santiago 7810000, Chile

Ignacio Aznar-Lou
Teaching, Research & Innovation Unit, Institut de Recerca Sant Joan de Déu, Esplugues de Llobregat, Parc Sanitari Sant Joan de Déu, 08830 Sant Boi de Llobregat (Barcelona), Spain
Centro de Investigación Biomédica en Red en Epidemiología y Salud Pública, CIBERESP, 28029 Madrid, Spain

Cristina Carbonell-Duacastella
Teaching, Research & Innovation Unit, Institut de Recerca Sant Joan de Déu, Esplugues de Llobregat, Parc Sanitari Sant Joan de Déu, 08830 Sant Boi de Llobregat (Barcelona), Spain

Ana Rodriguez and Inés Mera
Spanish Society of Community and Family Pharmacy (SEFAC), 28045 Madrid, Spain

Maria Rubio-Valera
Teaching, Research & Innovation Unit, Institut de Recerca Sant Joan de Déu, Esplugues de Llobregat, Parc Sanitari Sant Joan de Déu, 08830 Sant Boi de Llobregat (Barcelona), Spain
Centro de Investigación Biomédica en Red en Epidemiología y Salud Pública, CIBERESP, 28029 Madrid, Spain
School of Pharmacy, University of Barcelona, 08028 Barcelona, Spain

Tahsin Barış Değer
Directorate of Health Affairs, Söke Municipality, Söke, Aydın 09200, Turkey

Zeliha Fulden Saraç, Emine Sumru Savaş and Selahattin Fehmi Akçiçek
Geriatrics Section, Faculty of Medicine, Ege University, Bornova, Izmir 35100, Turkey

Isabel Salas Lorenzo
Department of Nutrition, Food Sciences and Gastronomy, Faculty of Pharmacy and Food Sciences, University of Barcelona, Av. Joan XXIII 27-31, E-08028 Barcelona, Spain
Institut de Recerca en Nutrició i Seguretat Alimentària de la UB (INSA-UB), 08921 Barcelona, Spain

Aida M. Chisaguano Tonato
Nutrition, Faculty of Health Sciences, University of San Francisco de Quito, Quito 170157, Ecuador

Ana Nieto, Florian Herrmann and Estefanía Dieguez
Centre of Excellence for Paediatric Research EURISTIKOS, University of Granada, 18071 Granada, Spain
Department of Paediatrics, University of Granada, 18071 Granada, Spain

Maria Rodríguez-Palmero
Basic Research Department. Ordesa Laboratories, 08830 Barcelona, Spain

Lisa D Hobson-Webb, Paul J Zwelling and Ashley N Pifer
Duke University Department of Neurology/ Neuromuscular Division, Durham, NC 27710, USA

Carrie M Killelea, Mallory S Faherty and Timothy C Sell
Duke University Department of Orthopaedic Surgery, Durham, NC 27710, USA
Michael W. Krzyzewski Human Performance Laboratory, Durham, NC 27710, USA

Amy M Pastva
Duke University Department of Orthopaedic Surgery, Durham, NC 27710, USA
Duke University Claude D. Pepper Older American Independence Center Durham, NC 27710, USA

Beatriz Olaya and Maria Victoria Moneta
Research, Innovation and Teaching Unit, Parc Sanitari Sant Joan de Déu, Carrer Doctor Pujadas 42, 08830 Sant Boi de Llobregat, Spain
Instituto de Salud Carlos III, Centro de Investigación Biomédica en Red de Salud Mental (CIBERSAM), Calle Monforte de Lemos 3-5, 28029 Madrid, Spain

Cecilia A. Essau
Department of Psychology, University of Roehampton, Whitelands College, London SW15 4JD, UK

Elvira Lara, Marta Miret, Natalia Martín-María, Darío Moreno-Agostino and José Luis Ayuso-Mateos
Instituto de Salud Carlos III, Centro de Investigación Biomédica en Red de Salud Mental (CIBERSAM), Calle Monforte de Lemos 3-5, 28029 Madrid, Spain
Department of Psychiatry, Instituto de Investigación Sanitaria, Hospital Universitario de La Princesa (IISPrincesa), Calle de Diego de León 62, 28006 Madrid, Spain
Department of Psychiatry, Universidad Autónoma de Madrid, Madrid, Calle Arzobispo Morcillo 4, 28029 Madrid, Spain

Adel S. Abduljabbar
Psychology Deparment, King Saud University, Riyadh 11451, Saudi Arabia

Josep Maria Haro
Research, Innovation and Teaching Unit, Parc Sanitari Sant Joan de Déu, Carrer Doctor Pujadas 42, 08830 Sant Boi de Llobregat, Spain
Instituto de Salud Carlos III, Centro de Investigación Biomédica en Red de Salud Mental (CIBERSAM), Calle Monforte de Lemos 3-5, 28029 Madrid, Spain
Psychology Deparment, King Saud University, Riyadh 11451, Saudi Arabia

Katarina Wilhelmson
Department of Health and Rehabilitation, Institute of Neuroscience and Physiology, The Sahlgrenska Academy, University of Gothenburg, 40530 Gothenburg, Sweden
Centre of Aging and Health-AGECAP, University of Gothenburg, 40530 Gothenburg, Sweden
Department of Geriatrics, The Sahlgrenska University Hospital, 40530 Gothenburg, Sweden
Region Västra Götaland, Sahlgrenska University Hospital, Department of Acute Medicine and Geriatrics, 413 45 Gothenburg, Sweden

Isabelle Andersson Hammar, Eva Holmgren and Synneve Dahlin Ivanoff
Department of Health and Rehabilitation, Institute of Neuroscience and Physiology, Sahlgrenska Academy, University of Gothenburg, 405 30 Gothenburg, Sweden
Centre for Aging and Health—AgeCap, University of Gothenburg, 405 30 Gothenburg, Sweden

Anna Ehrenberg
School of Education, Health and Social Studies, Dalarna University, 791 31 Falun, Sweden

Johan Niklasson
Department of Community Medicine and Rehabilitation Geriatric Medicine, Sunderby Research Unit, Umeå University, 901 87 Umeå, Sweden

Jeanette Eckerblad
Department of Neurobiology, Care Sciences and Society, Karolinska Institutet, 171 77 Solna, Sweden

Niklas Ekerstad
Region Department of Medical and Health Sciences, Division of Health Care Analysis, Linköping University, 581 83 Linköping, Sweden
Department of Research and Development, NU Hospital Group, 461 73 Trollhättan, Sweden

N. David Åberg
Region Västra Götaland, Sahlgrenska University Hospital, Department of Acute Medicine and Geriatrics, 413 45 Gothenburg, Sweden
Department of Internal Medicine, Institute of Medicine, Sahlgrenska Academy, University of Gothenburg, 405 30 Gothenburg, Sweden

Antoinette Broad
Community Services, Oxford Health NHS Foundation Trust, Oxford OX3 7JX, UK

Ben Carter
Department of Biostatistics and Health Informatics, Institute of Psychiatry, Psychology & Neuroscience, King's College London, London SE5 8AF, UK

Sara Mckelvie
Emergency Medical Unit, Oxford Health NHS Foundation Trust, Oxford OX3 7JX, UK
Primary Care Research Group, Faculty of Medicine, University of Southampton, Southampton SO17 1BJ, UK

Jonathan Hewitt
Division of Population Medicine, Cardiff University, Penarth CF64 2XX, UK

Junko Ueshima
Department of Clinical Nutrition and Food Service, NTT Medical Center Tokyo, Tokyo 141-0022, Japan

Keisuke Maeda
Palliative Care Center, Aichi Medical University, Aichi 480-1195, Japan

Hidetaka Wakabayashi
Department of Rehabilitation Medicine, Yokohama City University Medical Center, Yokohama 232-0024, Japan

Shinta Nishioka
Department of Clinical Nutrition and Food Services, Nagasaki Rehabilitation Hospital, Nagasaki 850-0854, Japan

Saori Nakahara
Department of Nutrition, Suzuka General Hospital, Suzuka 513-8630, Japan

Yoji Kokura
Department of Clinical Nutrition, Keiju Medical Center, Nanao 926-8605, Japan

Charmaine Childs, Jennifer Elliott, Khaled Khatab and Sally Fowler-Davis
College of Health, Wellbeing and Life Sciences, Sheffield Hallam University, Sheffield S10 2BP, UK

Susan Hampshaw
School of Health and Related Research (SCHARR), University of Sheffield, Sheffield S10 2TN, UK

Jon R. Willmott
Electronic and Electrical Engineering Department, University of Sheffield, Sheffield S10 2TN, UK

Ali Ali
Sheffield Teaching Hospitals, National Institute for Health Research (NIHR), Biomedical Research Centre, Sheffield S10 2JF, UK

Gwendolen Buhr
Duke Center for the Study of Aging and Human Development, Durham, NC 27710, USA

Carrissa Dixon
Duke Office of Clinical Research, Durham, NC 27710, USA

Jan Dillard and Elissa Nickolopoulos
Duke Outpatient Clinic, Durham, NC 27704, USA
Department of Case Management and Clinical Social Work, Duke University Medical Center, Durham, NC 27710, USA

Lynn Bowlby
Duke Outpatient Clinic, Durham, NC 27704, USA

Holly Canupp
Duke Outpatient Clinic, Durham, NC 27704, USA
Department of Pharmacy, Duke University Medical Center, Durham, NC 27710, USA

Loretta Matters
Duke University School of Nursing, Durham, NC 27710, USA

Thomas Konrad
Cecil G. Sheps Center for Health Services Research at University of North Carolina, Chapel Hill, NC 27516, USA

Laura Previll and Mitchell Heflin
Duke Center for the Study of Aging and Human Development, Durham, NC 27710, USA
Durham VA Geriatric Research, Education and Clinical Center, Durham, NC 27705, USA

Eleanor McConnell
Duke Center for the Study of Aging and Human Development, Durham, NC 27710, USA
Duke University School of Nursing, Durham, NC 27710, USA
Durham VA Geriatric Research, Education and Clinical Center, Durham, NC 27705, USA

Janine Overcash
The College of Nursing, The Ohio State University, 1585 Neil Ave, Newton Hall, Columbus, OH 43201, USA

Nikki Ford, Elizabeth Kress, Caitlin Ubbing and Nicole Williams
Stephanie Spielman Comprehensive Breast Center, The Ohio State University, 1145 Olentangy River Road, Columbus, OH 43121, USA

Index

Printed in the USA
CPSIA information can be obtained
at www.ICGtesting.com
LVHW080311230923
759035LV00008B/986